Also in the Variorum Collected Studies Series:

JERRY STANNARD
(Ed. Katherine E. Stannard and Richard Kay)
Pristina Medicamenta: Ancient and Medieval Botany

JERRY STANNARD
(Ed. Katherine E. Stannard and Richard Kay)
Herbs and Herbalism in the Middle Ages and Renaissance

ANDREW WEAR
Health and Healing in Early Modern England: Studies in Social and Intellectual History

NATHAN SIVIN
Medicine, Philosophy and Religion in Ancient China: Researches and Reflections

DANIELLE JACQUART
La science médicale occidentale entre deux renaissances (XIIe s.–XVe s.)

Y. TZVI LANGERMANN
The Jews and the Sciences in the Middle Ages

VIVIAN NUTTON
From Democedes to Harvey: Studies in the History of Medicine

DAVID M. KNIGHT
Science in the Romantic Era

WALTER PAGEL (Ed. Marianne Winder)
Religion and Neoplatonism in Renaissance Medicine

JOHN M. RIDDLE
Quid Pro Quo: Studies in the History of Drugs

FRANZ ROSENTHAL
Science and Medicine in Islam: A Collection of Essays

A. RUPERT HALL
Science and Society: Historical Essays on the Relations of Science, Technology and Medicine

VARIORUM COLLECTED STUDIES SERIES

Ancients and Moderns in the Medical Sciences

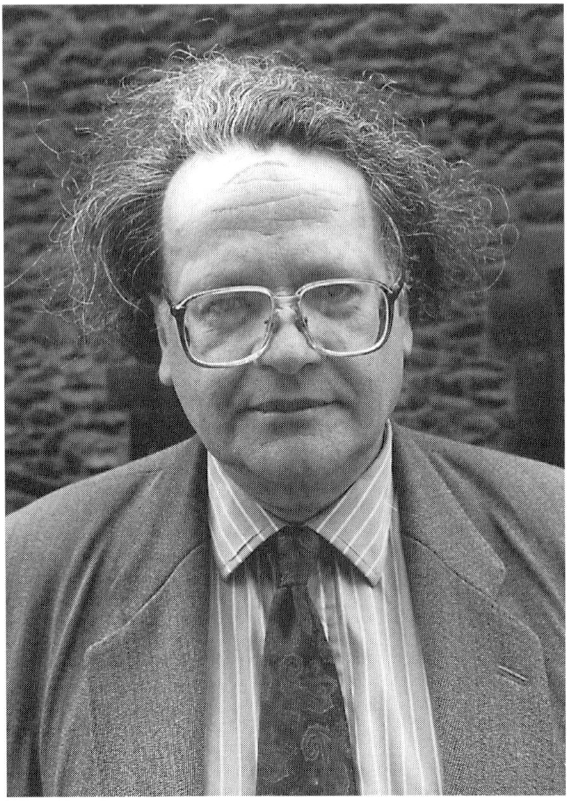

Dr Roger French

Roger French

Ancients and Moderns in the Medical Sciences

From Hippocrates to Harvey

Ashgate
VARIORUM

Aldershot · Burlington USA · Singapore · Sydney

Published in the Variorum Collected Studies Series by

Ashgate Publishing Limited
Gower House, Croft Road,
Aldershot, Hampshire GU11 3HR
Great Britain

Ashgate Publishing Company
131 Main Street
Burlington, Vermont 05401–5600
USA

Ashgate website: http://www.ashgate.com

ISBN 0–86078–834–2

British Library Cataloguing-in-Publication Data
French, Roger
Ancients and Moderns in the Medical Sciences: From Hippocrates to Harvey. – (Variorum Collected Studies Series: CS685).
1. Medicine–Europe–History. 2. Medical literature–Europe.
3. Medical education–Europe–History.
I. Title
610. 9' 4' 09

US Library of Congress Cataloging-in-Publication Data
Library of Congress Card Number: 00–100177

The paper used in this publication meets the minimum requirements of the American National Standard for Information Sciences – Permanence of Paper for Printed Library Materials, ANSI Z39.48–1984. ™

Printed by St Edmundsbury Press, Bury St Edmunds, Suffolk

VARIORUM COLLECTED STUDIES SERIES CS685

CONTENTS

This volume contains xxii + 280 pages

PUBLISHER'S NOTE

The articles in this volume, as in all others in the Variorum Collected Studies Series, have not been given a new, continuous pagination. In order to avoid confusion, and to facilitate their use where these same studies have been referred to elsewhere, the original pagination has been maintained wherever possible.

Each article has been given a Roman number in order of appearance, as listed in the Contents. This number is repeated on each page and is quoted in the index entries.

INTRODUCTION

The Scope of this Volume

A central part of the development of European medicine in the Middle Ages and Renaissance was the establishment and use of ancient texts. This is the theme of this volume. Its story is not a chronological history of medicine, but is about how successive generations of medical men and other scholars made use of what was seen as the pristine and authoritative knowledge of the ancients. Nor is this a story of how ancient knowledge was received (or how it 'diffused') across large temporal and geographical barriers. Hand in hand with the doctrine that the ancients were authoritative came the practice of actively seeking out their writings: if the authority of the ancients could be converted into Latin knowledge and into medical practice then, it was held, those who held that knowledge would be better doctors. Better doctors attracted more patients and more pupils, and better doctors made sure that in intellectual and institutional terms their superiority lay in their grasp and development of ancient knowledge.

We are concerned in this volume mostly with the career of ancient medical writings at the hands of medical men from late antiquity to the time of Harvey. It was only in Harvey's time that natural philosophers and medical men began to assert that there was no necessary virtue in following ancient authority. Aristotle's natural philosophy ceased to be taught in the schools, and the theory of medicine, which depended on it, collapsed.

The papers in this volume reflect the growth of a European civilization. That they do so is partly a natural result of the availability of historical sources (comparisons with non-European civilizations are in their early stages) and so to a certain extent it is a parochial story. But there are two things in particular we should note about it. The first is that the Europeans *chose* their intellectual ancestors. In the twelfth century and again in the early sixteenth they made (rather different) claims about the paternity of their technical subjects such as medicine and philosophy. When in the first half of the thirteenth century Oxford students were taught the whole range of Aristotle's natural philosophy, it was not a passive inheritance of an indigenous tradition, but one *imported* over considerable geographical and historical distance.

The second thing to note is that by the sixteenth century European culture was being *exported* to other and large areas of the world. Medicine was part of that culture and was characteristically European in being anatomical and dialectical. The medicine of other cultures did not have these features. When in later centuries medicine came to be seen as 'scientific', its basis was a development of European medicine.

Greek Authority

In European medicine the great ancient authorities were Hippocrates and Galen. The Hippocratic writings are in fact a collection made later than the historical Hippocrates, but one that seems to include some of the earliest written Greek medical works. 'Hippocrates' is therefore an invention, but was always seen as a person, for traditions rest more securely on Fathers than on historical accidents: it is supposed that it was an Alexandrian librarian who assembled the collection. In particular the *Aphorisms* of 'Hippocrates' remained central to European medical education down to the eighteenth or nineteenth century. It seemed to be a work of deep medical wisdom, entirely personal and based on no earlier written material (there may indeed have been none), expressed in a dense and somewhat oracular fashion. It thus demanded interpretation, and each successive generation of doctors interpreted it to their own satisfaction. One of the first of them was Galen, the Greek physician to Marcus Aurelius and Commodus in second-century Rome. By now Hippocratic language was out of date, and more important, Galen thought that Hippocrates' terse wisdom needed interpreting in the light of reason: that is, the discovery of the physical principles and logical processes that must have lain behind the wisdom of Hippocrates and which in any case lesser and later men needed in order to understand it. Galen found his physical principles and dialectic in the natural philosophy of Aristotle (who was in fact two or three hundred years later than many of the Hippocratic works). The medievals similarly found that Aristotle was useful in explaining Hippocrates (and Galen) and the search for their works was a joint one.

Arabic Medicine

A major sub-plot in the story of the search for ancient authority in medicine was the episode of the Arabs. From the seventh and eighth centuries the Arabs expanded rapidly into the eastern Mediterranean countries, North

Africa, up through Spain and even past the Pyrenees into what is now Southern France. They translated a great deal of technical ancient material including mathematics, astronomy/astrology and medicine. The first three items in this collection reflect the early beginning of this process, where the detail and complexity of the Greek works resulted in some of them being lost and others being condensed or reduced to diagrams. For example, Galen's big and most practical book on anatomy, the *Anatomical Procedures,* too complex to survive in Latin translation in the culturally depressed West, was partly lost even in Greek. The lost books were recovered from the Arabic at a very late date, but some of the Greek can be recovered from the early commentators. Galen's other major text, on 'anatomy' as form and function, was *On the Use of the Parts*, which was equally technical and even bigger. This was made intelligible in the early Middle Ages partly in the form of a very small Byzantine summary and more importantly by a rather corrupt and truncated paraphrase which originated somewhere where Arabic scholarship was assimilating Greek medicine.

In one such area, Alexandria, something is known of the compression of Galen's writings into a form suitable for the formal curriculum of a vocational school. The Alexandrian *summa* of Galen's works formed the basis for the medical education of the Greeks, Arabs and probably also Persians who followed. Some diagrams of parts of the body in even late medieval manuscripts derive ultimately from teaching-drawings of late classical Alexandria. The medieval diagrams typically consist of a group of five organ systems which reflect Galen's five brief anatomical texts as compressed in the *summa;* that on the bones preserves, through Latin, Persian and even Catalan, the Greek capitals that Galen used to illustrate the patterns of the sutures of the cranium. In Alexandria, too, the demands of a professional school led to the development of formal structures within teaching – such as the *accessus* – as devices to handle the content of the courses in medicine and natural philosophy.

The more distant West made contact with Islam later and in commercial and military enterprises. This was the background to cultural interchange between the Latins and the Arabs by which it became clear to the Westerners that there was medical authority in Arabic authors too. The Arabic material was largely Greek because the Arabs also saw authority in the ancients. But their translations, summaries and codifications of Greek material were not at first seen as derivative by the Latins. The great compilers and commentators – Avicenna and Averroes – were, on an ancient-modern timescale, practically contemporaries of the Latins enjoying the economic and cultural upswing of the eleventh and later centuries. That Arabic medicine seemed to them to be much the same as Greek meant simply, until the fifteenth century, that both truly represented the human body and its diseases.

Astrology, Prognosis and Reputation

One of the most exciting things offered by the new Arabic material was the possibility of foretelling the future. This was the purpose of astrology, long derided by modern historians of science as unscientific in comparison to the exemplary arch-science of astronomy. In fact astronomy may largely, perhaps, be seen as the theory needed to practise astrology; and in any case the terms were often interchangeable. The medical men were especially interested in astrology because it was very like prognosis in predicting what would happen to a person. Doctors in the Middle Ages were acutely aware of the professional advantages of correct prediction and in medieval medical and philosophical teaching Hippocrates was duly celebrated as 'glorious' in his skill in prognosis, with all its possibilities for an enhanced reputation. As a mathematical system for predicting the actions of the physical world, astrology was perhaps most credible before the adoption (in about 1200) of Aristotle's non-mathematical and qualitative cosmos. In the 1170s Roger of Hereford could represent astrology as the near-perfect and all-embracing art that stood at the head of God's creation. Even in the Aristotelian universities of the fourteenth century and later, astrology was sometimes (but not by any means always) taught in conjunction with medicine and its philosophical basis: the qualitative cosmos and its microcosm, the body, followed the nature and the cycles of the planets. The great Hippocrates was now reckoned an astrologer, and the doctrine of critical days was treated with the mathematics of lunar and solar cycles.

The Medieval Schools

Although some synthesis was achieved between the medical – astrological tradition and the Aristotelian – philosophical, they remained largely alternative rather than joint modes of argument. Before about 1200 only a few doctors in Salerno were accustomed to use Aristotle's physical works to understand their ancient medical texts. Men like Alfred of Shareshill, one of the first translators of Aristotle, considered themselves to be philosophers and looked down their noses at medical men as mercenary and manual practitioners of doubtful morality. The big historical change here was the appearance in Europe of schools large and elaborate enough to teach the whole range of subjects, and to students from a number of countries – the *studia generalia*. There had been schools in antiquity, and the Byzantine schools, for example, teaching Aristotelian texts, developed the *accessus* as a device for asking a rote of questions that related to the title and authorship of each work, its contents, structure and the part of philosophy it belonged to. Such devices were adopted also in the Western schools and became particularly useful in dealing with the works of Galen. Galen had written diffusely, promoting his own views, belittling those of others and covering a very large number of topics. The constraints of the medieval school, where the economics and formality of the situation meant that the teacher and students wanted to move quickly to a point where formal qualification was possible, encouraged routine devices of exposition.

To take a single example we can choose the *De Sectis* of Galen. This was an introductory text written by Galen to enable the beginner to distinguish and so choose between the medical sects of Rome. The utility of the text made it the first one to be studied in the medical course in Alexandria, and those teaching it chose to interpret Galen's discussion as a profound endorsement of the Rationalist position, that is, the use of Aristotelian-philosophical principles to explain how medical wisdom (such as that of Hippocrates) worked in practice. *De Sectis* and its Alexandrian commentary were known early in the Western Middle Ages, the medical teachers of which again interpreted it as a part of a Rationalist tradition that now began with Hippocrates and extended down to the contemporary schools. Part of this Rationalist tradition was *anatomical*, where the rationality consisted of knowing the nature of the parts of the body, from where reason would lead to cure of disorders. The parts were known – taught and learned – by means of an *accessus* focussed in the body, where a routine set of questions was asked, not of a text, but of the body itself. Answers to these questions produced a set of observable features of each part of the body: its shape, consistency, connections, number and so on. Although the context is the dissection and vivisection undertaken by Galen and the old Alexandrians, the commentary is written as though these practices were still being pursued. This literary device helped to justify, and then characterised, human dissection and animal vivisection that began in the West in the later Middle Ages.

Professional classroom teachers, then, whose business was with words, generally identified with the Rationalist sect as described by Galen. While Galen had given some weight to the value of empirical observation, the schoolmen of the Middle Ages, now with the power to exclude from the highest part of the profession those without licences to teach and practice, turned the latter into 'empirics', a pejorative title derived from the Empiricists of Rome.

The natural philosophy of Aristotle – the basis of the theory of medicine - rapidly became the principal part of the second half of the arts course (and Alfred of Shareshill's commentary on the apparently Aristotelian text on plants became a standard item of the curriculum). To take advantage of this, during the thirteenth century the doctors fought to Aristotelianise their subject, insert it into the universities and to claim that a university degree in medicine was the only proper qualification for practice.

By the end of the thirteenth century the doctors were succeeding in their aims by establishing medical faculties within the universities. They had convinced those who mattered that the theory of medicine was almost entirely Aristotelian, as expressed by Galen (which was partly justifiable) and that even Hippocrates was a rationalist philosopher (which had no justification at all). But medicine and philosophy could not agree on all things, and the interminable philosopher-physician debates are well known to historians. The doctors coexisted with the teachers of the arts within the university by means of the institutional framework of their different faculties. Intellectually, they agreed to differ by devices such as subalternation. This was an Aristotelian doctrine that set out the relationships between the branches of knowledge: for the medical man it established what he was obliged to accept from the philosopher and what was his own business. The point 'where the philosopher finishes and the physician begins' was the point of subalternated articulation.

It was not just an institutional and intellectual matter, but also a social and moral one. Social, because the faculties had many features of medieval guilds. The essence of the guild was that it was an association of practitioners of the same trade, recognised at law and exchanging an assurance of the quality of the product for some degree of monopoly. In other words these men were the acknowledged experts in their field and yielded to no one in their assessment of the nature of their own business. Guilds of teachers agreed on the heroes and texts of their discpline and no one else had the authority to question these. The authority of the teachers derived of course from them *agreeing* on the figures of, and the apparatus surrounding, Hippocrates and Galen (for the doctors) and Aristotle (for the philosophers). Such pressures kept the authors authoritative and their texts canonical for a long time.

The Classroom

Subalternation was also a moral matter because teachers urged on their pupils the duty to accept and follow what was taught. This was ultimately what had been taught by the ancients; and the teachers appeared at the same time to be defending a long medical tradition and insisting on the physical

– clinical – effectiveness of what was learned. *De facto* they were also defending the apparatus that gave stability and authority to the guild and hence to the practising doctor. In the middle of the fourteenth century Gentile da Foligno was teaching his students to follow the straight and narrow medical path: it involved giving faith to the ancients and delivering the most effective medicine to their patients. The two went hand in hand of course, and another part of the package was the moral duty never to question the rules of subalternation. The ultimate effect was to build a classroom culture of trust in which the teacher gave detailed rules and strategies for attacking other medical writers but at the same time drew fences around areas that could not be attacked.

The key-word in that classroom culture was 'faith'. The pupil has to believe what his master teaches him, or education is impossible. To grasp the attention of the listeners, and make them hear in an agreeable frame of mind what was being said, was a formal device of rhetoric. Medical teachers adopted it, recognising perhaps that it *was* a strategy, that faith was invited before the substance could be demonstrated. We shall see that when the hellenist Leoniceno attacked Pliny, when Vesalius attacked the great teacher of all medical men, Galen, and when Harvey abandoned Galenic teaching on the heart and blood, many of their contemporaries were shocked by the very blatant breaking of faith. The story of Vesalius is not retold in this book, but the earlier attack on Pliny by Leoniceno demonstrates the same issues. Many argued that it did not matter that Pliny was occasionally wrong, for he was so great an ornament of Latin culture that human error could be forgiven: what mattered was the faithless attempt to attack that culture.

Respect for the Ancients

Within the period covered by this volume, the reverence shown by medical men for the ancients was deep and enduring. It calls for special attention, not only because it directed their actions and words but because it is difficult to empathise with today. Indeed, in modern science and medicine everyone agrees that progress and improvement lie in the future, not the past. A scientific paper goes out of date in a comparatively few years – except, that is, for a handful of 'classic' papers which are still respected for being ahead of their time. In contrast, respect for moderns in the period we are dealing with was accorded for deep and masterly interpretations of the past: they were better at being behind their times.

What are the reasons for this respect for the ancients? One of the simplest is the sheer scale of ancient achievement. Especially in Italy there were very visible vestiges of Roman architecture and engineering. Specialists in the arts, such as law, knew of comprehensive systems of imperial scale. In natural philosophy, on which the theory of medicine rested, the range and subtlety of Aristotle's system had been revealed by the early thirteenth century. By the end of that century Aristotle's philosophy was the basis of man's understanding of the natural world and was the intellectual foundation of that part of Christianity that dealt with physical things. Princes ruled an Aristotelian world partly by means of an Aristotelian code of politics. In medicine, Galen supplied a largely Aristotelian theory of how the body worked, how it went wrong and how it could be put right.

But this is not a complete explanation. Aristotle was not the only ancient; and recovery of ancient works and life continued to a goal of scholarship and medicine. In writings of the Middle Ages and Renaissance one sometimes catches a moral or even religious flavour when the topic under discussion is the ancients and the respect due to them. There were other forces at work besides the comprehensiveness of such systems as Aristotle's. There was something that gave authority to the authors. Only the ancients were authors, because they invented or constructed the disciplines: their authority, 'authorness' (the question of *auctor* and *authoritas*) was as founders, while the moderns were commentators.

The men of the Middle Ages felt inferior to the ancients. There were a number of reasons for this. In the broadest terms Christian Europe had a linear view of history. While some Eastern religions involved for example a cyclical history in which individuals returned in different bodies, the European Christian believed that the world had been created, not so very long ago and out of nothing, by an omnipotent creator. The world was not expected to last forever and the final stage of the individual's existence was the general resurrection.

This linear chronology was matched by the career of man.The Fall from Paradise had rendered man incapable of knowing God directly and had deprived him of Adam's knowledge of things. A great deal of the effort that went into medieval scholarship was directed towards restoring prelapsarian knowledge, as far as possible and in light of the coming end of the world. The world was in fact old and accordingly (it was often thought) frail, like the race of men. When the medievals said they felt like dwarfs standing on the shoulders of giants (able to see a little further but only reason of the gigantic labours of the ancients) they were expressing a feeling that man and nature were in decay. Even in the Renaissance it could be argued (particularly by opponents of Vesalius) that the body of man had degenerated since the time of Galen and that its anatomy was now different. Most of the ancients were of course pagans, having lived before Christ, but they had been alive in the youth of the world and accordingly had powerful faculties. It was commonly said that Hippocrates was a man of such great natural gifts that he did not need the arts such as logic or philosophy – which had not then been invented – to practise medicine perfectly.

There were also institutional reasons for having figures like Hippocrates as heroes or founding fathers. The arts and trades of the high Middle Ages characteristically came to be pursued in groups. The essential model (as we have seen) was the guild, which existed for the mutual benefit of its members. It was allowed to exist on the condition first, that its trade or art was a real one and second, that the guild undertook to maintain the quality of the product. On both counts it was important for the guild to set out the pedigree of its business, establish its heroes and become the authority on the nature of its business.

Teachers also formed such guilds. Teachers of medicine defined its ancient sources and its history, and set up curricula of the proper books to be read and the proper way of reading them in order to qualify as a doctor: that is, to join the teacher's guild. They generally agreed that the Father of Medicine was Hippocrates, who had written down his deep medical wisdom in his *Aphorisms*. Just as Fallen man could not read God's word directly in the Bible, but needed the arts to grasp the literal and spiritual meanings of the sacred page, so the medical man of later ages needed logic and philosophy to understand the oracular wisdom of the *Aphorisms*. Authoritative knowledge came in big old books: the truest kind was revealed, and came in the Bible; imperial law came in the *Digest* of Justinian; and medical knowledge came in the works of Hippocrates and his great interpreter Galen, and most conveniently of all in the vast *Canon* of Avicenna.

Medical Faith and Medical Ethics

The practice of teaching medicine in the high Middle Ages and Renaissance reflects all this. Medicine was taught in the classroom to fee-paying pupils who wanted to become doctors and start practice as soon as possible. Because the faculty was like a guild, the students learned an agreed curriculum and performed requisite exercises to gain their licence to teach and practise. Busy teachers coping with pupils in a hurry encourage efficiency in the practice of teaching. The teacher's most important task was to secure the attention and indeed allegiance of the pupil. One way of doing this was to stress the greatness of the founders of the discipline. If they were touched by divinity, as medicine was said to have been handed down to mortals by Apollo, so much the better. The ultimate aim of medieval medical teaching was to hear the ancients as if they were sitting in the same room, 'talking to us', and this needed a great deal of earlier education in the arts and devices of commentary. From Gentile da Foligno to the time of Harvey the pupil responded in a moral way to the teacher's demand for allegiance: he was being invited to join the medical tradition, from its ancient and perhaps divine origins to the present. The Hippocratic Oath expressed much of this, demanding the allegiance of the incomer, the preservation of secret knowledge, the fraternal treatment of insiders.

The medical tradition was rather like the *translatio studii* of the theologians. This was a claim for the legitimacy and authority of their teaching. In practice an *ad hoc* medieval consortium of teachers, the theologians wanted to be able to claim at least intellectual descent in a tradition from ancient beginnings. In a similar way the first Holy Roman Emperors had *de facto* political and military power, but what they claimed was a *translatio* of power from the ancient emperors of Rome.

Respect for the ancient authors was not limited to restoring and understanding their texts. The founders of a discipline were those who had laid down its principles. Principles could be developed and ancient methods turned to new areas. Fundamental to medicine was the theory of complexion. A healthy body was one complexioned by a correct balance of the elementary qualities; food and medicine were complexioned; the environment of the patient – his airs, waters and places – directly affected his complexion. The doctrine had been developed by Galen from Aristotelian beginnings and had been even more systematised by Avicenna. Gentile da Foligno, the great commentator on Avicenna, further developed the doctrine, in line with the methods of quantification set out by the Mertonians in Oxford. The essential point of Gentile's vast treatment was the quantification of the elementary *qualities* that made up complexions, so that an enormous amount of mathematical elaboration appeared to give great precision in questions about the perfect complexion and departures from it. Gentile was aware that he and the doctors of Bologna had come a long way from Galen and even Avicenna in this mathematical enterprise. Gentile, putting his medical faith in Avicenna, even declared that Galen had been intellectually incapable of developing his own doctrines in this area. But this was unusual, and Gentile's regard for his students and their faith in the medical tradition is everywhere apparant.

Faith in the medical tradition and its teachers was expressed too by the doctors of the medical and guild-like incorporations, the faculties and professional colleges, in 'ethical' terms. The medieval textbook of medicine, the *Articella*, began in the fifteenth century to include Hippocratic 'ethical' works, and Renaissance editions of the collected Hippocratic works often begin with them, as though *the Oath, Decorum, Ancient Medicine* and so on were introductory. These works were ethical in the sense that, partly by protecting the patient, they clearly also protected the interests of the group of physicians that was their source. The ethical works are concerned with topics like who shall join the group, to whom knowledge shall be given and how unethical all the other groups are. This can be linked to the needs and circumstances of doctors in Hippocratic times. But characteristically the men of the middle ages and renaissance made these ancients texts part of their own medical context. Men who read Galen's *De Sectis* treated the Methodists, Rationalists and Empiricists as their own contemporaries; Galen's enemies became their enemies. Likewise what was ethical for Hippocrates became ethical for them.

But we can also see that the medical circumstances of the late middle ages gave rise to 'ethical' behaviour, and a few texts, that reflect the needs of the doctors of the time. The university-trained rational and learned physician was at the top of the profession, and took great care that the two facets of his reputation, his learning and rationality, should remain intact. He did so partly by means of his own teaching. A teacher like Gentile in the first half of the fourteenth century was essentially a 'heroic' teacher (like the great teachers of the twelfth-century schools) in attracting pupils. One of his attractions as a teacher was his ability to resolve disputed questions, a technique of teaching that had been added to the commentary. Gentile was known as the *speculator* because he could 'see further' into disputed questions (like the quantification of qualities) than his contemporaries. The faith that he required of his students was local to his classroom and his view of the medical tradition. To Gentile, teaching in Perugia, contemporary medical teachers in Bologna were competitors rather than colleagues: he had to resolve questions more authoritatively than they. There was little professional fellow-feeling between doctors of different studia in the fourteenth century, and they were in any case moderns, not ancients, and could be given little allegiance.

By the end of the fifteenth century a doctor like Gabriel de Zerbi recognised that all university-trained physicians would benefit from a common code of behaviour. It was paramount that such learned and rational men should never disagree in public, for when doctors disagree the layman loses all confidence. Zerbi's ethics dealt with topics such as how the doctor should handle money, his colleagues, his female patients, apothecaries and surgeons. Much is ethical in the sense that the doctor does the best for his patients, but it it is not a deeply-hidden message to his medical readers that a prime result of ethical behaviour is the enhanced reputation of the learned and rational doctor as a *kind* of practitioner.

Hellenists and Humanists

Respect for the ancient medical men grew, rather than diminished, in the Renaissance. There were two rather different groups of teachers who must briefly take our attention here. The humanists were men who taught the 'more human letters' such as literature. They developed techniques of evaluating their texts that explained features of those texts in terms of their circumstances, particularly historical. The humanists did not primarily study the technical subjects such as mathematics or medicine, but techniques of textual evaluation, including the historical, were adopted by the medical men and by the sixteenth century medicine in certain places had become as 'humanised' as a dialectical and philosophical discipline could.

Secondly, the hellenists were those who held that the pure medicine of antiquity was Greek, not Roman, and certainly not Arab. They gave their faith, like Leoniceno, to the Greeks. They held that the Arabs had purloined and debased Greek medicine, filling it with linguistic barbarisms: Greek alone was 'eloquent' and Latin was the language of mere commentators. Like the medieval scholastics, whom the Hellenists affected to despise, the Hellenists wanted to hear the voices of the ancients speaking directly to them, but they maintained that this could only be done by – effectively – *listening* in *Greek*, without the intermediate Latin interpretation, dialectical analysis and commentary. Leoniceno regarded Latin simply as the language of the schoolmen, scholars of the unfortunate period between the Greeks and the Hellenists themselves. This period soon came to be called the 'Middle' Ages, identified only by the virtues of the periods before and after it. The Hellenists were partly at least outside the universities and sneered at the dialectical and Arabist scholars within, using in a pejorative sense that still survives the term 'scholastic', which earlier was used by the scholars themselves to denote mastery of technical subjects such as medicine.

One of the things in favour of Greek medicine was that it was older than Roman. When Leoniceno attacked Pliny, it was because Pliny was Roman and misrepresented his Greek sources. When Vesalius attacked the Greek doctor of imperial Rome, Galen, part of his justification was that Galen had corrupted the human anatomy of the earlier Greeks, Herophilus and Erasistratus, by his use of animals. Some writers held that the arts had been given to mankind by the gods and had been more perfect in their original form. In this case the sources were older than the Greeks, and Hermetic wisdom looked valuable. Others espoused a 'translation' of studies that combined great antiquity with religious authority so that, for example, Moses could be held to have been the great law-giver but also a repository of natural knowledge that passed down to the philosophers.

But there was a limit to how far back one could go in searching for a pristine form of a discipline. Most people agreed that all the true arts had appeared long ago (and that preserving them was the business of the guilds). But while some held that the arts had originally been given to man by the gods, others thought that man had developed them himself, so that they had a history, from primitive beginnings. It was for example commonly held that anatomy had not been highly developed in Aristotle's time, and that this – and not a personal defect – was the cause of his mistakes, such as his declaration that the heart had three chambers. But even here, it was generally admitted that some sort of perfection had been reached before the end of the period of the ancients, for Galen was the master of those who knew anatomy.

Many of these new ways of looking at old medicine coexisted in the Renaissance. What you believed, as always, depended on who and where you were. A medically-trained surgeon such as Berengario da Carpi in the Bologna of the early sixteenth century was proud to call himself a scholastic. He had read just about every anatomical work available and felt justified in calling himself learned. He knew of the 'skilful hellenists' like Leoniceno, but suspected their business was with words, not things. His wide experience of human dissection and a surgical sensory epistemology led him to deny that the human body possessed a *rete mirabile*, an organ central to Galenic physiology. Yet he admitted to fear in denying Galen and exhibited great faith in the Teacher of Medicine. For all his empirical leanings, he chose to structure his text on anatomy on the model of the elaborate commentary form of the high Middle Ages.

New Medicine

Gentile, Leoniceno, Berengario and Vesalius differed from some of the ancient authorities but in a sense remained within the medical tradition, which after all contained a critical component. The loyalties that were tested in these adventures were intellectual, moral and even religious. Medical 'faith' was expressed or denied in terms that had a clear relationship with the testing times of the Reformation. While Vesalius disagreed with Galen on matters that retained the classical form given to them by Galen, anatomy after him became overtly religious. Just as both sides of the Christian divide could respond to discussion about the natural attributes of God, man and Creation, so the Vesalian question was subsumed in the new assertion that the human body was the Temple, or the Image, of God.

The new philosophers of the early seventeenth century likewise found that they could avoid conflicting systems of thought by treating the physical world as Creation. The system of thought they most wanted to avoid was that of Aristotle. The rejection of Aristotelianism produced a crisis in medicine. If the elements, qualities, form, matter, privation and so on were no longer the physical principles of the world, then medicine had no theory. Some doctors proclaimed that medicine was, after all, simply an Art and not a *scienta.* Galen's vast rationalising of Hippocrates' medicine, so important in the earlier period, came under criticism as the intellectual system of one man. (Hippocrates in contrast remained popular because he could be seen as non-rationalising, even empirical.) Many others, particularly in the schools and professional colleges, held tight to Galenism. Indeed, the professional colleges had defined their medicine as Galenic and quizzed candidates for the fellowship about the extent of their Galenic knowledge.

One of the men who did so, as Censor of the London College, was William Harvey, even after his discovery of the circulation of the blood. This discovery can be seen in the context of the attacks by Leoniceno and Vesalius on the ancients. It was an accidental result of applying a reformulation of a procedure first practised by an ancient, Aristotle: Harvey was no revolutionary in philosophy. It was an unphilosophical result, because Harvey could not 'demonstrate' it in the traditional way. Many of his contemporaries rejected it for this reason. Others rejected it because it broke the medical faith that all medical men should share in the ancient teachers: some said it felt like apostasy to accept the circulation. Students were delighted with the scandal it caused and many established teachers were horrified on the directly religious grounds that it denied the traditional action of the soul in the heart.

The controversy over the circulation of the blood was caught up in that over the new philosophy. Descartes adopted a form of circulation as a principal example of his new mechanical physiology, but others thought that mechanism was atheistic, and that blood moved as it had always been said to move. Those who attacked Harvey from positions within traditional medicine had a very considerable armoury of Aristotelian natural philosophy and dialectic, to which Harvey had a limited reply. The new philosophers, whether for or against Harvey, had like him a limited repertoire of argument for the promulgation of the new articles of faith, like the denial of 'attraction'. The sceptics, denying all 'systems', accepted only some experimental results as 'probable knowledge' about a world unified only by its being Creation.

These disputes took on recognisable national boundaries. Latin had been the learned language of all Europe since the Middle Ages and was the voice of traditional philosophy. But now the vernacular began to appear.

Descartes sometimes wrote in French, as did the sceptic Gassendi. Harvey's opponents, like the Englishman Primrose and the famous Parisian anatomist Riolan, continued to use Latin for its range and command of the traditional technicalities of medicine and philosophy. Harvey himself wrote notes to himself for his anatomy lectures mostly in Latin but partly too in English. The Latin covers all the weighty matter of his philosophy, the new Aristotelianism of Padua. No vernacular usage could have the import or connotations of the Latin terms. But Harvey used English where he needed a telling analogy or simile, mostly in connection with the particulars of sensory perceptions. Colours, images from the home or farm, well-known places, all could be supplied more vividly in English than in Latin. Harvey's Latin deals not with particulars, but universals, the general truths that Harvey held could be elaborated in the mind from particulars. In the schools, Latin continued to be used even for new formulations of philosophy. But the New Philosophy of the seventeenth century was practised mostly perhaps outside the universities. When Boyle wrote in English it was because the connotations of Latin terms were no longer needed.

The texts that are discussed in this collection of essays are conspicuously concerned with the theory of medicine. When traditional natural philosophy collapsed, so did the theory of medicine; the ancients had died. This meant the end of a Europe-wide latinate medical culture in which the comparatively small circle of élite and university-trained physicians used their traditional rationality and learning to defend their image and privileges. In time, other natural philosophies – and ultimately science – became available, and were used in the same manner and for the same purposes as traditional natural philosophy. But that is outside the scope of this collection.

ROGER FRENCH

Cambridge
November 1999

Errata and Note on Names

Proper names vary in appearance in the secondary literature, particularly over a period of time and when used in a second language. Rhazes and Rhasis have both been regularly used for the Arabic original, and both forms appear here. Fashions also change in rendering Latin names into their vernacular, especially when the latter is several centuries old. For example the Latin Fallopius sometimes appears as Fallopio, Falloppio or Fallopia. The Greek-to-Latin shift has produced both Chalcondyles and Chalcondylas. Read Collenuccio for Colenuccio, and Gabriele de Zerbi for Gabriel de Zerbis. Pietro d'Abano is to be preferred to Peter of Abano

ACKNOWLEDGEMENTS

Grateful acknowledgement is made to the following persons, journals, institutions and publishers for their permission to reproduce the papers included in this volume: Professor P.U. Unschuld, Editor, *Sudhoffs Archiv* and Sir Geoffrey Lloyd (I); The University of Chicago Press (II, V); Professor P.U. Unschuld, Editor, *Sudhoffs Archiv* (III); Professor W.F. Bynum, Editor, *Medical History* (IV); Cambridge University Press, Dr A.R. Cunningham, Professor Jon Arrizabalaga and Luis García-Ballester (VI); B. Sullivan, Managing Editor, *Viator* (VII); Kluwer Academic Publishers, Dr John Roche and Professor J.D. North (VIII); Dr Joanna Geyer-Kordesch and Andrew Wear (IX); Cambridge University Press (X); Routledge Publishers and Frank Greenaway (XI); Oxford University Press (XII).

I

Greek Fragments of the Lost Books of Galen's Anatomical Procedures

Introduction

Galen's major work on anatomy and the techniques of dissection, the Anatomical Procedures, narrowly escaped extinction during its long history. The single surviving Greek exemplar breaks off in book nine, which left, in the middle ages, some five and a half books unknown to the Latin West. This first half of the work, known in the middle ages as De Anatomicis Aggressionibus, and after *Guinter*'s translation as De Anatomicis Administrationibus, was a very important source of Galenic anatomy, but it did not include *Galen*'s account of the brain and spinal cord, the eyes and face, the larynx and other structures in the neck, the generative organs, the veins and arteries, and the cranial and spinal nerves. Chief among these are *Galen*'s accounts of his striking and sophisticated experiments involving sectioning the spinal cord and the nerves of the throat, in an analysis of nerve function and distribution.

It does not seem to have been noticed by recent historians that some fragments of the lost Greek books, 9–15, have been preserved in *Oribasius*. The entire Greek text was available to him, as it was to the Arabs. The Arabic text was published in 1906 by *Max Simon*, together with a German translation[1], and an English version, by *Duckworth*, appeared in 1962[2]. Neither *Simon* nor the editors of *Duckworth*'s translation make any reference to *Oribasius*'s Greek text, but the identity of the source of some of the fragments here considered was known to *Daremberg*, who presented the Greek text together with a French translation in 1858[3]. However, *Daremberg* had only a provisional and unsatisfactory translation of the second half of the Anatomical Procedures from Arabic, made by *Gustave Dugat* in 1854–5. He was unable to identify corresponding passages with any certainty, and was not in a position to shed light on the lost Greek text of the

[1] *M. Simon:* Sieben Bücher Anatomie des Galen, 2 vols. (Leipzig, 1906).

[2] *Galen:* Galen on Anatomical Procedures, trans. *W. Duckworth*, ed. M. Lyons and B. Towers (Cambridge, 1962).

[3] *Oribasius:* Œuvres d'Oribase trans. *Bussemaker* and *Daremberg*, 6 vols. (Paris 1858) vol. 3.

Galenic work. The same is true of *Raeder*, the text of whose edition is used here[4].

Daremberg did, however, analyse the sources in *Galen* of the other Oribasian passages. In the section of *Oribasius'* text considered here, the passages from the Anatomical Procedures are interspersed with some from De Usu Partium, and a comparison of *Oribasius'* Greek with that of the surviving Greek of the latter Galenic work provides us with a standard by which we can measure *Oribasius'* accuracy in copying from *Galen*. In general *Oribasius* did not condense the Galenic original, but copied out selected passages with great accuracy, and we can be fairly confident that the Greek he gives for the lost passages of the Anatomical Procedures represents well the Galenic text.

Oribasius achieved his compression of the original, then, by omitting certain kinds of passages. A parallel case is the Arabic (or Syriac) compression of De Usu Partium, known to the Western middle ages as De Juvamentis Membrorum. Here the editing translator, like *Oribasius*, omitted many of *Galen*'s technical descriptions of dissecting procedures, his attacks on his predecessors and his apostrophes to wise and beneficent Nature.

This paper presents those fragments of the lost Greek Galenic text that can now be found in *Oribasius*, on the basis of a comparison of the Greek of *Oribasius* with the reliable translation now available of the Arabic version of the Galenic work.

The renaissance Latin version of *Oribasius* in *Estienne*'s edition has been used as a check, as has the translation of book 24, chapter 3, published by *Cohen* and *Drabkin*[5]. It should be added that translation by way of the Arabic has a very close agreement to the form of the Greek in *Oribasius*.

The method of presentation (in the second part of the paper) is that the Greek of the fragments is given, each with a number and brief descriptive title. Each is followed by the English translation of the equivalent passage of the Arabic version. This is given in italics. The purpose of this paper is to place these fragments, with translations, in their context (again from the English translation) in order that they may be quickly located, and so that the reader may see what material *Oribasius* has omitted. Where the intervening context is too long to be given in this way, the fact is indicated within square brackets. A

[4] *Oribasius:* Collectionum Medicarum Reliquiae, ed. *J. Raeder* 3 vols. (Leipzig and Berlin, 1928) III, (1931).

[5] A Source Book in Greek Science, (Harvard, 1958).

similar indication is given where *Oribasius* paraphrases the original or introduces text from De Usu Partium: in these cases the Greek is not given. (Square brackets within the English translation are, of course, those of *Duckworth*). The bulk of these fragments, and the longest of them, come from the third chapter of book 24 of *Oribasius*' Medical Collection, and the first fragment stands at the head of that chapter. The rest of the fragments come from *Oribasius*' chapters 8 and 9 (7 to 15). Some of these consist only of a short sentence, and we can be perhaps less confident about the accuracy with which they represent their source. Finally, there is a substantial fragment, chapter 8 of *Oribasius*' 25th book.

The third part of the paper contains a commentary on the fragments. For example, we see that in several places, *Oribasius*' Greek clarifies the text. For example in fragment 4 *Oribasius* has κῶλα for those parts of the body paralysed by a certain incision of the spinal cord. The word means members of the body, particularly the legs. *Daremberg* has 'les membres' and *Estienne* 'artus omnes'. The English translation has 'feet', which is less appropriate, and perhaps reflects an error at the Greek-Arabic stage of translation. Likewise in fragment 10 there is nothing in the Greek to match the 'pulsating blood-vessels' of the English translation, which retains in addition the 'arteries' of the original Greek. The former phrase is certainly an Arabic gloss, for it was regularly used to translate the latter from the Greek in, for example, De Juvamentis Membrorum. Again, in fragment 9 the Greek speaks of the tongue's 'band of communication' expanding. This is rendered correctly by *Daremberg* and *Estienne*, but the English version has 'shrinks'. Likewise in fragment 4 *Oribasius* has nothing to match the pleonastic 'and arrests their movements' of the English. This may be an example of condensation on *Oribasius*' part, or perhaps an Arabic gloss. The fragment has not been divided on this account. It is possible that *Oribasius*' omission of '. . . so that when it is used for speaking . . .' from fragment 9 has a similar cause. Again, the fragment has not been divided. Other cases in which the English-Arabic version differs from the Greek are noted in the third part of the paper.

(II) The Fragments

1. The membranes of the spinal cord

Τὰς δύο μήνιγγας ὁ νωτιαῖος ἔχει, τήν τε παχεῖαν καὶ τὴν λεπτήν, ἀπὸ τῶν περὶ τὸν ἐγκέφαλον πεφυκυίας, αἷς δὴ καὶ ἥνωται· τρίτον δ' ἔξωθεν αὐταῖς περιβέβληται σῶμα, καθάπερ ἀμφίεσμά τι καὶ πρόβλημα τοῦ νωτιαίου μυελοῦ, τὴν ἀρχὴν τῆς ἐκφύσεως ἐκ τῶν κορωνῶν τῆς κεφαλῆς εἰληφός. ἔστι δ' ἡ φύσις αὐτοῦ τῇ τῶν συνδέσμων ἡ αὐτή, καθ' ὅ τι καὶ πέφυκεν ἐξ ὀστοῦ τοῖς συνδέσμοις ὡσαύτως· καὶ μέντοι καὶ συνδεῖ πως πρόσω σπονδύλων ἐγκαταβαῖνον τὸ σῶμα τοῦτο διπλοῦν ταῖς μεταξὺ χώραις αὐτῶν.

For the spinal marrow has two meninges which take their origin from the meninges of the brain. And wrapped around them the third structure, which serves the marrow as a preservative and a covering and a protection, surrounds both of them outwardly. The place from which this structure grows out, its site of origin, is on the skull, and its nature is that of a ligament, since it grows out from the bones, just as is the case with the outgrowth of the rest of the ligaments. Besides this, it binds together the vertebrae in front, since, folded up, it breaks in upon the spaces between them[6].

When you have cut away the bones from behind, at the place at which, as I said, lies the root of the dorsal ridge, and you see this ligament lying exposed to view, then insert at the place which you have laid open, a broad tool of the class of the instrument which one calls a spatula, between the third outer covering, of which I said that by its nature it is a ligament, and the vertebra enclosing it. Then place the so-called bone-breaking instrument upon it. When you have done that, you then cut freely loose, from whichever vertebra you please, by a smooth, rapid, cautious incision, that portion which extends as far as the vertebral basis. By the expression 'vertebral basis' I mean that part of it which is inclined forwards, there where I said that the ligament is folded up and breaks in between the vertebrae. And here, in accordance with the sequence of the vertebrae, the nerves spring out on both sides of them, and the nerve-roots pass out through perfectly rounded foramina, the width of each single foramen corresponding to the thickness of the nerve which passes out through it. In the cervical vertebrae, this foramen is formed by two vertebrae, each one of which has a semicircular groove forming one half of the foramen. In all quadrupeds the cervical vertebrae are seven in number just as is the case in mankind. But in the thorax, the first vertebra is somewhat more strongly curved than the one lying beneath it. That peculiarity becomes more marked towards the lumbar vertebral column until finally in the last vertebrae the whole nerve emerges solely through the foramen in the upper vertebra, which is always to be found at the root of the process at the side of each single vertebra.

[6] *Raeder*, III, 11, 24–31, *Duckworth*, p. 21.

When you have thus uncovered the spinal marrow, on whichever vertebra you please, then introduce a hook upwards and only superficially into the ligament described, so as to pierce it easily and by itself alone without cutting into any part of the meninx lying beneath it.

2. Incising the spinal ligament

τμηθεὶς δ᾽ οὗτος ὁ σύνδεσμος, εἴτε κατὰ μῆκος, εἴτε κατὰ πλάτος, εἴτε κατ᾽ ἄμφω, βλάβην οὐδεμίαν ἐργάσεται τῷ ζῴῳ, καθάπερ οὐδ᾽ ἂν ἡ σκληρὰ τμηθείη μῆνιγξ, κακώσει τὸ ζῷον,

Make the incision as you wish, either lengthwise or crosswise or in both directions. The cutting into this ligament brings no injury to the animal, just as it does not harm it at all if you distend and cut into the dura mater in the same manner[7].

Now assume that you have already done what is here described, so that the spinal marrow, protected only by the pia mater, lies exposed. Now this sheath is laid upon it absolutely tensely and intimately, and in it are numerous veins just as in the pia mater enveloping the brain. You see these veins in the large animals very clearly, plunging down into the substance of the spinal marrow, and sinking into the depth of it. Were you to expose this sheath round about the spinal marrow then no harm would befall the animal on that account.

3. Longitudinal incision of the spinal marrow

οὐδ᾽ ἂν τὸν νωτιαῖον αὐτὸν τέμῃς κατὰ τὸ μῆκος· πέφυκε γὰρ ἑκάτερον τῶν νεύρων ἃ κατὰ συζυγίαν ἐκφύεται τοῦ νωτιαίου κατὰ τὰς συμβολὰς τῶν σπονδύλων ἐκ τῶν πλαγίων, τὸ | μὲν δεξιὸν ἐκ τοῦ δεξιοῦ, τὸ δ᾽ ἕτερον ἐκ θατέρου.

or even if you made a longitudinal cut into the spinal marrow itself, since all the respective nerves branch off at the places where the vertebrae meet one another at the sides, the right-sided nerve on the right side, the nerve of the opposite side on the left[8].

Should you wish to bring the region below the incised portion into the paralytic state, and to arrest its movements, then carry the incision transversely . . .

[From this point in the text, *Oribasius* is presenting a paraphrase rather than a direct borrowing from *Galen*, and it finishes

[7] *Raeder*, III, 11, 32–35, *Duckworth*, pp. 21–2.

[8] *Raeder*, III, 11, 35–p. 12, 3. *Duckworth*, p. 22.

on line four, page 23, of *Duckworth*'s translation. *Oribasius* then omits a lengthy but important passage in which *Galen* gives technical instructions for performing, and the results of, serial section of the spinal cord. His borrowing from *Galen* begins again after the following sentence of page 25 of the English translation: . . . If now you know from their anatomy where the nerves of these muscles arise, then you also know for certain when any single one of these muscles will be paralysed.]

4. Transverse incision of the spinal marrow

νυνὶ δὲ τοσοῦτον ἔτι προσθήσω τῷ λόγῳ· ἡ μὲν ἐν τῷ μεταξὺ κεφαλῆς τε καὶ τοῦ πρώτου σπονδύλου τομὴ τοῦ νωτιαίου, τὴν σκέπουσαν μηνιγγα τὸ πέρας τῆς ὀπίσω κοιλίας ἐγκεφάλου διαιροῦσα, παραχρῆμα τὸ ζῷον ἅπαντος τοῦ σώματος ἀκρατές τε ἅμα καὶ ἀναίσθητον ἐργάζεται. κατὰ τοῦτο τὸ μέρος ὁρᾶτε καὶ τοὺς ταύρους τεμνομένους ἐν τοῖς ἱεροῖς ὑπὸ τῶν βουτύπων. ἡ δὲ μετὰ τὸν πρῶτον, οὐχ ὅτι ταύτης μόνης ἅπτεται τῆς κοιλίας, διὰ τοῦτο τὰ αὐτὰ συμπτώματα φέρει τοῖς ζῴοις, ἀλλ' ὅτι τά τε κῶλα παραλύει τοῦ ζῴου καὶ πᾶσαν ἀναιρεῖ τὴν ἀναπνοήν. ταὐτὸν δ' ὑπάρχει τοῦτο καὶ τῇ μετὰ τὸν | δεύτερόν τε καὶ τρίτον καὶ τέταρτον σπόνδυλον, ἐάνπερ αὐτὸν οὕτως ἀκριβῶς τέμῃς, ὡς τὸ κατὰ τὴν συμβολὴν αὐτοῦ τὴν πρὸς τὸν πέμπτον ἀποφυόμενον νεῦρον διατεμεῖν· τά γε μὴν πρῶτα τοῦ τραχήλου κινεῖται τοῖς οὕτω τμηθεῖσι ζῴοις. ἡ δὲ μετὰ τὸν πέμπτον τομὴ τοῦ νωτιαίου τὰ μὲν ἄλλα πάντα τοῦ θώρακος παραλύει, τὸ διάφραγμα δ' ὀλίγου δεῖν ἀπαθὲς φυλάττει καί τι βραχὺ τῶν ὑψηλοτάτων μυῶν. ἡ δὲ μετὰ τὸν ἕκτον τοὺς μὲν ὑψηλοὺς τοῦ θώρακος μῦς ὁμοίως παραβλάπτει, τὸ διάφραγμα δ' ἧττον ἢ πρόσθεν. ἡ δὲ μετὰ τὸν ἕβδομον, ἔτι δὲ μᾶλλον μετὰ τὸν ὄγδοον, ἀβλαβῆ μὲν ἅπασαν ἔχει τὴν τοῦ διαφράγματος κίνησιν,

But I should like to add more to what I have mentioned here, namely, that should the spinal marrow that lies between the skull and the first vertebra be severed, or the meninx which protects the end of the posterior ventricle of the brain be cut through, then at once the whole of the body of the animal becomes deprived of movement. It is just here that you will see, in the temples of the gods, the oxen receive the stab when the so-called sacrificers of oxen cut into them. But as for the incision which is made behind the first vertebra, it inflicts on the animal just the same manifestations, not because it lays open the first ventricle [*fourth* in modern terminology] but because it paralyses the feet of the animal and arrests the whole of its respiration. And this is found also with regard to the incision which is made behind the second, third and fourth vertebra, when in making the cut you go to work thoroughly so that you divide the nerve which springs off at its [the fourth vertebra's] junction with the fifth vertebra. However, the first [ie: upper] segments of the neck still move themselves in the animal on which the cut has been made in such a manner. Transection of the spinal marrow behind the fifth vertebra paralyses all the remaining parts of the thorax, and arrests their movements, but the diaphragm remains almost unscathed, and so does a small portion of the upwardly ascending part of the musculature of the thorax [*Mm. scaleni*]. The transection which takes place behind the sixth vertebra damages in the same way the upwardly ascending thoracic musculature, and the diaphragm meets with less damage than that which followed in consequence of the preceding cut. But after the transection which takes place behind the seventh vertebra, and more particularly after that made behind the eighth vertebra, the whole of the mobility of the diaphragm remains unscathed[9].

5. Further transverse incisions of the spinal marrow

ἀβλαβῆ δὲ σχεδόν τι καὶ τὴν τῶν ὑψηλῶν μυῶν καὶ τῶν τοῦ τραχήλου παντός, οὐ μὴν τῶν γε μεσοπλευρίων· ἀπόλλυται γὰρ ἅπασα, κατὰ πάντας ⟨τοὺς⟩ τοῦ τραχήλου σπονδύλους τῆς τομῆς γενομένης, ὅπου καὶ μετὰ τὸν | πρῶτον αὐτοῦ τοῦ θώρακος ὅλου τμηθέντος τοῦ νωτιαίου, οὕτως ἀπόλλυται πᾶσα τῶν μεσοπλευρίων μυῶν ἡ ἐνέργεια. παντάπασι δ᾽ αὐτῆς ὀλίγον σῴζεται, κατὰ τὸ δεύτερον μεσοπλεύριον τῆς τομῆς γενομένης· ἐφεξῆς δὲ κατὰ λόγον ἀεὶ τῶν μὲν ὑψηλοτέρων τῆς τομῆς μεσοπλευρίων μυῶν ἐνεργούντων, τῶν ταπεινοτέρων δὲ παραλυομένων.

Again the mobility of the upwardly extending musculature, and the mobility of the whole neck will remain quite free from damage, but the intercostal muscles do not at the same time remain uninjured thereby. For the mobility of this musculature is destroyed and becomes totally lost when one imposes the cut upon any one of the vertebrae of the neck, and the whole hind-brain is cut off from the first thoracic vertebra. Amongst the proofs of this is the fact that the activity of the intercostal muscles become totally lost when one carries through the spinal medulla behind the first thoracic vertebra a cut which completely divides it, whereas a slight proportion of this activity stays retained when the cut takes place behind the second vertebra. In connection with this there is the fully analogous point that those intercostal muscles which lie higher up than the situation of the incision preserve their activity, whereas the activity of the muscles lying below the site of the incision will be abolished[10].

(End of chapter 3).

(*Oribasius*, Chapter 8)

6. The internal lining of the mouth and throat

Ὁ χιτὼν τῆς γλώττης συνεχής ἐστιν ἅπαντι τῷ κατὰ τὴν τοῦ στόματος εὐρυχωρίαν ἄχρι τῆς φάρυγγος·

This covering is firmly united with the one which clothes [lines] the whole of the oral cavity uniformly as far as the fauces[11].

[9] *Raeder,* III, 12, 8–27. *Duckworth,* p. 25.

[10] *Raeder,* III, 12, 27–35. *Duckworth,* p. 26.

[11] *Raeder,* III, 18, 29–30. *Duckworth,* p. 54.

I

When I say fauces I understand by it that portion within the mouth up to which the head of the oesophagus and that of the larynx extend.

7. The same, continued

ὁ δ᾽ αὐτὸς οὗτος καὶ διὰ τοῦ στομάχου καὶ τῆς τραχείας ἀρτηρίας κατέρχεται, συνεχὴς ὢν ἑαυτῷ,

The same covering passes downwards into the oesophagus and the larynx as a continuous, firmly woven single structure[12], yet variable in its different parts.

Its essential structure does not change, and it differs only in respect of its thickness or attenuation. That is to say, the mucous lining, so long as it passes down in the oesophagus to the stomach, continues to increase in thickness, and when it comes to the stomach, there it is even thicker. For the inner one of the linings of the stomach is the one which is continuous and conjoined with that of the cavity of the mouth. And just as this layer becomes thicker than it was, so it diminishes in thickness gradually while it passes down through the fauces into the trachea. You know that it is the larynx which lies between the fauces and the trachea, and it is through the larynx that that lining passes to the trachea. Its position is

8. The position of the internal lining

πάντων, ὡς εἴρηται, τούτων ὑπάρχων κοινός, γλώττης καὶ στόματος παντὸς ἐπιγλωττίδος τε καὶ φάρυγγος καὶ στομάχου καὶ γαστρὸς καὶ λάρυγγος καὶ τραχείας ἀρτηρίας.

as I have described it, that is to say, it is common to and envelops all these organs, namely the tongue, the whole oral cavity, the epiglottis, the fauces, the larynx, the trachea, the oesophagus, and the stomach[13].

Because of the position of this covering, it is best that you should cut away the mandible as a whole . . . [Here again *Oribasius* omits *Galen*'s technical instructions for dissection, and his details of the extrinsic muscles of the tongue. He takes up *Galen*'s words again after the sentence in the English translation ending . . . how scanty is the amount of blood in it.]

[12] *Raeder*, III, 18, 30–32. *Duckworth*, p. 54. Note that there is no Greek equivalent of 'single'.

[13] *Raeder*, III, 18, 32–34. *Duckworth*, p. 54.

9. The *frenulum* of the tongue[14]

τὸ δ' ἐν τῷ στόματι μέρος τῆς γλώττης ἄνωθεν μὲν ὅλον φαίνεται, κάτωθεν δ' οὐχ ὅλον, ἀλλ' ἐκεῖνο μόνον ὅσον ἐκτός ἐστι τοῦ πρὸς τὴν γένυν δεσμοῦ κατὰ τὸν ἔξωθεν αὐτῆς χιτῶνα γινομένου. καὶ πολλάκις γε μέχρι πλείονος ὁ δεσμὸς οὗτος ἐκτεταμένος οὐκ ἐπιτρέπει τῇ γλώττῃ πολυειδῶς κινεῖσθαι, καὶ διὰ τοῦτο ἀναγκαζόμεθα τέμνειν τε τὸν δεσμὸν ἀπολύειν τε τῆς δέσεως τὴν γλῶτταν, ὡς χαλαρὰν γενομένην ἐκτείνεσθαι πρός τε τὴν ὑπερῴαν καὶ τὰ πλάγια πάντα τοῦ στόματος μέρη. παρὰ δὲ τὸν δεσμὸν τοῦτον ἑκατέρωθεν ἐκ τῶν πλαγίων μερῶν εὑρήσεις ἀγγείων στόματα τῶν σιαλοχόων ὀνομαζομένων,

10. The salivary ducts[15]

ταῦτα τὰ ἀγγεῖα τὴν ἀρχὴν | ἔχει κατὰ τὴν ῥίζαν τῆς γλώττης, ἔνθα καὶ οἱ ἀδένες αὐτῆς εἰσιν· ἐξ ἐκείνων γὰρ ἐκφύεται παραπλήσια ταῖς ἀρτηρίαις ὄντα τὴν ἰδέαν,

That part of it which lies in the mouth reveals itself freely and visibly in its entirety from above, but from below you do not view it as a whole, but you see only that part which is outside its band of communication with the mandible (*frenulum*) which is found in its outer covering. This band frequently shrinks considerably, and then does not permit the tongue to perform its various movements. Because of this defect we are forced to cut the frenulum and subsequently liberate the tongue, so that when it is used for speaking it can extend itself and reach to the uppermost part of the hard palate and the sides of the mouth. On both sides of this band (*frenulum*) you will find the orifices of ducts called salivary (*ducts of Bartholin or Wharton*). [Oribasius here condenses the following sentence: On the tongue of an ox a thick sound (probe) may be able to penetrate into any one of these orifices, but with the tongues of small animals, the use of a fine sound is required for that purpose.] The origin of these ducts in near the root of the tongue, where the spongy flesh [glandular mass] attached to the tongue lies, since the origin of these ducts is from that part. Their aspect is that of the pulsating blood vessels, that is, the arteries.

[*Oribasius*' Greek now is taken from *Galen's* De Usu Partium, and copied down faithfully. This is followed by two passages of uncertain origin, and *Oribasius* returns to the Anatomical Procedures at the beginning of his chapter 9, corresponding to line 33, page 68 of the English translation.]

[14] *Raeder*, III, 18, 34–p. 19, 6. *Duckworth*, p. 60.

[15] *Raeder*, III, 19, 7–9. *Duckworth*, p. 60.

I

244

11. The larynx

Τὸ ὑπὸ τῇ κάτω γένυϊ κατὰ τὴν μέσην χώραν τῶν πρώτων τοῦ τραχήλου ʹμερῶν τεταγμένον σῶμα, προπετὲς εἰς τὸ πρόσω φαινόμενον, ἅπαντες ἴσασί τε καὶ καλοῦσι λάρυγγα,

I say, then, that the body lying beneath the mandible in the mid-line of the first part of the neck, that is to say the part projecting forwards, is a body which everybody knows and designates by the name larynx [16].

[*Oribasius* then condenses the sentence: Among wrestlers, one will often be thrown by the other when the latter grips that structure and dislocates and fractures it, when the two competitors are exerting themselves violently in wrestling a fall and one slips in below the armpit of the other.]

12. The passage of air

πνίγεται γὰρ παραυτίκα θλασθέντος αὐτοῦ τὰ ζῷα, στενοτάτης κατʼ αὐτὸ τῆς διεξόδου τῷ κατὰ τὴν ἀναπνοὴν ἀέρι γινομένης.

When this structure is ruptured or crushed, the animal is choked forthwith because the passage of the air through which it passes here, being expelled or breathed in, is very narrow [17].

[*Oribasius* here returns to De Usu Partium, and then takes up the Greek of the Anatomical Procedures as follows.]

13. The cartilages of the throat

τὰς γὰρ ὁριζούσας τὰ πλάγια μέρη πλευρὰς τοῦ θυρεοειδοῦς θεάσει διὰ παντὸς ὁμιλούσας ταῖς πλευ|ραῖς τοῦ δευτέρου χόνδρου, τό τε κάτω μέρος ὅλον τῷ κάτω διὰ μυῶν ἡνωμένον. τὸ δʼ ἄνω πέρας ἑκατέρου τῶν χόνδρων ἀντιτέτακται,

You see that of its margins those which mark the limits of its two flanks [*lateral thyroid laminae*] continuously adjoin the margins of the second cartilage [*cricoid cartilage*]and you see that the whole of its lower portion is fastened to the lower part of that [second] cartilage, and is connected to it by means of muscles. But as for the upper ends of both cartilages, that of the one stands opposite to that of the other [18].

[At this point *Oribasius* slightly condenses *Galen*'s analogy with two shields.]

At this place is a third small cartilage, seated upon the second, the shape of which is like that of a drinking vessel. Consequently it derives

[17] *Raeder*, III, 19, 23–25. *Duckworth*, p. 69. [16] *Raeder*, III, 19, 20–22.
[18] *Raeder*, III, 19, 33–36. *Duckworth*, p. 71.

its name from the name 'drinking vessel', and it is called the drink-vessel-like or drink-vessel-shaped.

When you have seen all these things which I have described, and those things also which I wish subsequently to describe after you have removed the whole larynx, then your understanding and comprehension of the dissection of which I am about to tell you will be clearer. The things of which I said I wished to speak to you are as follows.

14. The thyroid cartilage

τεττάρων δ' οὐσῶν τοῦ θυρεοειδοῦς γωνιῶν κατὰ τὰς συμβολὰς τῶν ὁριζουσῶν αὐτὸν τεττάρων γραμμῶν,

I say that the thyroid cartilage has four angles [*cornua*] at the meeting places of the four lines which bound it[19].

Those two angles which lie below are attached by an articular ligament to the second cartilage.

15. The hyoid bone

αἱ μὲν κάτω δύο συμφύονται διὰ νευροχονδρώδους δεσμοῦ τοῖς κάτω πέρασι τῶν ταπεινῶν πλευρῶν τοῦ λαβδοειδοῦς· ἐπίκειται δὲ τοῦτο τῷ ἄνω πέρατι τοῦ πρώτου χόνδρου, τὴν μὲν εὐθεῖάν τε καὶ μέσην ἑαυτοῦ γραμμὴν κατ' εὐθὺ τῆς τε ῥάχεως ἔχων τοῦ θυρεοειδοῦς καὶ τῆς ἐν τοῖς κάτω μέρεσι τῆς γλώσσης γραμμῆς, τὰς ταπεινὰς δὲ δύο πλευρὰς ἐπὶ τὰς ἄνω γωνίας ἐκτείνων τοῦ πρώτου χόνδρου· θυρεοειδῆ γὰρ λέγειν ἢ πρῶτον, οὐ διοίσει.

[but] the two upper angles are united to the lower margins of the lower [ie: greater] ribs [*cornua*] of the bone which resembles the letter Λ of the Greek script [*hyoid bone*] by a ligament of which the nature [substance] is intermediate between tendon and cartilage [*cartilago tritice in the thyrohyoid ligament*]. For the hyoid bone lies above the upper margin of the first cartilage [*thyroid*] and its vertical median line stands opposite to the median line of the underlying parts of the tongue. But its two lower ribs [*cornua*] go back towards the two upper angles [*cornua*] of the first cartilage: it is the same whether you call this cartilage 'first' or 'thyroid'[20].

16. The hyoid, continued
(*Oribasius*, book 25, chapter 8)

Τὸ λαβδοειδὲς ὀστοῦν τὴν ἰδέαν ἐστὶ τοιοῦτον· τὸ μὲν μέσον αὐτοῦ μέρος, ὃ κατὰ τὴν οἷον διχοτομίαν τοῦ τραχήλου ἐστὶ καὶ παντὸς τοῦ σώματος,

[19] *Raeder*, III, 19, 38–p. 20, 1. *Duckworth*, p. 71.
[20] *Raeder*, III, 20, 1–8. *Duckworth*, p. 72.

ὀστοῦν ὄψει βραχὺ μὲν καὶ τῷ μήκει, τὸ δ' οὖν πλάτος τε καὶ βάθος οὕτως ἔχον μικρὸν ὡς καὶ τοῦ μήκους ὑπάρχειν ἔλαττον· ἐκ δὲ τῶν πλαγίων μερῶν τοῦ κάτω πέρατος αὐτοῦ δύο ἀποφύονται πλευραὶ πρὸς τὰς ὑψηλὰς γωνίας, ὡς ἔφην ἄρτι, τοῦ θυρεοειδοῦς ἐκτεινόμεναι λοξαί. τὸ δ' ἄνω πέρας τοῦ λαβδοειδοῦς ὀστοῦ τοῦδε δύο ἄλλας ἔχει πλευρὰς ἀποφυομένας παραλλήλους ταῖς κάτω, λεπτὰς καὶ στενὰς καὶ περιφερεῖς ὡς βελόνας παχείας ἢ γραφίου τὸ πέρας. ἡ δ' οὐσία τῶν πλευρῶν τούτων, λοξῶν καὶ αὐτῶν, ἀτρέμα εἰς τὸ κάτω νευουσῶν, ἀκριβὴς χόνδρος ἐστί, καί τις στρογγύλος οἷάπερ τὰ νεῦρα σύνδεσμος ἀπὸ τοῦ πέρατος ἑκατέρας αὐτῶν ἐκφυόμενος ἐπὶ τὰς γραφιοειδεῖς τῆς | κεφαλῆς ἀποφύσεις ἐκτείνεται, πέρας καὶ ταύτας ἐχούσας ὁμοιότατον αὐταῖς ταῖσδε ταῖς ὑψηλαῖς πλευραῖς τοῦ λαβδοειδοῦς· τῇ τε γὰρ οὐσίᾳ χόνδροι εἰσί, καὶ τὸ σχῆμα ταὐτὸν ἁπάσαις ἐστίν· τῷ μήκει δ' ἀπολείπονται τῶν πλευρῶν τοῦ λαβδοειδοῦς αἱ γραφιοειδεῖς ἐκφύσεις.

I say, then, that you find in these animals, and particularly in those apes which most closely resemble Man, the constitution of this bone [*hyoid*] as follows. You will find its middle portion [*body*], that is the portion across which runs the line which divides into two halves [R. and L.], the neck and the whole of this bone, of small length. You will find it deficient also in breadth and depth, a deficiency which is even greater than that of its length, as you will find when you compare its three dimensions[21]. Two ribs spring from the two sides of its lower margin, which pass in a sloping direction towards the upper angles [*cornua*] of the thyroid cartilage, as I have described previously. And on its upper margin this hyoid bone has two other 'ribs' which grow outwards parallel to the lower 'ribs'. Now these two upper ribs are slender and cylindrical like two stout needles, or the ends of two awls, and the substance of these two ribs, which are likewise slanted and inclined slightly downwards, is pure cartilage. From the end of each of the two [*lesser cornua*] goes a cylindrically shaped ligament [*stylohyoid ligament*] like a nerve, and each of these two [ligaments] extends itself to one of the two processes of the skull which are called 'awl-like' [*styloid processes*].

These two processes also have two margins which resemble the upper ribs of the hyoid bone. For their substance is cartilaginous and the form of them all is one and the same. But as to the length, here the two styloid processes are shorter than the two ribs [*?lesser cornua*] of the hyoid bone[22].

(III) Commentary

1. The membranes of the spinal cord

Note that the version from the Arabic source is in some respects condensed, in omitting τήν τε παχεῖαν καὶ τὴν λεπτήν ('both the thick and the thin', ie: the dura and the pia mater) and αἷς δὴ καὶ ἥνωται

[21] This last phrase of the sentence has no counterpart in Greek.

[22] *Raeder*, III, 55, 6–22. *Duckworth*, p. 72–73.

('it is indeed with those that it [the spinal cord] is united'). On the other hand, where the Greek has κορωνῶν (condyles) the Arabic-English is less specific '. . . is on the skull'.

The Greek of the last sentence of the fragment in *Daremberg*'s text (⟨τὸ⟩ πρόσω ⟨τῶν⟩ σπονδύλων) gives what *Cohen* and *Drabkin* render as '. . . seems to bind together the anterior surfaces of the vertebrae . . .'. *Raeder*'s text, though slightly more difficult, might yield '. . . binds together somehow further into the vertebrae . . .' or perhaps '. . . in front of the vertebrae . . .'.

The first and third of these readings do not appear very satisfactory anatomically. It is possible that the Arabic version was based on a sounder Greek text; the English has '. . . binds together the vertebrae in front . . .' which if taken to imply in front of the spinal cord and its meninges, the object of Galen's attention, suggests the posterior longitudinal ligament, which, together with the ligamenta flava, is identified by *Duckworth* as *Galen*'s 'third structure'. This interpretation is perhaps strengthened by *Galen*'s later reference (in the Arabic-English text) to the place where the third structure is 'folded' as that where the nerves emerge from the cord, ie: towards its anterior. The reference to folding appears to be an Arabic interpretation of the Greek, which indicates that the membrane is double. Conceivably *Galen* was looking at the posterior longitudinal ligament lying over the ligamentous external surface of the intervertebral discs, which do indeed bind together the vertebrae.

4. Transverse incision of the spinal marrow

Note that the first two incisions mentioned as separate operations in the English are identical in the Greek. The 'first ventricle' of the English, which *Duckworth* identifies with the fourth of modern terminology, is referred to in the Greek simply as 'this ventricle', ie: the posterior already referred to. The discrepancy between 'feet' in the Arabic-English version and κῶλα in the Greek, has already been noted, p. 3 above.

5. Further transverse incisions of the spinal marrow

This fragment calls for special comment. The Arabic-English version is generally fuller than the Greek, but it is not clear whether *Oribasius* has condensed *Galen*'s words or the Arabic expanded them. Thus in the second sentence, where the Greek has 'is totally destroyed', the Arabic has the repetitive 'is destroyed and becomes totally lost'. It is probably therefore an Arabic addition, but the same is unlikely to be true of what follows: '. . . and the whole hind brain in cut off from the first thoracic vertebra . . .', which appears to be a technical note of the further explanation omitted by *Oribasius*. The following 'Amongst the proofs of this is the fact that . . .' is matched simply by ὅπου, ie: 'since' or 'whereas' in the Greek, and it appears to be an Arabic attempt to grapple with a rather technical point made in the flow of *Galen*'s argument. *Galen*'s whole discussion is centred on the progressive nature of the paralysis and loss of sensation in the body as the sectioning of the spinal cord moves upwards. It follows that as the total activity of the intercostal muscles is destroyed by a section behind the first thoracic vertebra, this paralysis is subsumed in that which follows section at a higher point, ie: between any cervical vertebrae. *Galen* has in mind that since, in his opinion, all motor nerves arise from the posterior part of the brain, and some of them descend through the spinal canal, if they are damaged by an inferior section of the cord, they will certainly be damaged by a superior.

In translating *Oribasius*' text at this point, *Cohen* and *Drabkin* have 'Even when a complete section of the spinal cord is made just below the first vertebra of the chest, the activity of the intercostal muscles in completely suppressed'.

However, the Greek more easily gives a meaning which follows *Galen*'s argument as outlined above: '. . . for it is all destroyed when a cut is made at any of the vertebrae of the neck, *since* when the spinal cord is completely cut through after the first vertebra of the thorax itself the entire activity of the intercostal muscles is *thus* destroyed', (ie: destroyed in the same way).

10. The salivary ducts

It has been noted above, p 3 that the frenulum is said to expand in the Greek, while the Arabic-English has 'shrinks'. The latter, however, seems to make the better sense in the context. Reference has also been made, p 3 to the use of the term 'pulsating blood vessels' in the Arabic-English.

15. The hyoid bone

Daremberg's reading, with ἄνω in the first line of this fragment, corresponds to the Arabic-English version. One might conjecture that the Greek of Raeder's text has arisen from a haplography. The Arabic-English version clearly distinguishes between (A) 'Those two angles which lie below . . .' and (B) 'the upper two angles'. If eg: αἱ μὲν κάτω δύο originally stood for (A) and αἱ δ' ἄνω δύο for (B) a scribal eye may have jumped from the first to the second δύο omitting the intervening material.

Note that the Arabic-English version has omitted τῆς τε ῥάχεως ἔχων τοῦ θυρεοειδοῦς, in: the median line of the hyoid is aligned also with the spine of the thyroid.

16. The hyoid, continued

Note that the opening flourish of the Arabic-English version has no counterpart in the Greek, which begins directly with a description of the bone. In the second line of the fragment, the Greek has 'body' where the English has 'bone'.

De Juvamentis Membrorum and the Reception of Galenic Physiological Anatomy

GALEN'S MOST IMPORTANT WORK on functional anatomy is *De usu partium.* It is complementary to the work on morphology and the techniques of dissection, *De anatomicis administrationibus,* and to that on the biological forces which were the basis of his physiology, *De naturalibus facultatibus.* All three works give us the theoretical background of Galen's biomedical system; in particular *De usu partium* deals with the form and function of the body in the context of Galen's natural-philosophical worldview. The transmission of this text through subsequent ages is therefore of considerable interest.

Galen's position at the height of Hellenistic culture was not regained by those who followed. In the absence of a comparable figure able to assimilate and transcend Galen's achievement, progress in anatomy and physiology was not made. The three major Galenic works remained in the library at Alexandria, but teaching depended on a single work, *Minor Anatomy,* compiled from Galen's short introductory works on the five tissue systems (nerves, veins, arteries, muscles, and bones).[1] It is probably as a result of this arrangement that Arabic and early medieval Western medical education gave little attention to anatomy. The two major Galenic anatomical works were rendered intelligible to the less sophisticated ages that followed Galen by the production of summaries and abstracts: *De usu partium* was compressed into a very small compass by the Byzantine Theophilus Protospatharius, and Oribasius' extracts from *De anatomicis administrationibus* (4th century) are all that remain from the lost Greek of the second half of that work.

After this period *De usu partium* was the sole vehicle of physiological anatomy as applied to man and therefore of use in a medical context. The surviving first half of *De anatomicis administrationibus* was not widely known before Latin versions were produced by Chalcondylas and Guinter in the earlier sixteenth century, and the techniques of dissection that Galen describes within it are clearly applied to apes, not man. Although Aristotle's works on animals had been known in the Middle Ages in the translations by Michael Scot and William of Moerbeke, Aristotle had admitted that the inside of *man* was one of the most unknown of all things, and medical use of the zoological works was limited. Moreover, Aristotle's anatomical and physiological

*Wellcome Unit for the History of Medicine, University of Cambridge, Cambridge CB2 3RH England.

[1]A. Z. Iskandar, "An Attempted Reconstruction of the Late Alexandrian Medical Curriculum," *Medical History,* 1976, *20*:235–258; p. 250.

descriptions were often less detailed and consistent than those of Galen, largely because the fruitful Alexandrian period occurred between the lives of the two men. In particular Aristotle's descriptions of the "nerves," of the heart and its vascular connections with the lungs, were powerfully criticized by Galen. In contrast, *De usu partium* claims to be dealing with human structure and function and was addressed equally to physicians and philosophers. It was an immensely important work for the future of medicine and biology in the West. It is the only classical authority quoted extensively by William Harvey in *De motu cordis,* and it was the physiology of the work that he and the discoverers of the pulmonary transit had to overcome. In the absence of a complete version of *De anatomicis administrationibus, De usu partium* was the most important anatomical work available to Vesalius, whose anatomical exposition was guided entirely by his classical predecessor and chosen opponent.

THE TRANSLATION OF DE USU PARTIUM

For the reasons mentioned above it is of interest to look at the history of the translation of *De usu partium*. Its importance was soon realized in the East, and it was first rendered into Syriac by Sergios in the sixth century. Hunain, in the ninth century, tells us that this version was unsatisfactory, and he himself produced a Syriac version. He also had access to an incomplete and imperfect Arabic version by his nephew Hubaish, which he completed and corrected in that language.[2] The medieval Latin West recovered the full text from the Greek in the early fourteenth century. However, before this version was available, a Latin translation was made from an incomplete and (if we may judge by the Latin text) unsatisfactory Arabic version,[3] possibly that of Hubaish. This Latin version is known as *De juvamentis membrorum,* and by reason of its small size and freedom from much of the complexity and technicalities of Galen's thought, it remained much more popular than *De usu partium* until well into the Renaissance. There are many more manuscripts extant of the shorter work,[4] and two hundred years after Nicholas of Reggio produced the full text from the Greek, *De juvamentis membrorum* was being printed alongside it in the collected works of Galen, for example, in the edition of Pavia, 1515–1516 and that of Venice, 1528. This popular but corrupt and incomplete text misinformed its readers of many of Galen's ideas and kept them in ignorance of others. It is the purpose of this paper to illustrate the results of this situation. We may first look at the text itself,[5] and then examine some particular uses of it by medieval authors.

[2]Max Meyerhof, "New Light on Hunain ibn Ishaq and His Period," *Isis,* 1926, *8*:685–725; p. 695.

[3]It is of course possible that this Arabic version is itself a translation of a late Hellenistic summary, although known Hellenistic compressions of Galen's anatomical works achieve their brevity without misrepresenting or misunderstanding Galen's text: see R. K. French and G. E. R. Lloyd, "Lost Greek Fragments of Galen's Anatomical Procedures," *Sudhoffs Archiv* (in press); Theophilus' compression of part of *De usu partium,* although very short, does not distort the original (the Latin versions only have been compared): Theophilus Protospatharius, *In Galeni de Usu partium epitome* (Paris, 1540). A hint as to the translator of *De juvamentis membrorum* is given in MS BN 14389, "translatus a Iohannitio filio Ysaac." "Joannitius" is a name that has been taken to indicate the translator Hunain, where Joannitius appears as the author of the *Isagoge,* the first work of the medieval medical curriculum.

[4]D. Campbell, *Arabian Medicine and Its Influence on the Middle Ages,* 2 vols. (London, 1926), Vol. II, p. 43.

[5]The Pavia edition of 1515–1516 is the principal source of the text as used in this paper, with frequent reference to the Venice edition of 1528. On specific points two MSS have been consulted: Peterhouse 33 in Cambridge and Balliol 231 in Oxford. The version of *De usu partium* used for purposes of comparison in the medieval context is that printed in Paris in 1528, in which the text of Nicholas of Reggio's translation, which was available in the period we are discussing, has not suffered the improvements of Renaissance Latinists. It should also be noted that there is another version with a different Latin style, including a

Since *De juvamentis membrorum* is most probably in its original form an Arabic compression of the Greek and not a Latin compression of an Arabic version of *De usu partium,*[6] we can tell by comparing the two texts exactly how the Arabic translator shortened the Greek original,[7] or in other words what in one instance the Arabs were looking for in the incoming Greek science. We can see the technical difficulties of making a translation from Galen's sophisticated Greek into the culturally unprepared languages of Arabic and in turn Latin, and we can follow in detail the degeneration of the anatomical and physiological ideas of the original. The use of *De juvamentis membrorum* in the West supplies us with an example of how the reception of Greek science and its development were hindered by textual problems.

DE JUVAMENTIS MEMBRORUM AND ARABIC SCIENCE

We have already seen that *De usu partium* was too big and complex to be used in medical teaching, and it was no doubt the desire to render the work intelligible and convenient that led to the production of the shortened text we are now considering. The translator compressed twelve of the seventeen books of *De usu partium* into ten (some manuscripts have nine) of *De juvamentis membrorum*. We do not know whether it did not serve the translator's purpose to continue his summary to the last five books or whether he stopped for other reasons; perhaps part of his summary has been lost. However, we do know by comparing the texts that his compression of the original was on the whole not paraphrastic and depended instead on the omission of certain kinds of passages, with the result that other passages remain more or less intact from the original.

By this method of condensation the editing translator hoped to pick out the essence of Galen's anatomy and physiology. He consequently omitted first from his translation those passages in which Galen passionately and extensively refutes many of the opinions of his predecessors. Thus where Galen draws from Plato a notion of causality to explain the anomalous structure of the pulmonary blood vessels,[8] the Arabic translator omits Galen's brief reference to Erasistratus and his vigorous and lengthy attack on Asclepiades' reasons for the structure of these vessels.[9] Second, the Arabic translator was apt to ignore Galen's frequent references to the rationality of a personalized and benign Nature, the creator of the body. The whole purpose of *De usu partium* was to give a "reasoned account" of the structure and function of the body, relating them to the rest of natural philosophy and metaphysics; in fact, so pervasive is Galen's teleology that the whole work is almost an exercise in natural theology. Galen's sentiments, however, were either irrelevant to the translator or

---

different incipit and explicit, known as *De utilitate particularium,* which is also attributed to Nicholas of Reggio; see, e.g., the collected works of Galen in 1528 (Venice). There is considerable confusion in the secondary literature over the relationship of the two versions of *De usu partium* with each other and with *De juvamentis membrorum,* but the former question does not affect the argument of this paper.

6 Campbell, *Arabian Medicine,* Vol. I, p. 23, claims that there are Arabic MSS extant, but it appears from Diels, Campbell's source, that at least one of these, Escurial 850, actually contains *De usu partium*; Hermann Diels, *Die Handschriften der griechischen Ärzte* (Berlin: Akademie der Wissenschaften, 1905–1906). See also Manfred Ullmann, *Die Medizin im Islam* (Leiden: Brill, 1970), p. 41.

7 For the purposes of a Greek-Arabic comparison the English translation of the Greek is a convenient guide to the published Greek texts (Galen, *De usu partium libri XVII,* ed. G. Helmreich, 2 vols. Leipzig: Teubner, 1907–1909); see Galen, *On the Usefulness of the Parts of the Body,* trans. M. T. May, 2 vols. (Ithaca: Cornell University Press, 1968).

8 Galen, *On the Usefulness,* Vol. I, p. 307.

9 *De juvamentis membrorum* VII 3.

opposed to his religious ideas, so we cannot find in *De juvamentis membrorum* Galen's admiration for nature's positioning of the esophagus (it should be in VII 1) nor his introductory remarks on nature's foresight in arranging the organs of respiration (VII 2).[10]

Galen's use of comparative anatomy did not always interest the translator either, for example Galen's reference to the number of lobes of the lung and the reasons why fish do not have lungs.[11] Galen was a champion of the observational method and often advises his readers to consult, by means of dissection, nature as the ultimate arbiter in disputed questions of anatomy. His advice fell upon deaf ears until the Renaissance in the West, and the Arabic translator omits many of Galen's recommendations to perform dissections to understand, for example, the structure of the lung,[12] which should be at the beginning of the eighth book of *De juvamentis membrorum*. In questions of physiology the observational method extended its role in Galen's methodology into vivisection and experiment. Part of his reasons for conducting experiments was to prove by appeal to the senses that someone else's opinions were wrong, but this was apparently both too practical and too close to Galen's vituperative style of argument for the translator of *De juvamentis membrorum*. He did not, for example, share Galen's pleasure in inflating the lungs of a dead animal to observe the movement of the tracheal cartilages[13] and consequently omitted the experiment from the first chapter of Book VIII.

Often when Galen is describing a dissection technique or an experiment he is obliged to refer to other works, such as the more severely practical *De anatomicis administrationibus,* or to preliminary or introductory works of his own, which he expects his readers to be familiar with. In these cases Galen is most often elaborating a point already made in the text of *De usu partium,* not uncommonly by reference to practical techniques. The translator was content with the simple statement of Galen's viewpoint, without its elaborate cross reference or practical proof. Thus in the discussion on the functioning of the organs of respiration (*De juvamentis membrorum* VIII 1) the translator has not included Galen's references to *De voce* or to a lost work on the motion of the thorax and lung.[14]

Lastly we need not be surprised that the Arabic translator condensed Galen's expansive style of writing wherever he could, whether by omitting recapitulations and repetitions or by ignoring Galen's rhetorical questions. Perhaps we may also put into this category Galen's remarks on his own methodological superiority (which often take on a personal tone) and the extended arguments in which Galen displays his powers. The Arabic translator preserved in many cases only Galen's conclusions.

We have listed above some seven or eight categories of textual material omitted from the Greek text of *De usu partium* by the Arabic translator and compiler of *De juvamentis membrorum,* and although only one or two examples have been given in each case, they could be multiplied almost indefinitely. The impression gained from the resulting text is that at this comparatively early stage in the reception of Greek science into the Arabic language (that is, before the great synthesizers such as Avicenna) the Arabic writers were interested in Galen's concrete statements about the structure and function of the human body and less interested in the relationship between these ideas and the rest of Hellenistic culture, whether historically (through

[10]Galen, *On the Usefulness,* Vol. I, pp. 287, 290.
[11]*Ibid.,* pp. 285, 341.
[12]*Ibid.,* p. 335.
[13]*Ibid.,* p. 339.
[14]*Ibid.,* pp. 338, 339.

Galen's predecessors) or philosophically (through Galen's worldview and modes of argument).[15]

DE JUVAMENTIS MEMBRORUM IN THE WEST

It is likely that the work was translated into Latin in the twelfth century, but we cannot be certain of the date or translator; Burgundio of Pisa seems an unlikely suggestion.[16] Whatever its immediate source, it is clear that it was available before the full text of *De usu partium* had been translated from the Greek. During its earlier history in the West, *De juvamentis membrorum* was the only identifiable source of Galenic physiological anatomy, for while most of the Arabic medical writings available were Galenic at root, the identification of this source was a question for future scholarship.

The most important of the Arabic works was the *Canon* of Avicenna, translated by Gerard of Cremona sometime after 1170 and of considerable influence in the following century. Aristotle's influence is seen to a greater extent in the *Canon* than in the other, earlier, Arabic systematic medical treatises, and we must see *De juvamentis membrorum* as the only alternative, extended in form and known to be by Galen, to the anatomical and physiological ideas of Aristotle. These ideas appeared in the West at a comparatively early date: sometime between 1210 and 1225 Michael Scot translated Aristotle's *De partibus animalium* and *Historia animalium* from the Arabic, in which language they were regarded as parts of a single work, the *Liber animalium*.[17] Michael Scot also translated Avicenna's treatise on animals, which is usually regarded as a summary of the combined Aristotelian zoological treatises[18] but which in fact contains a considerable amount of anatomical information and argument from Galen, although in a fragmentary form. For example, it contains both the Aristotelian and Galenic accounts of the structure of the heart.[19] Michael Scot interpolates such phrases as *dixit Medicus maximus* and *dixit Philosophus* to distinguish the opinions of Galen from those of Aristotle. The zoological works of Aristotle were translated from the Greek by William of Moerbeke about 1260. That the West now had a more or less complete account of Aristotle's zoology, with much more details of physiology and comparative anatomy, emphasizes the importance of *De juvamentis membrorum* as the only classical work in an extended form that

[15]We may compare the criticism of earlier anatomical texts offered by Haly Abbas in composing the *Liber regius*. Galen's anatomical texts were considered too diffuse, repetitive, and given to excessive criticisms of others and lengthy justifications of Galen's own opinions in the face of criticism. Haly also criticizes the fragmentation of Galen's writings into many short treatises; Haly himself tried to produce a comprehensive coverage. P. de Koning, *Trois traités d'anatomie arabes* (Leiden, 1903). See also Lucien Leclerc, *Histoire de la médecine arabe* (Paris: Leroux, 1876), Vol. I, p. 384, and E. G. Browne, *Arabian Medicine* (Cambridge: Cambridge University Press, 1921), p. 55.

[16]May, in *On the Usefulness*, Vol. I, p. 6, and George Sarton, *Galen of Pergamon* (Lawrence: University of Kansas Press, 1954), p. 57. Burgundio was not known for translations from the Arabic; see George Sarton, *Introduction to the History of Science*, Vol. II, Pt. 1 (Baltimore: Williams & Wilkins, 1931), p. 348, and M. Steinschneider, "Die Europaischen Übersetzungen aus dem Arabischen bis Mitte des 17. Jahrhunderts," *Sitzungberichte der philosophisch-historischen Klasse der Kaiserlichen Akademie der Wissenschaften*, 1905, *149* and 1906, *151*.

[17]Francis E. Peters, *Aristoteles Arabus* (Leiden: Brill, 1968), p. 47.

[18]See, e.g., S. D. Wingate, *The Medieval Latin Versions of the Aristotelian Scientific Corpus with Special Reference to the Biological Works* (London: Courier Press, 1931), p. 84, and M. Steinschneider, "Die Arabischen-Übersetzungen aus dem Griechischen." *Beihefte zum Centralblatt für Bibliothekwesen* (Leipzig, 1893–1894).

[19]Avicenna, *De natura animalium* in *Opera* (facsimile reprint of the 1508 ed., Frankfurt-am-Main, 1961).

claimed to be dealing with *human* structure, and therefore was useful in medicine, and which formed an alternative to Aristotle's ideas.

DIFFICULTIES IN TRANSLATION

The loss of the force of Galen's text by the omission of parts of it was inevitably furthered by difficulties of translation. Both at the Greek-Arabic and Arabic-Latin stages the recipient language was technically ill-equiped to receive the complex ideas and terminology of the work, and the translator faced the double difficulty of understanding and of expressing the original in his own language. There were normally two alternatives: if the translator understood the original technical term, he might find that there was nothing comparable in the recipient language and be obliged to use a word of general application in a technical sense; if he did not understand the original, then he would probably transliterate it. There is abundant evidence of both procedures in the Latin of *De juvamentis membrorum*.

The process whereby the translator sought out words of general application to use in a technical sense inevitably weakened the force of the original and introduced the possibility of confusion. For example, where Galen uses *thorax* for "chest,"[20] the meaning was transmitted through the Arabic to the Latin, which had no such precise word, and the translator was obliged to use *clibanus,* "oven" or "vessel in which bread is baked," to denote the chest as a rigid, hollow structure containing the heat-producing heart.[21] As examples of the second procedure, *taharib* is a transliterated Arabic word without a gloss, meaning perforated or spongy bone, *alrafila* is the conjunction of two brain ventricles, and *derezi* and its variants (*derec, darz*) is a suture of the cranium.[22] These words, entirely strange to the Western copyists and incapable of the normal Latin declension, were constantly misspelled by them, becoming corrupt as well as foreign.

THE HEART AND VESSELS

The organs contained within the *clibanus,* the spiritual or respiratory organs of Galen, furnish us with a good example of the textual degeneration of Galen's ideas. It is an important example because it was an area where Galen and Aristotle were irreconcilable and also because it was in resolving the difficulties of the ancient accounts that physiological progress was first made in the discovery of the pulmonary and systematic circulations.

There is no need to emphasize the part played in these discoveries by a considera-tion of the action of the valves. Yet the *idea* of a valve as we (and Harvey) understand it, and the word we use to express it are quite recent in origin. Galen, rather, discusses the action of the membranes, *hymenes,* which for us are merely parts of a valve. Galen held that one set of these, as part of their normal function, did not close their orifice completely. His ideas are only to be understood by reading the text in which he lays out the function of the membranes in their every situation, and in which he uses such explanatory analogies as he can. *Hymenes* is not a word used in a technical sense to encapsulate the meaning of a valve, for it applies to membranous structures

[20] Galen, *Opera omnia,* ed. C. G. Kühn, 20 vols. (Leipzig, 1821–1833), Vol. III (1822), p. 410.
[21] VII 1; the sentence in which the word occurs survives otherwise intact from the Greek. See Galen, *On the Usefulness,* Vol. I, p. 278.
[22] *De juvamentis membrorum* X 2, IX 6, X 6.

in general (Aristotle used it for the meninges). Consequently, when the text of *De usu partium* suffered in the construction of *De juvamentis membrorum,* so did Galen's idea. The medieval Latin translator used the term *coopertorium* for "membrane" in a general way (it is used also in Book IX for the meninges). In the language of the time it meant a "cover," anything from a lid of a pan to a suit of armor. The shortened text does not give enough support for the use of this word in the technical sense of "valve"; perhaps in the twelfth century there was no analogous mechanical contrivance well enough known to the reader of *De juvamentis membrorum*. Nor does the Arabic translator seem to have had an idea of a valve to guide him in his selection of which Galenic passages to retain in order to make clear the action of the heart. For example, in Book VII, Chapter 7 the action of a cardiac valve is entirely omitted; and in Chapter 4 the vagueness of the text fails to make clear the mechanical absurdity of the action of the mitral valve which so affronted Harvey in the full text of *De usu partium*.

The task of the translators and their readers in attempting to understand Galen on the action of the heart was made even more difficult because the Arabs did not use a word that corresponded to *arteria* in Greek.[23] They consequently used the phrase "pulsating vein" to express the Greek word, and the Latin translator of *De juvamentis membrorum* translated this directly as *vena pulsatilis*. Now, it is well known that the pulmonary vein for Galen looked like a vein but functioned as an artery and was consequently called the "venous artery," and that for the reverse reasons the pulmonary artery was called the "arterial vein." Such terminology was not available to the Arabic translator, who was obliged to use the clumsy "the pulsatile vein that looks like a nonpulsatile vein" and its reverse, translated directly by the Latin translator. Further difficulties arose because Galen said that the pulmonary vein, the "artery that looks like a vein," actually pulsated, *but* with a unique motion, following the movement of the thorax and not that of the heart; and the pulmonary artery ("the nonpulsatile vein that looks like a pulsatile vein" of the Arabs) did *not* pulsate in Galen's view because it functioned as a vein. The unfortunate reader of *De juvamentis membrorum* was faced with a nonpulsatile vein that looked like a pulsatile vein and which Galen said did not pulsate, but which in fact did. Moreover the omission of *non* from a phrase like *vena non pulsatilis* was a frequent copyists' error.[24]

DE JUVAMENTIS MEMBRORUM AND PETER OF ABANO

The greater availability of the shortened work at an early date and its greater popularity during the fourteenth century and later meant that it figured more largely than *De usu partium* as a source for the medical writers. Their anatomical and physiological knowledge correspondingly suffered; in particular the difference between the views of Aristotle and Galen on several important issues did not appear with the clarity that might stimulate progress in the later period.

Indeed, it is well known that many attempts were made to reconcile the differences between the two classical authorities during the Middle Ages, and the best-known author to make the attempt was Peter of Abano. His "conciliations" between the two

[23] The distinction between arteries and veins was made long after there was a word in Greek, Arabic, and Latin meaning "blood vessel," so *phleps* and *vena,* like the English *vein,* could mean either kind of blood vessel in a nontechnical context.

[24] One such error is printed in the 1515 ed., VII 2.

normally have an Aristotelian bias, but he knew enough of Galen's superior anatomy to find himself in difficulty when attempting to give credence to Aristotle on such questions as whether the brain or heart was the origin of the nerves and whether the vena cava arose in the liver or heart, questions much discussed in the Middle Ages. Peter ultimately decided in favor of the Aristotelian position in the dispute over the origin of the nerves. His proof of his conclusion consists of rejecting the arguments of others on the basis of close definition of terms, and in the course of this he systematically sets out the medical and philosophical positions. So corrupt was the text of *De juvamentis membrorum* that Peter was able to enlist its aid in defense of the Aristotelian view that the nerves arise in the heart. Certainly Peter was arguing principally on philosophical grounds that the heart was the prime organ of the body and that all other organs and faculties arose from it either embryologically or in an essential but not necessarily material way, but he was also making a morphological statement that exacerbated rather than conciliated the dispute.[25]

Two questions arise from this instance of Peter's use of *De juvamentis membrorum*: how can this Galenic text be taken to support an Aristotelian position and why did Peter rely on it to such a great extent? The dispute was essentially a medieval not classical question, because Aristotle did not have a clear notion of what a nerve was—the discovery of the central nervous system was the result of the work of the Alexandrians.[26] Before that time Greek writers used the word *neura* to include a number of fibrous structures some of which were nerves and some of which were the "sinews" of the joints which, it was a common Greek opinion, were one of the agents conveying motion to the limbs. It was Galen's view that Aristotle described the *neura* within the heart which Galen (but not Aristotle) saw were associated with the cardiac valves, and it was possible for those seeking to defend Aristotle to relate the cardiac *neura* and the *neura* of the joints. In fact *neura* (and the Latin *nervus*) had become a technical term for "nerve" drawn from wider usage, as the work of the Alexandrians became known. This specialist use of the word might well be unknown to a translator in a culturally unprepared language, and he would naturally translate it by another nontechnical word of wide application, thus reintroducing old confusions. For example, late classical accounts of anatomy in Latin are almost totally ignorant of the work of the Alexandrians and use *nervus* as "fibre."[27] Confusion was reinforced in Latin by the translation of *De juvamentis membrorum*: Galen thought of the heart as consisting of the ventricles only, the auricles being *fibrous* (we might say "sinewy") expansions of the veins. The word used to cover this meaning emerged in Latin as *nervus*. By another degeneration of Galen's text in the same sentence his "heart" had become "auricle." So the entire passage, in which Galen describes the sinewy expanded vessel connecting the heart to the vena cava, had degenerated into a description of a large *nerve* growing out of the auricle and joining the vena cava in the middle of the chest. Hence Peter of Abano had textual grounds for enlisting Galen in defense of Aristotle.

The passage from *De juvamentis membrorum* in question illustrates many features, discussed above, of the work as a whole:

[25]Peter of Abano, *Conciliator controversiarum, quae inter philosophos et medicos versantur* (Venice, 1565), p. 62v (Diff. 41).

[26]See Friedrich Solmsen, "Greek Philosophy and the Discovery of Nerves," *Museum Helveticum*, 1961, *18*:150–197.

[27]Translators' use of a word for "blood vessel" to translate technical terms for "artery" and "vein" likewise reintroduced old confusions. Cf. n. 23.

Et utilitas istius vene ample in corpore est magna utilitas sicut declaravimus; et propter hoc necessario ascendit[28] ad diafragma, et ascendit ad cor illa vena et ex corde etiam ascendit ad pulmonem, quare indiget etiam custodia in istis locis. Et etiam indigent ut custodiantur rami qui ex ea dividuntur ut non impediantur a motibus dorsi et cordis, et diafragmati et pulmonis. Quare creator ingeniabatur ponere illam venam et suos ramos in coopertoriis. Istud ergo est universale isti vene et aliis. Sed quod est proprium isti vene et cuilibet partium ejus sunt tria:[29] quorum unum est nervus fortis et oritur ex auricula dextra cordis, et occurit ipsi vene in medio pectoris et adjuvant ipsum. (VII 1)

And the use of this *vena cava* to the body is a great one, as we have said; and on account of it this vein necessarily rises to the diaphragm and then to the heart, and from the heart it ascends to the lung: and because of this it needs support in these places. Likewise the branches which arise from it need support lest they be disturbed by the motions of the back, the heart, the diaphragm and the lung. For this reason the creator contrived to place this vein and its branches in covers. This vein has that in common with others, but what relates to this vein alone is threefold: the first of which is a strong nerve, and it arises from the right auricle of the heart, and it runs up to this vein in the middle of the chest and assists it.

In the Greek, Galen had used the phrase *νευρώδη τε και ἰσχυρὰν ἀπόφυσιν*,[30] "a sinewy and strong outgrowth." In translating from the Greek Nicholas of Reggio has *nervosam et fortem apophysin et producionem*,[31] adding the last word as a gloss to *apophysin*, which clearly presented a stumbling block to both the Latin and Arabic reader: in *De juvamentis membrorum* it was omitted entirely, the associated adjective becoming a noun. The full text of *De usu partium* goes on to explain that the function of the *apophysis* will shortly be explained, that is, where Galen describes the action of the auricle, but the reference cannot apply in the text of *De juvamentis membrorum* (because *apophysis* is now *nervus*) and is consequently omitted.

A parallel case occurs at the beginning of the quoted passage, where the *vena ampla* is said to reach the diaphragm, heart, and *lung*. Galen had used *σφαγή*[32] to indicate the part of the throat that was cut in sacrificing animals. The context does not elucidate the meaning of the word, and it was probably transliterated in the Arabic translation. The word remained unintelligible to the Latin translator, who guessed that "lung" was indicated, thus introducing unnecessary confusion over the relations of the pulmonary vessels, which cannot have helped to clarify the confusion discussed above.

The medieval reader who chose *De usu partium* over *De juvamentis membrorum* would have encountered the full passage as quoted below.[33] This is followed by an English translation from the *Greek* for the benefit of the modern reader who will be able to form a notion of Galen's thought on the matter and compare the original with the medieval versions.

Concavam igitur venam, maximas utilitates animali praebentem (sicut in libris prioribus ostendebatur) necessarium quidem fuit per medias phrenas ad cor deferri,[34] et rurus inde ad vocatae σφαγῆς[35] hoc est iuguli regionem ascendere, sicut et hoc monstrabitur. Cumque moveatur semper cor ipsum, et pulmo, et phrenes, et totus thorax: non erat tuta[36]

[28] Balliol 231 and Peterhouse 33 have *descendit.*

[29] The wording of the beginning of this sentence differs in Balliol 231.

[30] Galen, *De usu partium,* ed. Helmreich, Vol. I, p. 306.

[31] *De utilitate particularium,* ed. Nicholas of Reggio (1528), p. 159 (VI 4).

[32] Galen, *On the Usefulness,* Vol. I, p. 283 and n. 12.

[33] Galen, *De usu partium corporis humani* (Paris, 1528), p. 158.

[34] *De utilitate . . .* (1528) has *referri.*

[35] *Ibid.,* has *sfagis* and omits the explanatory *hoc est iuguli regionem.*

[36] *Ibid.*

per medium eius spacium, nisi aliqua extrorsum auxilia natura excogitasset: per quae auxilia, quamvis agitetur semper vena concava, et quasi sit suspensa, ad haec resistat, et si violentur cadat aliquando supra dorsum vel pectus animal, vel ab aliquo externo percutiatur,[37] maneat salva et sana et nihilo sua tunica, (quam et unicam et tenuem habet) minus tuta sit, quam arteria, multiplici et crassa.[38] Quae igitur industriae ad vix patiendum, ipsi venae a natura inventae sunt, iam dicendum. Communes quidem omnium ipsius venae non solum partium: sed etiam explantationum praedictae tunicae existunt, enatae cum omnibus ipsis explantationibus, ut et eas colligent simul adiacentibus continue particulis, et totam molam tunicae efficiant robustiorem. Ipsam autem concavam hae deferunt a phrenibus usque ad iugulum.[39] Quod vero est per singulas eius venae partes auxilium, trifariam distributum est. Per media enim thoracis, velut manum quandam, cor ei praebet nervosam et fortem apophysin et productionem.

Well then, the vena cava, which is of the greatest use to the animal, as I have shown in earlier books, must pass up through the middle of the diaphragm to the heart, and, as I shall likewise show, it must also ascend from the heart to the region called σφαγή. Since, however, the heart itself, the lung, the diaphragm, and the whole thorax are in constant motion, a route through the midst of the open space of the thorax was not safe unless Nature devised some additional assistance by means of which the vena cava, though suspended, so to speak, and continually shaken, holds steady. Even if the animal suffers a bad fall on its back or breast or is struck by some external object, the vein remains safe and sound thanks to this assistance, as well protected in spite of its one thin tunic as an artery whose tunic is as many times as thick.

I must now tell what devices Nature has invented to make this vein resistant to injury. Those that are common to all parts of the vena cava and to its ramifications as well are the tunics I have just mentioned, which grow out together with them all to bind them to the parts on both sides and to make the whole mass of the tunic stronger. They accompany the vena cava from the diaphragm to the throat. Assistance is provided in three ways to the various parts of the vein: in the middle of the thorax the heart extends towards it a strong, sinewy outgrowth like a hand; . . .[40]

Our second question about Peter of Abano and the philosopher-physician dispute was why he relied to such a great extent on *De juvamentis membrorum,* even preferring it to the evidence of his senses, as we shall see below. It is clear from his text that he was familiar with *De usu partium,* which he often simply refers to as "the book in Greek"; in these cases we can identify the work through the quotations he excerpts from it. Moreover, he tells us himself that he was aware of the fact that *De juvamentis membrorum* was an abbreviated version, containing in nine books twelve of the original seventeen.[41] Finally, he claims to have translated *De usu partium* from the Greek.[42] He must therefore have been aware of the detailed differences between the two texts, and he might have guessed, from the very different terminology, that the abbreviated version had a history of translation including passage through Arabic; he might even have guessed the source of confusion over *nervus*. In his argument, however, he makes no use of the idea that *De juvamentis membrorum* had become textually corrupt, but he is ready to capitalize on the fact that Galen appears to contradict himself. For example, Book IX of *De juvamentis membrorum* retains much of the force of the argument by which Galen in the larger work established the brain as the source of the nerves. Either we accept that Galen contradicts himself,

[37] *Ibid.* omits *vel . . . percutiatur.*

[38] *Ibid.* has *et in nullo pro eo quod habet unam tunicam subtilem deficiat infallacia a multiplici secundum grossitiem arteria.*

[39] *Ibid.* has *sfagem.*

[40] Galen, *On the Usefulness,* Vol. I, p. 283.

[41] Peter of Abano, *Conciliator,* p. 71r (Diff. 47).

[42] See Lynn Thorndike, "Translation of the Works of Galen from the Greek by Peter of Abano," *Isis,* 1942, *33*:649–653.

argues Peter, or *De juvamentis membrorum* (or parts of it) is not Galenic; in either case Galen is made to appear a less authoritative source than Aristotle. We can conclude that, at best, Peter used *De juvamentis membrorum* in preference to *De usu partium* because of its smaller size and greater simplicity, and at worst he used it because its inconsistencies and corrupt text allowed him to maintain an Aristotelian position at the expense of not admitting that the two Galenic texts had a common origin in the Greek and that the shorter should simply be dismissed as a less accurate report of Galen's thinking.

Let us take one more example from the *Conciliator,* which introduces a new topic that leads us on to the next author to be considered. In *Differentia* 47 Peter argues the parallel question to the one already discussed, namely whether the liver or the heart is the source of the veins. Here again he tries to show that parts of Galen's scheme, at least, agreed with Aristotle, by referring to the passage in Book VII of *De juvamentis membrorum* where the text says that the nonpulsatile vein that serves the lung is one vein at least that arises in the heart. Peter may have had in mind the first part of the passage quoted above from the first chapter of Book VII, where the text says that a branch of the vena cava reaches the heart and then comes out of it again to proceed to the lung: *et ex corde etiam ascendit ad pulmonem*. As we have seen, this was not what Galen said. Alternatively Peter may have been referring to the nonpulsatile-vein-that-looks-like-a-pulsatile-vein (the pulmonary artery) but *according to Peter,* the nonpulsatile vein in question is said (in the corrupt text) to arise from that part of the heart that gives rise also to the pulsatile veins of the whole body. The text of *De juvamentis membrorum* does not say this, for it is the *pulsatile*-vein-that-looks-like a-nonpulsatile-vein that is here said to arise from the same (right) ventricle as the aorta. What is abundantly clear, however, is that a great deal of confusion has been introduced by Peter's use of the pulsatile-vein nomenclature of *De juvamentis membrorum* in place of the "artery" of *De usu partium*.

It is also clear that Peter was referring to Book VII, Chapter 2, where this matter is discussed and where Galen is considering the comparative nobility of the parts of the heart. It is part of Peter's argument for the heart as the origin of veins that the heart is the most noble of all organs, and that the point of attachment of the veins is the most noble part of the heart. In Aristotelian fashion, one reason for the nobility of the heart is that it is the first organ to come into being in the developing embryo; correspondingly it is the last organ to die. Its motion is evidence of its life, and so we can judge the most noble part of it by observing the last part of it to stop moving. Peter writes:

> Many times while anatomizing, I have noted this by sight, that while the motion of the heart is stopping (and with it life, since it is maintained by motion) the motion of the left ventricle ceases little by little, even while the right moves regularly, until finally the motion (as it were) arrives at the mid-point where the hollow vein is attached to the heart; and so this very clearly appears to be the point where every motion of life ceases.[43]

Later in the same *differentia* he says more directly:

> . . . the part from which life and motion last depart will be the most noble and foremost. This is the right, for, motion and life leaving the left ventricle, they can be perceived for a little while in the right. Thus I have many times perceived in vivisections—since they end in death—that motion leaves the left ventricle for the right; this by close and constant

[43]Peter of Abano, *Conciliator.* p. 69v.

> examination of what was moved and what was immobile around it, until at length [the motion] reached that place where this vein arises from the heart.[44]

Now the point where the vena cava is attached to the heart is the right auricle, precisely where the ghost "nerve" of *De juvamentis membrorum* should have appeared, and Peter as a dissector was in an excellent position to solve a traditional problem, to throw light on a text, or to make an empirical anatomical description. It is clear that his purposes lay in none of these things, but rather in giving weight to an opinion that was for him already established.

DE JUVAMENTIS MEMBRORUM AND MONDINO

The *Conciliator* is said to have been finished in 1303,[45] and so Peter must have been dissecting in the late thirteenth or early fourteenth century. As he claims to have translated *De usu partium,* we cannot ascribe his use of *De juvamentis membrorum* to the fact that his writing was complete before the appearance of Nicholas of Reggio's translation of the former in 1317. Mondino, the second of the authors to be considered in this paper, was also dissecting in the early fourteenth century, and like Peter, he made extensive use of *De juvamentis membrorum* (it was his most frequently quoted source, along with a version of Galen's *De locis affectis* known as *De interioribus*). Unlike Peter, however, he had no access to the full text of *De usu partium;* his *Anathomia* of 1316 missed the completion if not publication of Nicholas' translation by as little as a year. Mondino was the most important anatomist of the Middle Ages, at least in the Italian tradition, and his text formed the basis of anatomical teaching for more than two centuries. Berengario da Carpi, probably the most important of the pre-Vesalian anatomists, laid out his own anatomical work as a commentary on Mondino in 1521, and Curtius was still teaching from the old text in the lectures that accompanied Vesalius' demonstrations in Bologna in 1540. It is thus of considerable historical significance that Mondino relied so heavily on the short and corrupt Galenic text. His attention to it (he also wrote a commentary on it, which does not appear to have survived) served to increase its popularity because of the popularity of his own text, despite the new availability of *De usu partium.*

One of Mondino's reasons for writing was to provide a descriptive anatomy for surgeons. He therefore found *De locis affectis* important, for here Galen describes disorders of the body in relation to structure, and Mondino was of course bound to describe human anatomy, for which *De juvamentis membrorum* was still the sole source. So although we might expect to find that Mondino was more of *medicus* than a *philosophus,* nevertheless the incomplete state of his Galenic sources obliged him to give some credence to Aristotle's biological ideas. These may have come to him through William of Moerbeke's translation of *De partium animalium,* through Avicenna, or in part through the Salernitan anatomies.

Again, the heart and vessels supply us with an example of the difficulties caused by the state and availability of the sources used by the medieval writers. Mondino tells us that the heart has three chambers.[46] This Aristotelian idea got to Mondino at secondhand (but not through Avicenna), and he attempted to reconcile it with the

[44] *Ibid.,* p. 71v.

[45] Lynn Thorndike, *A History of Magic and Experimental Science,* Vol. II (New York: Columbia University Press, 1923), p. 876.

[46] The text used here is that given by Berengario da Carpi, *Commentaria cum amplissimis additionibus super Anatomia Mundini* (Bologna, 1521), p. cccxxxii^r.

Galenic anatomy of *De juvamentis membrorum* by equating the "third ventricle" with the pores that Galen said existed in the septum between the two cardiac ventricles.

Mondino turns to Galenic anatomy of *De juvamentis membrorum* for his account of the vascular connections between the heart and lungs, and the phrase he uses in describing the reciprocal service paid by the heart to the lungs—transmitting blood to them in exchange for the lung's service in sending air to the heart—comes with little verbal change from the medieval Galenic work.[47] Had Mondino had the full text of *De usu partium,* he would have seen that the passage he quotes is preceded by another in which Galen discusses the number of ventricles in the hearts of different animals and consequently refutes Aristotle's opinion.[48] This latter passage was omitted by the translator of *De juvamentis membrorum,* and its absence contributed to the persistence of a false idea in Mondino's text.

Again, Mondino necessarily turns to the Galenic work when discussing the cardiac valves. He thought of the auricles as maintaining a reserve capacity in case of excessive production of blood or spirit in the ventricles. This implies a lack of a clear notion of the unidirectional function of the valves' action, and again we may suppose that the vague term *coopertorium* and the imprecise context of *De juvamentis membrorum* contributed to Mondino's confusion. Further evidence of this is that Mondino misinterprets the Galenic scheme of bloodflow from the liver. He says that blood arriving at the heart from the liver through the *vena chilis* (the Arabic term for *vena cava*) enters the right ventricle past an inward-looking valve. After some concoction the blood is sent partly across the septum, in part to the lungs, and the remainder leaves the heart through the *same orifice* as it entered. For this reason, says Mondino, the inward-looking valve does not completely close. Galen's description of the incompletely closing valve of the *left* side of the heart survives in *De juvamentis membrorum,* and Mondino may have transferred the description to the *right* side of the heart, or he may have taken it from another source.[49] In the full text of *De usu partium* Galen is clear about the motion of blood on the right side of the heart, but the account in *De juvamentis membrorum* is confused.

The Aristotelian primacy of the heart is maintained by Mondino, who calls the heart the "source and ultimate root of all organs."[50] Perhaps Mondino, like Peter of Abano, understood by this that the heart in Aristotle's scheme was the *embryological* precursor and determinant of the other organs. Galen believed on the contrary that the primordium of the liver and its vegetative faculty was the first to appear in the developing embryo, since the higher faculties and their organs depended in turn upon this; but Galen's views on generation were lost to the West until the full text of *De usu partium* had been translated.

To summarize what has been said about Mondino, he missed Nicholas of Reggio's translation of *De usu partium* by a very short space of time, with consequent damage to his discussions of anatomy. Unlike Peter, he had no access to or could not use the

[47]VII 2.

[48]Galen, *On the Usefulness,* Vol. I, p. 295.

[49]Possibly the Hippocratic *De corde:* F. R. Hurlbutt's translation, "Peri kardies," *Bulletin of the History of Medicine,* 1939, 7:1104–1113, makes this point clearly enough, but creates confusion over the terminology of the vessels. However, *De corde* is thought not to have been known in the West until the 16th century.

[50]Quoted from Charles Singer's translation in his introduction to Johannes de Ketham's *The Fasciculo de Medicina* (Florence: Lier, 1925), p. 82. Mondino's words are *princeps et prima radix omnium membrorum* (Berengario da Carpi, *Commentaria,* p. cccxxxi).

Greek version of the work. With his medical interests it is likely Mondino would have adopted Galen's work more readily than Peter, but he was obliged to draw upon Aristotelian sources already available. His interest in *De juvamentis membrorum* also had the effect of popularizing it and so lengthening its period of circulation. In particular Mondino's ideas on cardiac physiology suffered as a result of the corrupt text of *De juvamentis membrorum* and as a result of Aristotle's ignorance of the valves and the nature of the pulmonary vessels. An understanding of what Galen had said was essential for an understanding of the true nature of the heart.

HUMAN DISSECTION AND PROGRESS IN ANATOMY AND PHYSIOLOGY

To appreciate the importance of the state of, or the absence of, certain texts in the Middle Ages, the relationship between observation and textual authority should be made clear. Vesalius argued that his predecessors had not advanced anatomy because they did not personally dissect, and indeed there was a period of apparent stagnation in anatomy after Mondino, when the anatomy teachers sat in a high professorial chair reading the text of Galen or Avicenna while the *ostensor* performed the actual dissection. The result—that any discrepancy between the appearance of the body and the words of the text went unnoticed by the professor (who could not see the details of the body) or the *operator* (who could not understand the professor's Latin)—can be contrasted with Mondino's method of personal involvement in dissection. However, Mondino was not on the point of breaking with the ancient authors by the introduction of the new technique of observation of the corpse. On the contrary, his reliance on authority was extreme, and he was not yet at the point where he had available all the necessary texts or where he understood properly those he had; there is even a spurious air of reality about some of his anatomical observations.

The reasons for writing the *Anatomia,* said Mondino, were to satisfy friends, to serve as a mental exercise, and to remind the reader what he had learned. It was not the purpose of the book or the dissections it described to confirm what the old text said, still less to question it. The purpose of dissection was in fact inimical to anatomical progress in serving to emphasize with visual images the verbal descriptions of the authorities.

Anatomy and physiology did not make serious progress in the West until the practice of human dissection, begun as a teaching device in the Middle Ages, became a research device in the fifteenth and sixteenth centuries. This change in the role of anatomy was not complete until the classical and Arabic texts had been subjected to full scholarly investigation, and indeed it began partly as a means of establishing the true reading of corrupt passages and then as a means of judging between the different opinions of the authorities thus revealed. The particular value of studying the history of *De juvamentis membrorum* is that it is a corrupt summary of a very important Galenic work, *De usu partium*: by comparing the use to which the two texts were put we can sketch some of the characteristics of early scholarship, and by comparing the texts themselves we can see how Galen's ideas lost their force in transmission from culture to culture, how the writers of the time were misled, and how they tried to remedy the situation.

III

An Origin for the Bone Text of the 'Five-Figure Series'

The 'five-figure series' is a series of anatomical figures and text in medieval manuscripts, first described by *Sudhoff*.[1] Since then new members of the family have been discovered[2] but historians have been able to say little about their origins.[3] *Sudhoff* postulated an Alexandrian source, but no textual evidence could be found to support this. In the most recent examination of the problem *O'Neill* justly calls the series a "bridge to the unknown".[4]

To reach the unknown we need some signposts from the known. These in fact seem to be provided by what we know of the fate of Hellenistic medicine and by what is presented to us by the manuscripts themselves. Firstly it is clear from the texts that the anatomy they represent is, at root, Galenic. Not only is *Galen* cited at the beginning of the text, but we can see the mangled remains of his description of the *rete mirabile* in the *anaphusa* of the artery-man and of his description of the hepatic origin of the veins.

Indeed a Galenic text would be the natural place to look, not only because of *Galen's* pre-eminence as an anatomist but because we are learning more about the use of his works in late antiquity and in the Arab world.[5] Can we cross the bridge into the unknown by postulating that the five figure series represents some ultimate result of the kind of compression of Galenic works that we know went on in medical teaching in late antiquity and the early middle ages?

Looking at the problem in this light, we are at once struck by the fact that *Galen* wrote introductory texts on five anatomical topics, the arteries and veins (put together in one treatise) the nerves, the muscles and the bones. These treatises formed part of the so called 'sixteen books of *Galen*' as used in the school of Alexandria. According to *Hunain*[6] the Alexandrians divided the single treatise on arteries and veins into two, and gave the single title 'On anatomy for students' to the collection of five treatises.

It is helpful to see these texts in an educational context. The second 'grade' of the Alexandrian curriculum – the beginning of the full course of instruction – began with the Galenic 'naturals': the elements, temperaments, faculties, organs, etc. In other words it located the structure and function of the body in the natural world as a whole. This was a very natural introduction to the purely medical course that followed and for the same reason was used by almost every subsequent medical text.

[1] *Sudhoff, K.*, "Anatomische Zeichnungen (Schemata) aus dem 12. und 13. Jh. und eine Skelettzeichnung des 14. Jhrs." *Studien zur Geschichte der Medizin I*, Leipzig 1907, 49–65. Recently re-issued (Hildesheim, 1964) is *Sudhoff's Ein Beitrag zur Geschichte der Anatomie im Mittelalter*. Leipzig, 1908. *Sudhoff's* subsequent discoveries are listed by *Hill* et al (see notes 2 and 3).

[2] *Hill, B. H.*, "Another new member of the Sudhoff Fünfbilderserie – Wellcome MS 5000". *Sudhoffs Archiv Gesch. Med. 43* (1959) (1) 13–19; *Mackinney, L. C., and Hill, B. H.*, "A new Fünfbilderserie mansucript – Vatican Palat. Lat. 1100". *Sudhoffs Archiv Gesch. Med. 48* (1964) 323–330.

[3] See *O'Neill, Y. V.*, "The Fünfbilderserie reconsidered," *Bill. Hist. Med. 43* (1969) 236–245; and "The Fünfbilderserie – a bridge to the unknown". *Bull. Hist. Med. 51* (1977) 539–549.

[4] See note 3. *O'Neill* (1969) postulates an unknown medieval translation of *Galen's De Placitis Platonis et Hippocratis* and comparison of the figures alone have led other authors to suggestions of Chinese and Tibetan sources.

[5] See for example *Iskandar, A. Z.* "An attempted reconstruction of the late Alexandrian medical curriculum." *Medical History 20* (1976) 235–258.

[6] *Iskandar* (1976) 246.

We should notice particularly that in this process of introducing the student to the nature of the human body, the parts of the body to be treated first are the most elementary parts, those closest in their nature to the external elements. These were the fundamental and irreducible 'similar' parts of *Aristotle*, the lowest rung on a hierarchy of structure described by *Galen*, and the first stage in the formal and theoretical exposition of anatomy of a large number of teachers since.[7]

They were also the five subjects of the Galenic 'On anatomy for students' and the five subjects of the 'five figure series'.[8] Since *Sudhoff's* time it has become clear that the full complement of illustrations for the series is nine, not five, but it is no accident that *Sudhoff* first recognised the first five as a group. Figures six to nine are of a different kind: they are the next group in *Galen's* hierarchy of structure, the *organic* parts, built up of the similar parts, having 'function' in place of mere 'action', discrete rather than systemic in morphology; and taught to students after the similar parts.[9]

In one case, textual evidence is there to provide a link between *Galen's* text and the five-figures series. Taken as a whole, the series has two versions of the bone-text. Characteristic members of what *Sudhoff* recognised as five related figures have five short texts accompanying the figures. Other members of the family have, instead, a long bone-text and a skeleton which seems more closely related to that of the Persian examples of the series than to the simple bone-man of the original *Fünfbilderserie*. The distribution of the texts and illustrations among individual manuscripts is complex, and requires further analysis; but for our purposes it is enough that it is clear that the long bone-text and its figure are part of the series.

To begin with, we should note again the strong similarity between the 'long bone text figure' of the western manuscripts and their Persian counterparts.[10] A striking feature of resemblance is the inverted heads of these figures. The text accompanying the Persian figures has not been studied by specialists, but on account alone of its length cannot be a version of the Western long bone text; most of the Persian texts are in any case that of the late 14th century Mansur anatomy. But the Persian texts, Mansur's anatomy included, contain a characteristic series of diagrams representing the sutures of the head.[11]

These suture diagrams are widely spread in Arabic and Persian sources. The occur in *Ibn Jamī*ʿ*'s* treatise on the skeleton,[12] in *Haly Abbas*[13] and even survive in western printed versions

[7] *Aristotle* opens the *Historia Animalium* (486a) with a discussion of the similar parts; and the first chapter of *Galen's De Usu Partium* distinguishes the similar from the organic. The idea is practically universal in renaissance anatomies.

[8] The number of similar parts has varied somewhat in anatomical commentary. Fat and blood were often included, and sometimes categories like 'membrane.' But the five discussed are always the principal, and the only ones to build up into systems.

[9] Persian examples like India Office 2296 distinguish the similar from the complex parts. In general anatomy was taught theoretically, by the 'synthetic' method beginning with elements, qualities and similar parts to organic parts, which was said to follow nature in her construction of the body. Practical anatomy was 'analytic' and followed the sequence of dissections, in which the similar parts were (in theory) the final product.

[10] India Office, *Ethé* 2296; Vatican Palat. Lat. 1110; Bodleian Fraser 201; Munich 13042; Basel D, II, 11.

[11] E. g. Bodleian Fraser 201, where the illustrations are on the fly leaves. For the anatomy of *Mansur* see *Schullian* and *Sommer, A Catalogue of Incunabula and Manuscripts in the Army Medical Library*. New York, (n.d.), p. 335.

[12] *C. Rabin, "Ibn Jamī*ʿ on the skeleton". In: *E. Ashworth Underwood, Science, Medicine, and History*, 2 vols., Oxford University Press, 1953; vol. 1, pp. 177–202.

[13] See *P. de Koning, Trois traités d'anatomie Arabes*, Leiden, 1903, p. 110.

of *Avicenna's Canon.*[14] The common source of these is probably the Arabic 'compendium of the works of *Galen*',[15] that is, the Arabic version of the *Summaria Alexandrinorum.* This Arabic 'Abridgement'[16] of the works of *Galen* contains the suture figure, but the text of *Galen* on which this section is based, *De Ossibus,* does not.

To complete this link between *Galen's* text and the long bone text, we need to look at both in detail.

In *De Ossibus,* after discussing the nature of bony articulation, *Galen* lists the articulations – the sutures – of the bones of the head. First he lists the coronal, *stephaniaia,* at the front, and second the lambdoid at the back, named from the Greek letter *lambda. Galen* uses the adjective λανδοεδῆ)[17] but uses the capital Λ to illustrate the shape of the suture without using the noun.

Next *Galen* says that the shape of the sutures together (coronal and lambdoid) is like the shape of the Greek capital H. This time he supplies the capital without using noun or adjective. Then he gives the shape of the remaining sutures by means of the capital Γ, once more without name. Finally he observes that in certain skulls these sutures cross in the manner of the capital X, again without using the name of the letter.

Galen's terse description would have been perfectly intelligible to Greeks, but the text obviously was open to misunderstanding when translated. Even *Oribasius* in gathering Galen's description into his medical collection introduces the possibility of confusion by omitting Galen's capitals and writing out the name of the letters[18]: it was not now clear that *Galen* had been referring to the capital forms of the letters. (*Oribasius* in other respects adheres closely to *Galen's* text).

So the Greek capitals ΛΗΓΧ form a distinctive pattern at this point in *Galen's* text. *Galen's* description then proceeds to two non-sutured joints proceeding on either side of the head from back to front. He summarises by listing the five sutures of the cranium, the lambdoid, coronal, "straight" (sagittal) and two longitudinal squamous or false sutures.

To judge by the *Summaria*[19] *Galen's* text was somewhat compressed (omitting some details of variant skull shapes) and slightly altered (a description is given of the first *three* sutures taken together, not the first *two*).[20]

But no gloss is supplied, and *Galen's* Greek capitals *have been transcribed into the Arabic manuscript, retaining their illustrative shape but lost to the Arabic reader as letters.* The only exception is the diagram of the lambdoid suture, where alone *Galen* had used an adjective, and where as a result the Arabs and later translators recognised *Galen's* intention. (This seems to be the reason for the survival of *lambdoid* as a term).

So *Galen's* capital Λ became) or] and his H became)—(or (—(in which the Arabs saw a similarity to a bow and arrow: *Galen's* "straight" suture became "arrow like", *sahmi,* which

[14] See for example the edition of Venice, 1533, p. 9r. or the text of the commentators, such as *Primus (et secundus) Avicennae Canonis . . .una cum lucidissima Gentilis Fulginatis expositione.* Venice, 1520, p. 65r, col. 1 (Book 1, fen 1, doctrine 5).

[15] British Library Add. 23407, fol. 32; British Library Arundel Oriental 17, folio 60v.

[16] See *Rabin* (1953) and the *Catalogus Codicum Orientalalium qui in Museo Britannico asservantur.* (British Museum).

[17] *Kühn,* II 740.

[18] *Oribasius, Œuvres d'Oribase,* trans. *Bussemaker* and *Daremberg.* 6 vols., (Paris 1858), vol. 3, p. 395.

[19] See note 15 and the text appended to this article. I am deeply indebted to *Dr. Penelope Johnstone* for the translation.

[20] See Appendix.

reached Latin as *sagitale*.[21] The completed suture diagram was used editorally in the *Summaria* to illustrate the *Ars Parva*[22] where *Galen* describes the best shape of the head. Thus the sutures diagram appears twice in later Arabic and Persian medical works.

The long bone-text in Provençal published by *Sudhoff* does indeed have some remnants of diagrams within the text at these points. *Sudhoff* represented them typographically in his text, but unfortunately the associated photograph does not make clear the relevant section of text.[23] Although the Latin text as published by *Mackinney* and *Hill*[24] contains no indication of diagrams, the photograph shows the single composite suture diagram with which the Arabic sources conclude the description of the sutures.

The second link we have to make is between the long bone text and these Arabic sources. First, it is clear that the text shows traces of Arabic anatomy. The terms *oluvium [Elluvium* in the Provençal] for the sacrum is a variant of *alhavius* from the Arabic.[25] Likewise, the text opens with the statement that the number of bones in the body is 248 *praeter ossa cisamina*. 248 is an Arabic total of the *Abridgement*, not derived from *Galen*.[26] The excepting of the sesamoid bones from this list is found in the *Abridgement*, *Rhazes* and *Ibn Jamīʿ*.[27]

The bone text then turns to the bones (not sutures) of the head and lists the *coronale*, *sagittale* and the third *quod assimilatur laudae letterae graecorum et constituunt verticem per hunc modum*. It is precisely at this point that the *Abridgement* and *Haly* provide the figure generated from the vestiges of *Galen's* capitals and representing the first three sutures. Such a figure would make sense of the hanging *per hunc modum*.

In a very similar way the long bone text then describes the bones at the side of the head much as *Haly's* and *Ibn Jamīʿ*'s texts and concludes the sentence *et si cum aliis conjunguntur capitis orbitam constituunt per hunc modum*. Again, *hunc modum* strongly suggests a missing diagram, and at just the point where *Haly*, *Ibn Jamīʿ* and the *Abridgement* provide the composite figure of all the sutures.

In more general terms, the sequence of topics dealt with in the long bone text is very close to that of *Galen's De Ossibus*, allowing for the compression the latter went through in the *Summaria*. There must of course be a similarity between any two bone texts that work *a capite ad calcem*, but the similarity seems too great to be explained merely on that basis. Compare the *short* bone text: not even its obscurity can hide the fact that it is nothing like the long, or the Galenic text.

In short the text of the 'long-bone text' tradition of western MSS contains the suture-diagrams found in a tradition of Arabic and Persian diagrams[28] based ultimately on *Galen's* text; it contains Arabic terminology and bone-totals. The skeleton is clearly related to Persian illustrations. Given that the suture diagrams and sequence of exposition of the text in both western and oriental MSS can be traced to *Galen's de ossibus* we are bound to enquire into the circumstances of transmission.

21 See *Rabin* (1953) p. 199.

22 See the *Catalogus Codicum* . . . (note 16).

23 *Sudhoff* (1908/1964) p. 32. The text is appended to this article.

24 (1964) The photograph is appended to this article.

25 *MacKinney and Hill* (1964) p. 329; *Sudhoff* (1908/1964) p. 32; *A. Fonahn, Arabic and Latin Anatomical Terminology*, Kristiania, 1922.

26 Rabin (1953) p. 192 n. 72.

27 *Koning* (1903) p. 23; *Rabin* (1953) p. 182.

28 Fraser 200, p. 19.

Most historical attention has been given to the role of the Arabs in the transmission of sicence to the west, but here we are struck by the number of Persian MSS.[29] We should not of course expect Arabic representation of the body to appear in MSS (but it is notable that fine examples of the illustrations are attached to a copy of *Avicenna's Canon*),[30] but this prohibition clearly did not apply to *diagrams* one of which was originally recognised as a simple Greek capital, which is why we find the suture diagram in the Arabic sources.

We should not expect then, that the Persian examples are derived from Arabic originals. It seems more likely that the route of transmission was from Greek directly to Persian. For four and a half centuries, from about the time when *Galen* died to the spread of Islam, the 'neo-Persian' empire abutted the Greek world of the eastern mediterranean and Greek was replaced by Pahlavi (middle Persian) and Aramaic. The story of the cultivation and assimilation of Greek medicine at Jundishapur and Edessa is well known in outline and provides a route for the transmission of Hellenistic anatomy to Iran and the Persian language. Subsequent Arabic domination as easily provides a background for the appearance of the Arabic versions. Undoubtedly the long bone text and skeleton of the west has come from the orient.

[29] A review of the secondary literature provides a total of 26 known MSS. that have one or more features of the 'five figure series'. Of this total a dozen MSS are in Latin, 8 Persian, 2 'Islamic' without further qualification, and one each Arabic and Provençal.

[30] Wellcome OR. 155.

APPENDIX

1. Texts

1. The long bone text (The bones of the head)

   a. Vat. Palat. Lat. 1110 and Dresden C310.
   From MacKinney and Hill (1964):

" The treatise on bones which accompanies the skeleton is almost identical to that of Dresden MS. C 310 (14th c.), but in Dresden the text does not appear on the same page as the figure. In Basel MS. D.II.11 (13th c.), however, the text (in Provençal) appears with the illustration, and is distributed on the page exactly as it is in Vatican: one paragraph at upper left, another at upper right, and a third between the parted knees.

Below is the bone text *De ossibus corporis* from Dresden MS. C 310[2]. The corresponding words of Vatican which are too smudged to be deciphered are marked off in brackets. Vatican deviations from Dresden are shown in the notes. Some of SUDHOFF's internal punctuation has been omitted, and the following spelling differences have been ignored: ch for c, v for u, and e for ae. SUDHOFF's parenthetical comments have also been omitted. "

[Omnia] ossa corporis humani sunt numero .cc.xlviij[3]. praeter ossa cisamina. Ossa capitis sunt xv.[4] primum [vocatur. coronale] superius [in vertice. secundum] sagittale. [tertium quod assimilatur. landae litterae graecorum et constituunt verticem] per hunc modum. In dextra [autem] parte in sinis[tra][5] duo ossa [vocata sunt petrosa] ubi sunt foramina aurium [secunda] ad modum semicirculi et [si cum] aliis [coniungatur] capitis orbi[tam] constituunt per hunc modum. [In parte autem interiore] versus os[6] quod assimilatur landae literae est aliud os quod est os occipi[7] [cij.] Postea sunt duo [versus sagittale postea .iiij. versus timpora. postea] os quod assimilatur [canulae] quod ligat os frontis cum manubula[8] superiori..

Variants: [3] cc quadraginta [4] quin decim? [5] *after sinistra*: hinc [6] *after os*: coronale est os si... versus os [7] ocipitis [8] mandibula [9] quod [10] singua [11] sicut [12] cibi. [13] xiiij. [14] ex xvij den-.

b. Basel D II, 11. From Sudhoff (1908)

¶ totz los osses del cors son en nombre cc. xlviij. estiers los. assamina.

¶ los osses del. cap so .xv. lo primier sapela coronale de sus en la testa. lo .ij sagilitale lo iij. que es semblans a lande hen grecorum que constituinson la testa. per aytal maneyra un C›› In dextra part e senestra .a.ij os apelatz petrosa on son los traucz de las aurelas fayts ayssi C›› en la part empro dauant vays los coronal es los. del front .x. potrius uays los que sembla lande litre. et an autre os que es os de occiput. pueys. an .ij. vays lo sagitale pueys. iiij. uays las templas. pueys los que sembla canila que lia. los trontis ab la maychela de sus. pueys.

2. The Summaria Alexandrinorum (B.L. Add. 23407).
I am greatly indebted to Dr. Penelope Johnstone for this translation from the Arabic

242 a. The forms of the head are four: one natural and three non-natural. The natural form
1.5 is the circular, which has a prominence in the front and in the back . . . It has five sutures, three of them truesutures and two not. There are two called the Scaly sutures, which extend along the length of the head above the ears; the distance of each one is from the suture which goes along the centre of the head, lengthwise . . .

1.11 As for the tree true sutures, one of them is in the front of the head, where the crown is placed, and it is called the coronal, being of this shape: ⊐ The other is in the centre of the head, going lengthwise and it is called the straight or the sagittal: >—< and the third is at the back of the head, its shape is like that of the L in the Greeks' alphabet, which is this (margin): > When the shapes of the three sutures are put together, they look like this: >—<

242 b. As for the three shapes which are not natural, which are the shapes of the – (?) head . . . one of them is the shape of head which does not have a prominence in front, and when the head is like this it lacks the suture in the front of the head, which we have said is called the coronal; and it does have two sutures, one of them which goes straight along the length of the head and the other the lambdoid; the shape of its sutures is thus: ɔ——

The other is the shape of head which has no prominence in the back, and when the head is like this, it lacks the lambdoid suture, but there are found two sutures, one the straight, going lengthwise, and the other the coronal; the shape of its sutures is thus: ɔ——

1.10 The third: the shape of head which has no prominence in the front nor in the back, and when the head is like this it lacks the coronal suture and the lambdoid, but it has two sutures which cut each other at right-angles, being like this: X

2. *The Suture Diagrams*

The elements (derived in most cases from *Galen's* capitals) of the complete suture diagram are indicated by arrows.

British Library ms Add. 23407, fol. 242 a u. fol. 243 b

fol. 242 a

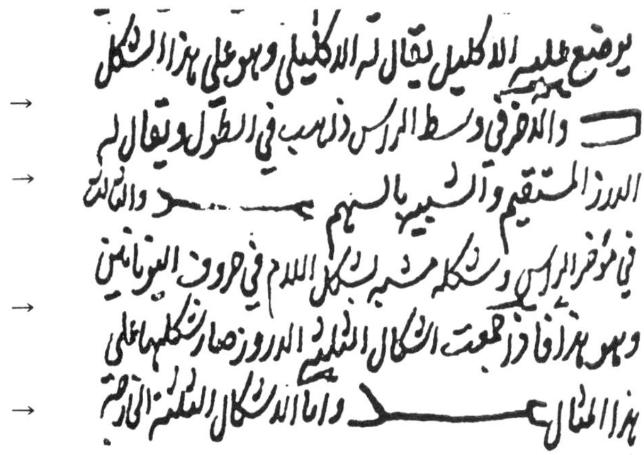

يوضع عليه الاكليل يقال له الاكليلي وهو على هذا الشكل
والاخر في وسط الراس ذاهب في الطول ويقال له
الدرز المستقيم والشبيه بالسهم والثالث
في موخر الراس وشكله مشبه بشكل اللام في حروف اليونانيين
وهو هذا فاذا جمعت الاشكال الثلثة الدروز صار شكلها على
هذا المثال واما الاشكال الثلثة الاخر

fol. 243 b

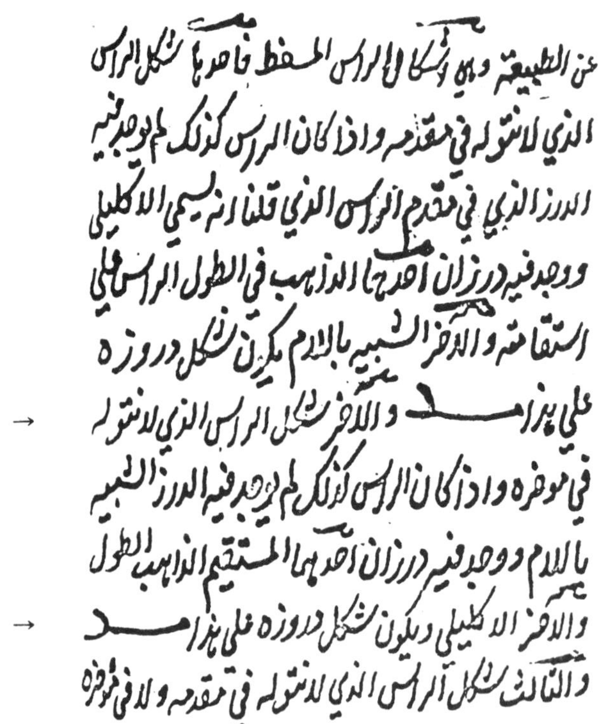

عن الطبيعة وهي اشكال الراس المسفط فاحدها شكل الراس
الذي لا نتو له في مقدمه واذا كان الراس كذلك لم يوجد فيه
الدرز الذي في مقدم الراس الذي قلنا انه يسمى الاكليلي
ووجد فيه درزان احدهما الذاهب في الطول الراس على
استقامته والاخر الشبيه باللام ويكون شكل دروزه
على هذا والاخر شكل الراس الذي لا نتو له
في موخره واذا كان الراس كذلك لم يوجد فيه الدرز الشبيه
باللام ووجد فيه درزان احدهما المستقيم الذاهب الطول
والاخر الاكليلي ويكون شكل دروزه على هذا
والثالث شكل الراس الذي لا نتو له في مقدمه ولا في موخره

واذا كان الراس كذلك لم يوجد فيه الدرز الاكليلي ولا الدرز
الشبيه باللام ووجد فيه درزان متقاطعان على زوايا
→ قائمة على هذا المثال X دروز عظم الراس وهي الشؤون
منها ما هو خاص للراس وحده وهي تلك الخمسة التي
ذكرناها قبل ومنها ما هو مشترك للراس وغيره وهما درزان
احدهما الدرز الذي يفصل ما بين الراس واللحي الاعلى والاخر
الذي يفصل بينه وبين العظم الشبيه بالوتد وعظام الراس
سبعة منها ستة هي له خاصة ومنها واحد مشترك له

British Library, Arundel Oriental 17, fol. 60 v

وهذا الشكل له درزان منها الفشريان وهما ممدان في طول الراس من
فوق الاذنين ومنها الدرز الاكليلي وهو في مقدم الراس موضع الاكليل
ومنها في وسط الراس ويقال له الدرز الشبيه بالسهم ومنها درز في موخر
→ الراس وهو الدرز الشبيه بلام اليونانيين وهذا صورته ٨ واشكال
→ هذه الدروز اذا ركبت على هذه الصوره [shape] فهذا هو الشكل الطبيعي
فاما الاشكال الخارجه عن الاعتدال فالراس الذي لا نتو له في مقدمه ولا يوجد
له الدرز الاكليلي ويوجد فيه الدرز السهمي واللامي ويكون على هذا المثال [shape]
والراس الذي لا نتو له في موخره واذا كان كذلك لم يوجد له الدرز الشبيه
باللام ويوجد له الدرز الشبيه باللام ويوجد له الدرزان السهمي والاكليلي
مثل هذا الشكل [shape] والراس الذي لا نتو فيه لا في مقدمه ولا موخره
→ فهو الذي يفقد فيه الاكليلي واللامي ويبقى له درزان اعني السهمين متقاطعان

Ibn Jamīʿ, *Irshad*, fol. 8 b und 8 c (*Rabin*)

fol. 8 b

في الاصابع كل اصبع ثلثه والذي في الرجلين اثنان في الخذب واثنان على مفصل
الركبتين وتسميان الرضفتين واربعة في الساقين وستة وعشرون في القدم من
عقب وكعب وزورقي واربعة في المشط وخمسة في الرسغ واربعة عشر في الاصابع
كل اصبع ثلثة ظاهرة واثنان خفية فاحد العظام منها يقال له الاكليلي وهو يتقدم
→ ينفصل بين عظم الراس والجبهة مقوس هاكذا ⊂ والاخر في طول الراس هاكذا — يقال له
→ سفودي واذا اعتبر باضافته الى الاكليلي حتى يصير هاكذا — قيل له سهمي لانه
يشبه قوسا في وسطه سهم والثالث ينفصل بين الراس من خلف وبين قاعدته

fol. 8 c

→ يقال له لامي لانه يشبه اللام في كتاب اليونانيين هاكذا Λ واذا اجتمعت الثلاثة صارت
→ هاكذا — والاثنان الحقيقيان مارّة في طول الراس من الجانبين ويسميان قشريين
→ واذا اتصلا بالثلثة الاخر صار الجميع هاكذا […] وهذه الدروز تكون بحيث
→ يكون الراس على شكله الطبيعي وينقص مع عدم احد النتوئين الفصل الثامن
في الغضاريف ه الغضاريف هي الاجسام الشبيهة بالعظام في المنظر الا انها الين
→ منها واصلب من سائر الاعضاء الاخر فهي لذلك قابلة للانثناء والانعطاف فمنها
الغضروفان اللذان في مجاري الاذنين والغضروف الذي في ارنبة الانف والثلثة
غضاريف التي في الحنجرة الدرقي والطرجهاري والذي لا اسم له وطرف قصبة الرئة

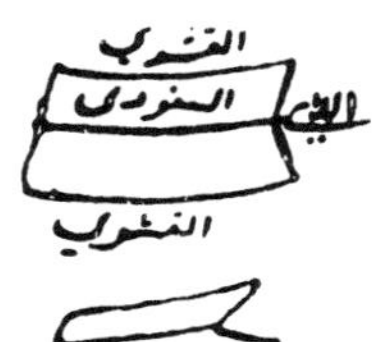

'Ali Ibn Al-'Abbās, Liber Regalis: the description of the sutures with figures, as published by *Koning*.

110

ى a للدماغ مواضع يتعلّق بها b ويرتبط لينشال c عن جرم الدماغ

الرابعة ليكون متى حدث بواحد d من عظام القحف آفة لم تسر

اجزائه والخامسة لانّ العظم الّذى فى مقدّم الرأس احتيج الى ان

ما والّذى فى مؤخّره احتيج f الى ان يكون صلبا ولم يمكن ان تجتمع

واللين فى عظم واحد. والدروز الّتى فى عظم d الرأس خمسة وتنقسم g

ظام القحف الى ستّة اعظم منها درزان ليسا دروزا بالحقيقة h يقال لهما

القشريّان وثلاثة هى دروز بالحقيقة واحد هذه الثلاثة الدروز فى مقدّم

الموضع الّذى يوضع عليه الاكليل ويقال له الدرز الاكليلىّ وهو على

→ ل) والثانى درز فى وسط الرأس مارّا i بالطول ويقال له الدرز المستقيم

→ بالسهم وهو على هذا المثال ——— والثالث الدرز الّذى فى مؤخّر الرأس

→ شبيه بشكل اللام فى كتابة اليونانيّين وهو هكذا k > فاذا اجتمعت هذه

→ الدروز كان منها شكل على هذا المثال 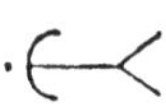. فامّا الدرزان الآخران

درزان من الجانبين فوق الاذنين l يأخذان من m الدرز الاكليلىّ فى نزول

الى قريب من الدرز الشبيه باللام فى كتابة اليونانيّين ويبعد كل واحد

ذين الدرزين عن الدرز الشبيه بالسهم بعدا سواء فاذا اجتمعت هذه

→ ز الخمسة كان منها شكل على هذا المثال n 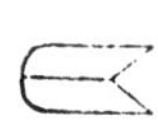 وهذا هو شكل الرأس

بعى وما كان خارجا عن هذا الشكل فليس بطبيعى. وعظام القحف

سم الى سبعة اعظم o فمنها عظمان فى وسط p الرأس يفصل q بينهما الدرز

بيه بالسهم ويقال لهذين العظمين عظما اليافوخ وهما مربّعا الشكل رخوا

The suture diagram and neighbouring letters from the text of Basel D II 11. See below, bone figure III, and above, text b from Sudhoff, 1908.

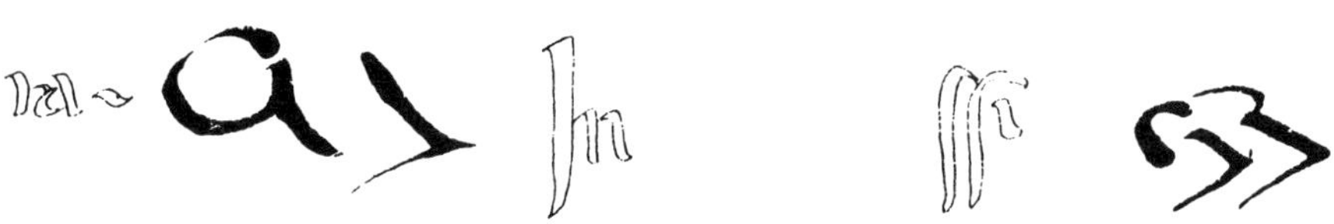

III

154

Avicenna, Canon, Venice, 1533, p. 9 r.

nem sūt posite: ⁊ sic oz vt nō coangustet̄. Et duas
hz eminētias ante ⁊ retro vt neruos defendat q de
scēdūt ꝑ ſ ad frōtē ⁊ ad nucha. | Et hec qdē figura
tres veras hz adorē, ⁊ duas hz mēdosas. Et in pri
mis vna adorē fronti est cōicans arcualis hoc mō.
→ C. ⁊ vocat̄ coronalis. Et alia adheret adorem
q̄ directe trāsiens in lōgitudinē diuidit caput i duo
media, ⁊ p se ɔsiderata vocat̄ sagittalis, ⁊ in ɔ̄ztuz
est ɔtigua coronali: vocat̄ neruealis. Et hꝰ qdē figu
ra arcui similat̄, in cuiꝰ medio linea recta sicut ppē
→ dicularis est recta, que est hoc mō. ϵ Et adorem
tertia iter occiput ⁊ basim ipsiꝰ cōis existit, cuiꝰ pū/
cto, cū ipsa sit sm figurā anguli, extremitas sagit/
talis ɔtinuat̄, ⁊ vocat̄ adorē laude, eo ꝙ laude lr̄e
→ grece silis existat que est ita. ᐸ Cūq3 duabꝰ ado/
rem q̄s prius noiauimus ɔiūgit̄ figura talis ϴ ᐸ
→ due xo adorē mendose sm capitis lōgitudinē sunt
ꝓtēse vtrinq3 eqdistātes sagittali, que ꝓfūditate i/
tegra in ossibꝰ nō ꝓfundant̄. Et he due corticales
vocaut̄.ª ┼ ┌

]Nō nāles aūt capitis figure
sunt tres: vna est vt anterior eminētia minuat̄: ⁊ ꝓ/
pterea de adorem, amittatur adorem coronalis.

Auic. b

ꝓ A. ab vtrisq3 la
teribꝰ seu ꝑtibꝰ.

q ┼ A. ⁊ quum cō
tinuant̄ cum cō/
missuris veris
efficiūt figuram
isto modo ϴ ᐸ ←
⁊ hec figura ē ca
pitis nālis co n
pleta ꝑ cōmissu/
rarum.

3. The Bone Figures

1. Munich MS. Codex Lat. Monacensis 13042

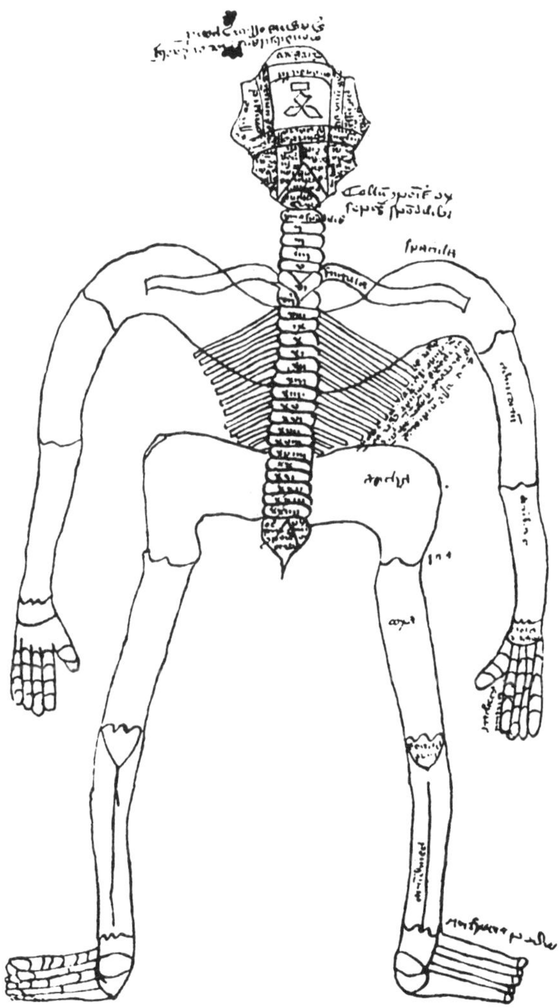

4. Fraser 201, fol. 1012
Oxford Bodleian Persian ms 1576
(A.D. 1722), Bone man

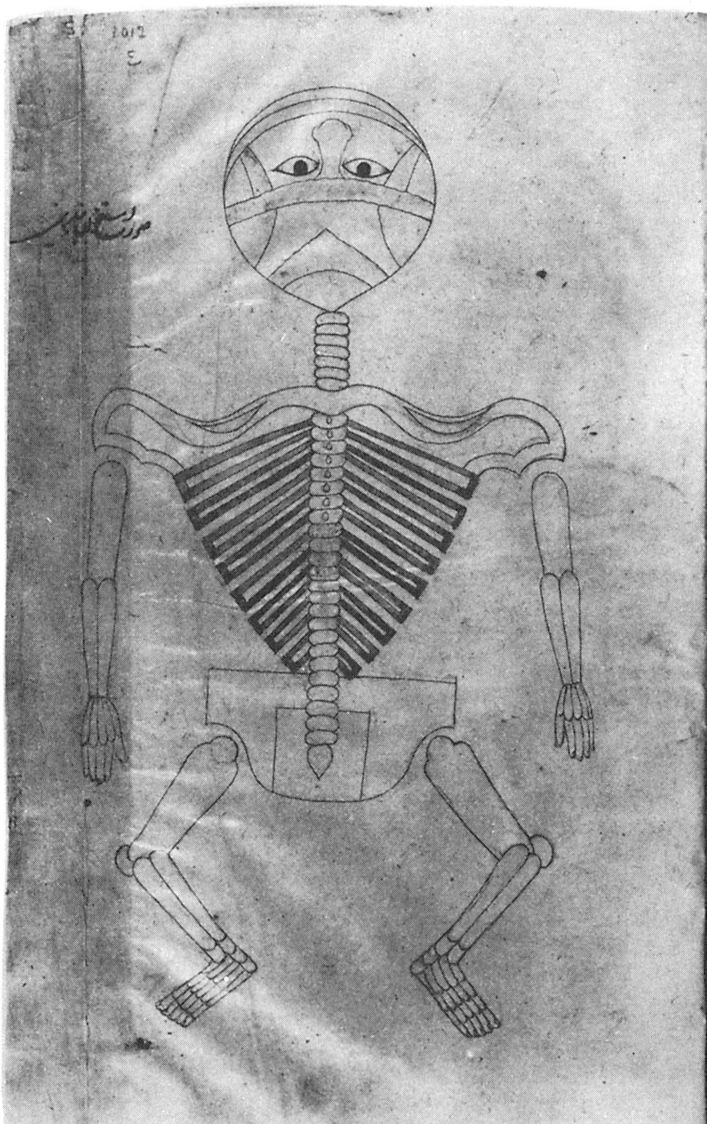

2. Vatican Palat. Lat. 1110 (14[th]C.), fol. f. Bone man
From MacKinney and Hill (1964). The suture diagram is indicated by arrows.

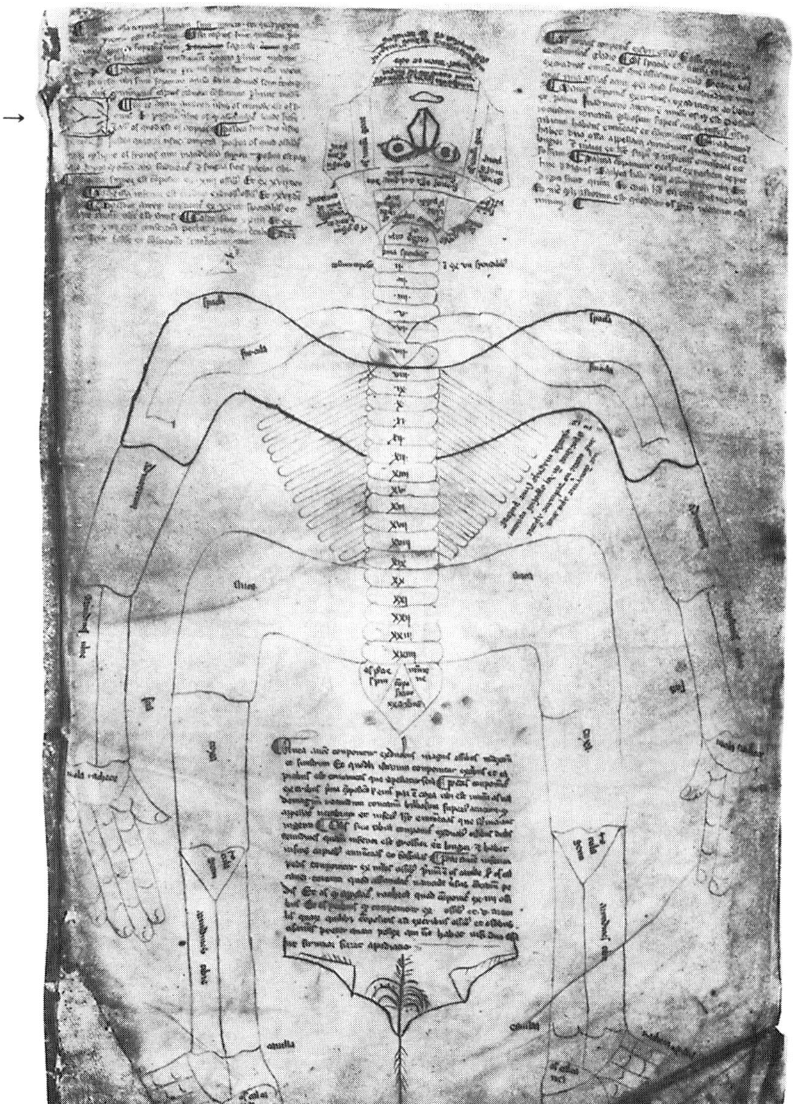

III

3. Basel ms D II 11

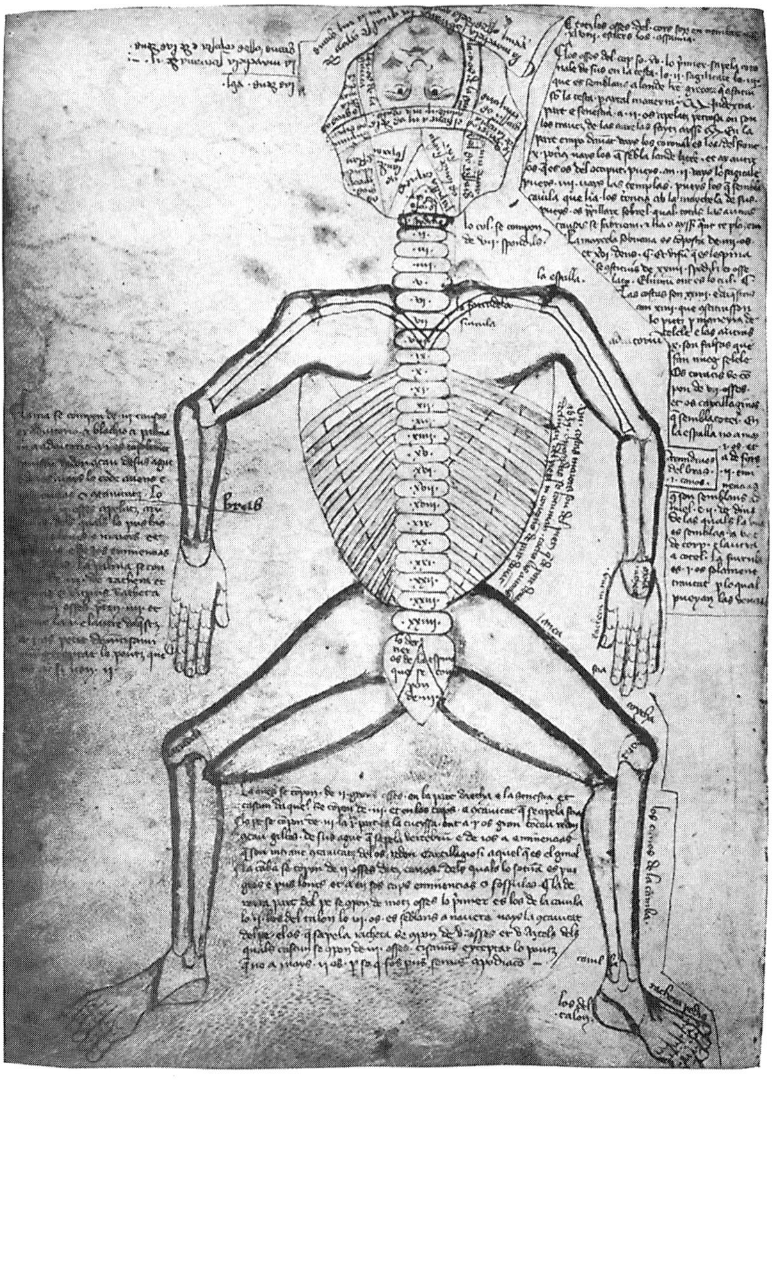

IV

A NOTE ON THE ANATOMICAL ACCESSUS OF THE MIDDLE AGES

In commenting on the classical authors the medieval commentators very often used a formal introduction setting out a number of topics to be treated in the commentary upon the text. This *accessus ad auctores* has been discussed by Quain,[1] who lists a wide variety of branches of study in which the *accessus* was used; the only significant omission from this list is medicine. Medical examples, however, have been pointed out by Temkin,[2] and the topic as a whole has been dealt with in medicine by Cunningham.[3] It is the purpose of this note to draw the attention of historians to the use of a form of *accessus* in anatomy and to make some tentative suggestions about the relationship between the *accessus* and the beginning of human dissection in the West.

The *accessus* is traced back by Quain to Ammonius, the fifth-century commentator on Aristotle. Ammonius was a mathematician, astronomer, philosopher, rhetorician, and grammarian: like Aristotle, he did not write anything on medicine, and the medical use of the *accessus* was borrowed from these other fields of study. The philosophers used the format of the *accessus* more rigorously than the rhetoricians, grammarians, and lawyers, and from the examples given below, it appears that the medical use of the form was even more flexible. The "school" of Ammonius includes all those who were interested in Aristotle from the fifth to seventh centuries, and it was, then, as a means of understanding Aristotle that the *accessus* developed. (At this point it should also be noted that the late classical and early medieval commentators gave much attention to the *Categories*[4] of Aristotle. The results of this are suggested below.)

The medical *accessus* was an elaboration of the last of ten questions which were considered mandatory by the philosophers in an introduction to any work of Aristotle.

*Roger French, M.A., D.Phil., Wellcome Unit for the History of Medicine, University of Cambridge, Free School Lane, Cambridge CB2 3EL.

[1] E. A. Quain, 'The medieval accessus ad auctores', *Traditio*, 1945, **3**: 215–264. I am grateful to Dr. A. R. Cunningham of the Wellcome Unit for the History of Medicine, Cambridge, for bringing Quain's article to my attention and for valuable discussions on the topic of the *accessus*.

[2] O. Temkin, 'Studies in late Alexandrian medicine. 1: Alexandrian commentaries on Galen's *De sectis ad introducendos*', *Bull. Hist. Med.*, 1935, **3**: 405–430.

[3] A. R. Cunningham, 'Two legacies of the later Alexandrian school: the preliminary questions in commentaries; the theory/practice division of medicine', *Proceedings of the second International Conference on the Comparative History of Medicine, East and West*, Tokyo (in press).

[4] Boethius, an important figure in the transmission of the *accessus* technique, included it in his commentary on Porphyry's introduction to Aristotle's *Categories*. See Cunningham, op. cit., note 3 above.

Medical History 23 (London, 1979), pp. 461–468.

These ten questions were:

1. The names and number of the philosophical sects.
2. The division of the works of Aristotle.
3. The works to be read first in studying Aristotle.
4. What is Aristotle's purpose in his philosophy?
5. How can the modern reader achieve this purpose?
6. The character of Aristotle's work.
7. Why Aristotle chose to be so obscure in his exposition.
8. The proper attitude of an Aristotelian commentator.
9. The proper attitude of an Aristotelian reader.
10. How many items, and what kind of items, should be considered in the introduction to the works of Aristotle, and for what reasons?

It is clear that these ten topics or questions are those that need to be raised by whoever wished to understand Aristotle's philosophy as a whole, and their formulation into a rigid programme suggests an institutional background of teaching and learning, two important points when the anatomical *accessus* comes to be discussed. The topics of the medieval *accessus*, developed from the last of these Aristotelian questions, can be listed as:

1. The life of the author;
2. the title of the work;
3. the intention of the writer;
4. the matter of the work;
5. the use of the work;
6. to what part of philosophy the work belongs.

The *accessus* became popular by the twelfth century and was represented in most parts of the school curriculum. Quain quotes from Conrad of Hirschau, who gives us the only known theoretical discussion of the form: in Conrad's case it is clear that it is a technique for elementary students, and he has two rather different forms of the *accessus* for ancient and for modern authors. For ancient authors one must know also the order of the books composing the work and their number, the character of the work, and an explanation of it, while the *matter* of the work, the *intention* of the author and the philosophical relations of the work are transferred to the list that relates to modern authors. The list *as a whole* therefore contains at least three of the topics that had been included in the original list of ten questions that related only to Aristotle's works. The *accessus* form was clearly flexible, accommodating new authors and new teaching circumstances. Most important for our point of view, the list for *modern* authors (in Conrad's account) includes the final cause of the work, a topic taken from the Aristotelian apparatus of fourfold causality.

One of the first appearances of the *accessus* in the medical literature is in John of Alexandria's commentary on the Hippocratic *Epidemics*,[5] where he gives some, but by no means all of the topics listed above. (He does not discuss his use of the form, but simply follows the rote, which suggests that this was the customary practice.)

[5] C. D. Pritchet (editor), *Johannis Alexandrini Commentaria in sextum librum Hippocratis Epidemiarum*, Leiden, Brill, 1975, pp. 1–6.

For the purposes of this note, we may call this list of topics the "literary *accessus*" to distinguish it from two further types discussed below. The first and fundamentally important of these other two types is the "anatomical *accessus*" which John of Alexandria uses in his commentary of Galen's *De sectis*. Now, *De sectis* is Galen's account of the different medical sects of his day and the arguments that arose between them; one of the most important of these arguments was whether a knowledge of anatomy was unnecessary and the process of dissection disgusting, as the Empirics said, or fundamental to a knowledge of how the body worked, as the Rationalists claimed. Moreover, there were those who claimed that vivisection was an invaluable aid to understanding the body's *function*, not merely its morphology. *De sectis* was the first book to be studied in the post-classical Alexandrian medical curriculum,[6] and so, apart from its complexity, it posed special problems for the inexperienced reader, and as a result it attracted much commentary.

John of Alexandria's commentary reflects all this.[7] His purpose is to make the work intelligible in as short a time as necessary (since life is short and the art is long) and he repeatedly refers to his task of making the task of learning easier for his listeners. In his proemium John discusses the nature of art, and points out that medicine, like carpentry, has both the material with which to work (the human body and wood respectively) and the finished product (health and a door or window). The proemium ends with eight items of a conventional literary *accessus* directed to *De sectis*. In the first comment John links these two ideas, the *accessus* and "art" by considering under the *accessus* topic "order of exposition" Galen's opening of chapter 1 where the subject matter and the purpose of medicine (the body and health) are discussed. John elaborates this into a complete scheme of Aristotelian causality, with a material, efficient, formal, and final cause. Aristotelian causality could be used to examine more than a single topic of the *accessus*, and was used later to replace the *accessus* by serving the same purpose, i.e. the examination of an entire work.

In his eleventh commentary, arising in the middle of Galen's fifth chapter, where Galen is discussing the reasoning with which the Empiricists and Dogmatists argue against and for anatomy, John says there are two kinds of anatomy (*artificiosa incisio*): of the living and of the dead. The anatomy of the living is vivisection, which Celsus tells us was defended by extreme Rationalists on the basis of the benefit accruing to medicine and the health of future generations, and in vivisection, says John, we must distinguish between Operation and Necessity, that is, some organs have an operative Faculty and others do not, but are necessary adjuncts of the Faculty of the other: this can only be seen in the living body. In the dead body anatomy is concerned with six *occasiones:*

1. The number of the organs (two kidneys, for example, or one liver).
2. The character of the part (whether bony, fibrous, or cartilaginous).
3. The position of the part (the liver on the right, the spleen on the left).
4. Size (the liver is larger than the kidneys or heart).
5. Shape (*scema:* the liver is concave interiorly, like the moon).
6. Anatomical relations (the liver is connected to the gall bladder at a certain point).

[6] A. Z. Iskandar, 'An attempted reconstruction of the late Alexandrian medical curriculum', *Med. Hist.*, 1976, **20:** 235–258.

[7] Galen, *Primum Galeni volumen quarta impressio ornatissima . . .*, Pavia, 1515, f.vir.

John has sided with the Rationalists and decided that anatomy is necessary to medicine: he has therefore to teach it in a convenient way, and to do so he has produced an *accessus* type of rote that applies to each of the body's organs in turn. He was in the same position as other teachers who were seeking a way into complex texts on their students' behalf, but he was faced with a complex description of a *body* rather than a reasoned text. Although the anatomy he is discussing was that of the Rationalists who in Alexandria at least dissected the human body, John's immediate sources are of course textual, and he is using a literary scholastic technique. It is a technique that seems to go back directly to Aristotle, rather than by way of the more normal form of *accessus*, for the six *occasiones* of the anatomy of the dead are very close to Aristotle's *Categories*, the source, as we have said, of much post-classical commentatorial interest. The categories may be summarized as follows:

1. Substance.
2. Quantity. Discrete quantity (as opposed to continuous) is number; comparable to the first of the anatomical *occasiones*.
3. Quality. The "character" of the second of the anatomical *occasiones* is a sub-category within Aristotle's third. Perhaps an additional *rationale* was that the anatomical "qualities" are reducible to the elementary qualities of the "similar" parts (e.g. bone, "fibre", and cartilage) of which the organs are composed. Aristotle's "quality" also includes "shape", and the fifth anatomical *occasio*.
4. Place. Aristotle deals with this category simply, with the example "in the Lyceum"[8] which has obvious anatomical counterparts: the third *occasio*.
5. Relation. Aristotle is principally concerned with the necessary relation of the greater and smaller, and to judge by John of Alexandria's example, this also seems to be what was meant by the fourth of the anatomical *occasiones*, "size". Relation for Aristotle also included "position" in relation to other things, so that we may compare this category also to the last of the *occasiones*.

These categories are not in Aristotle's order, which has been changed for convenience of comparison. The categories also include "time", which can have no counterpart in the anatomy of the dead, and "action" and "affection". If, like later commentators, we take John of Alexandria's two topics from the anatomy of the living as an extension of his anatomical *occasiones*, then we have his "necessity" and "operation" both as equivalent to Aristotle's "action". Later commentators added to John's list a last "affection", no doubt directly from Aristotle, but considered in a medical context: *passiones*, which came to be a vehicle for discussion of pathology. The two final things we need to note about the comparison between these two lists is first that Aristotle's category of "substance" is not represented, because largely inapplicable, in the list of *occasiones;* and second, that the last *occasio,* anatomical relations, although sharing something with Aristotle's "position", recalls more strongly the "to what part of philosophy it relates" topic of the literary and philosophical *accessus*. In general the styles and details of the *accessus* were flexible and interchangeable, and later commentators added to the list of *occasiones,* in first place, the name of the part. This had parallels both with the "title of the work" and "author" categories which were second and first on the literary *accessus* list, and with the etymological

[8] *Categories,* 11b. See also the discussion by G. E. R. Lloyd, *Aristotle: the growth and structure of his thought,* Cambridge University Press, 1968, p. 113.

interest in anatomy of writers such as Varro and Isidore, which was taken up by the medieval encyclopedists and anatomical writers.

So far, then, we have distinguished three formal sets of questions of the *accessus* type which were designed to be asked of different kinds of texts and which were related and ultimately derived from Aristotle and his early commentators: the literary or philosophical *accessus,* the categorical or anatomical, and the causality *accessus.* These three forms came to be known by writers on medicine and anatomy in the Western middle ages during a period when the study of anatomy changed from being purely literary to the practical study of animal anatomy and then to human dissection. The earliest anatomical writings of the West were compilations and translations, and probably the most important translation was Constantine's *Pantegni,* a version of the *Liber regius* of Haly Abbas. Constantine prefixed a literary *accessus* to his work, but the influence of this is not felt in the first accounts of animal dissection in the West, the Salernitan "demonstrations". The *Anatomia porci* is an uncomplicated account of the dissection of a pig in about 1150, depending partly on the *Pantegni* but also showing evidence of a survival of some as yet unknown Greek source. Later demonstrations show a much more scholastic approach, but rely on no further sources of information. The whole group of demonstrations suggests an active programme of assimilating new sources of knowledge with the old by means of dissection in an institutional framework of teaching.[9]

Despite a new translation of the *Liber regius* by Stephen of Antioch,[10] in 1127, the idea of using a formal rote of questions in relation to anatomy does not seem to have occurred again until *human* dissection began in the second half of the thirteenth century. The *accessus* then used was the categorical-anatomical, taken from John of Alexandria's commentary on *De sectis.* In other words the *literary* device of exploring, explaining, and teaching a difficult and perhaps previously unknown book was transferred to the *physical* dissection, explanation, and memorizing of the human body. Apart from other advantages this *accessus ad corpus,* as we might call it, was useful training in preparation to observe as much as possible in a rapidly decomposing body.

Both the use of this kind of *accessus* and human dissection seem to have begun in the circle of Taddeo Alderotti. His pupil Mondino[11] took the *accessus* directly from John of Alexandria, and followed the *occasiones* for every organ in the body. To the six original *occasiones* he added the two derived from vivisection (necessity and operation) and ninth "disease", which it was the purpose of his (surgical) anatomy to uncover, Bertruccio's pupil Guy de Chauliac following suit.[12] His book formed the basis of later anatomy teaching and commenting, at least in Italy.

[9] The texts of the Salernitan demonstrations are given by G. W. Corner, *Anatomical texts of the earlier middle ages,* Washington, Carnegie Institute, 1927. See also Y. V. O'Neill, 'Another look at the "Anatomia Porci",' *Viator,* 1970, **1**: 115–124.

[10] Printed as Haly Abbas, *Liber totius medicinae . . .,* Lyons, 1523.

[11] Mondino's *Anathomia* has been translated by C. Singer, in J. Ketham, *The fasciculo di medicina* (*Venice 1493*) edited by Charles Singer, part 1, Florence, R. Lier, 1925. It is also worthwhile following Mondino's text in Berengario da Carpi's commentary, because Berengario makes useful criticisms and discusses the use of the *accessus* as taken from John of Alexandria and the propriety of adding more *occasiones* from vivisection, and a ninth, "disease". Berengario da Carpi, *Commentaria cum amplissimis additionibus super anatomia Mundini,* Bologna, 1521, ff. vr., xxxxvr.

[12] Berengario da Carpi tells us that it was Guy who first added *aegritudines* that were suffered by

Another early dissector was William of Saliceto,[13] whose surgical anatomy text of 1275 expressly rejects scholastic principles (and therefore the *accessus*) but whose practice of dissection may owe something to Taddeo. Bartolomeo da Varignana, who refers to post-mortem examinations, and Henri de Mondeville, who performed human dissections in teaching, were also pupils of Taddeo. Taddeo himself used both the causality and philosophical *accessus* in his commentary on the *Isagoge* of Joannitius;[14] perhaps somewhere he uses also the categorical-anatomical, for he must have known of John of Alexandria's commentary on *De sectis*. Gentile da Foligna was another of Taddeo's pupils, and had read or heard Mondino: Gentile refers[15] to the use of the *accessus* in his own commentary on the *Ars parva*, and mentions John of Alexandria's use of the different kinds of *accessus* in commenting on the *Epidemics* and on *De sectis*. Gentile mentions also its use by Haly Abbas, that is, the *accessus* of Constantine or the sequence of topics of the *Liber regius;* Gentile describes all three as causality *accessus*, but in fact none of them is. His discussion, nevertheless, is of the *accessus* in general, and perhaps he had in mind that form of it favoured (so it appears from his own words)[16] by his teacher Taddeo, the causality form. As a medical Aristotelian, Taddeo was concerned to relate medicine to the rest of natural philosophy and to justify its study; and he was caught up in the institutionalization of his subject in Bologna. This last detail poses a minor problem for Siraisi[17] in looking for its significance in intellectual history or the history of science. There is one possible answer to this problem which is of the greatest significance: the possibility that these circumstances led to the introduction of human dissection. Taddeo and his circle had to justify the importance of their subject in the face of opposition from the old-established legal faculty of Bologna; they defended its status as a science and as an art; they analysed its ancient texts with the care and scholastic techniques that were used on legal texts (the legal *accessus* has a long history) and as an Aristotelian Taddeo seemed to favour the causality *accessus* and could hardly have been ignorant of the categorical form; the categorical *accessus* was an ideal form to borrow from literary sources for use in a real situation, that of human dissection, a practice which in the form of the post-mortem examination had almost certainly already begun in the legal faculty; only within the discipline of the (newly) institutionalized medical

---

the various parts, and that Mondino adopted this suggestion. Da Carpi also held that Mondino's list of *occasiones* had been wrongly set up by the printers of the early editions. For Guy de Chauliac see for example B. Wallner, 'The Middle English translation of Guy de Chauliac's anatomy', *Lunds Universitets Arsskrift* N.F. Ard. 1, 1964, **56**, which includes the text of a Latin MS.

[13] William of Saliceto, *Cyrurgia*, Piacenza, 1476. A facsimile of a MS. has been produced by G. Caturegli, *L'anatomia di Guglielmo da Saliceto*, Pisa, Giardini, 1969. William's book is dedicated to Taddeo Alderotti's son-in-law, and we may guess at some communication between Taddeo and William.

[14] Thaddeus Florentinus (Taddeo Alderotti), *Expositiones in . . . subtilissimum Joannitii Isagogarum libellum*, Venice, 1527, ff. 343r–344r.

[15] 'Gentilis fulginatis medici clarissimi expositio & quaestiones subtilissimae super primo libro microtechni Galeni', in Turisanus Florentinus, *Plusquam commentum in parvam Galeni artem*, Venice, 1557, f.221v.

[16] "de mea consuetudine in primo cuiuslibet libri perquirro": Taddeo, op. cit., note 14 above, fol. 343r.

[17] N. G. Siraisi, 'Taddeo Alderotti and Bartolomeo da Varignana on the nature of medical learning', *Isis*, 1977, **68**: 27–39.

teaching could the unnatural practice of cutting up the body of a dead person flourish; theoretical considerations taken from Galen and Aristotle urged that anatomy was the fundamental medical study, and that dissection was the proper way to reveal to the sense of observation the structure of the body; this teaching need had been felt in the professional but less theoretical medical school of Salerno, and had been answered by dissecting the pig, but to be of use in medicine the new teaching at Bologna had to use the human body.

At all events it is clear that interest in the *accessus* technique of analysis of texts was at its height when human dissection was first undertaken as a teaching device in a university medical faculty. Thereafter the categorical-anatomical *accessus* became a style of exposition that dominated anatomical exegesis until the sixteenth century. It was used by Niccolo Bertruccio, pupil of Mondino and teacher of Guy de Chauliac, who also used it, and it clearly became the standard mode of teaching, and was absorbed by later anatomists so thoroughly that they do not discuss the form, nor its original purpose: and the sequence of topics, although strict, is sometimes almost submerged in new discussions about morphology and function. Until Vesalius' influence had completely turned anatomy back to an older style of exposition (that of Galen, dominated by the philosophical implications of function) the categorical-anatomical *accessus* survived in a surprising range of writers, particularly in teaching texts: Benedictus,[18] Guinter,[19] Vasse,[20] Sylvius,[21] Berengario da Carpi,[22] Zerbis,[23] Achillini,[24] and Paré.[25]

[18] A. Benedictus, *Anatomice, sive de hystoria corporis humani, libri quinque,* Strasburg, 1528, p.6r: Benedictus uses the categorical form in the introduction.

[19] J. Guinter, *Institutionum anatomicarum . . . libri quatuor,* Paris, 1536: Guinter uses the categorical form in the prefatory epistle.

[20] L. Vasseus, *In anatomen corporis humani tabulae quatuor,* Paris, 1540.

[21] In agreement with most traditional anatomists, Sylvius argued that antomy began with the fundamentals of the Aristotelian world-picture, the elements and qualities. The "similar" parts of the body are composed of these and are the simplest constituents of the body. He has in mind the two ways of teaching anatomy, the analytic and synthetic, at the opposite poles of which are the complete and functioning body, and its simplest components: this involves a whole different field of theoretical considerations, but Sylvius links it with the one discussed in this paper by assuming that the "similar" parts, when arranged in the set of relations defined as *occasiones* by John of Alexandria, become "instrumental" parts, and a further similar arrangement creates instrumental parts of the second order that have purposeful action and not merely use or quality. These remarks are contained in his extremely short introduction to his edition of *De usu partium* of Galen, Paris, 1543.

[22] Da Carpi follows Mondino's use of the categorical *accessus* as a mode of exegesis throughout his work. See notes 11 and 12 above.

[23] G. de Zerbis, *Liber anathomie corporis humani,* Venice, 1502. Here the categorical *accessus* dominates the text, which is broken up into paragraphs each with a heading of one of the *occasiones,* even when inapplicable (such as the number of obviously single organs).

[24] A. Achillini, *Anatomical notes* (1520), in L. R. Lind, *Studies in pre-Vesalian anatomy,* Philadelphia, American Philosophical Society, 1975. Achillini discusses the use of the categorical form in his introduction in a manner similar to that of da Carpi, questioning the propriety of some of the *occasiones* and suggesting an otherwise unknown medieval source for the discussion, Francis of Piedmont.

[25] A. Paré, *Anatome,* for example in P. Uffenbach, *Thesaurus chirurgicae,* Frankfurt, 1610; or see Paré, *Les oeuvres,* Paris, 1579. As a surgeon, Paré did not have a regular medical education, and it seems probable that when he came to write his short text on anatomy he sought advice from a physician. The result is that he dutifully runs through all the standard, contemporary, and introductory "theory of medicine" from the "orders" of the *Ars parva* to the *occasiones* in a slightly naïve way that well reveals the educational source of these ideas.

SUMMARY

In commenting on the classical authors the medieval writers very often used a formal introduction setting out a number of topics to be dealt with in the commentary. Recent discussions of this *accessus ad auctores* do not adequately discuss its use in relation to medical topics and in particular its use in commentaries on anatomical texts has been ignored. This note sets out three kinds of *accessus* found in medieval medical writings, the philosophical, the categorical, and the causality *accessus*. There is the interesting possibility that the *accessus* technique, designed to explore and teach a text unknown to the student, was also used to explore and teach the unknown structure of the body when human dissection came to be practised in the medieval university.

V

Foretelling the Future

Arabic Astrology and English Medicine in the Late Twelfth Century

ROGER OF HEREFORD HAS BEEN KNOWN TO HISTORIANS since the work of C. H. Haskins. Subsequent discussions have only just begun to concentrate on the content of Roger's work. The most important of these is Jennifer Moreton's discussion of his *Compotus* in a recent issue of *Isis*. Even now, medieval astrology attracts less attention than that of the Renaissance; in the earlier period, Roger deserves more attention. He worked in the western borders of Norman England, an area that is increasingly being recognized as important in the mathematical and other arts.[1] He flourished at an important time in the West—the last quarter of the twelfth century—when schools in northern Europe, which had often depended on the fame of a teacher, were turning into universities where the masters formed corporations rather than competed. It was a time, too, when Arabic and Greek knowledge was being sought and incorporated into teaching. Aristotle's natural philosophy was coming to be used in Salerno to comment on medical texts (when Roger was young) and in Languedoc to fight heresy (perhaps while he was still alive), but it was not widely known in his lifetime.[2]

* Cambridge Wellcome Unit for the History of Medicine, University of Cambridge, Free School Lane, Cambridge CB2 3RH, England.

[1] C. H. Haskins, "The Reception of Arabic Science in England," *English Historical Review*, 1915, *30*:56–69; and Jennifer Moreton, "Before Grosseteste: Roger of Hereford and Calendar Reform in Eleventh- and Twelfth-Century England," *Isis*, 1995, *86*:562–586. Until Moreton's recent detailed account of Roger's work in the *Compotus*, little attention had been paid to him since Josiah C. Russell, "Hereford and Arabic Science in England about 1175–1200," *ibid.*, 1932, *18*:14–25; rpt. in Russell, *Twelfth Century Studies* (New York: AMS, 1978), Ch. 10, pp. 142–154. On the importance of the Hereford region see especially Charles Burnett, "Mathematics and Astronomy in Hereford and Its Region in the Twelfth Century," in *Hereford: Medieval Art, Architecture, and Archaeology*, ed. David Whitehead (British Archaeological Association Conference Transactions, 15) (Leeds, 1995), pp. 50–59.

[2] On Salerno see Danielle Jacquart, "Aristotelian Thought in Salerno," in *A History of Twelfth-Century Western Philosophy*, ed. Peter Dronke (Cambridge: Cambridge Univ. Press, 1988), pp. 407–428. Toulouse was a center of the Cathar heresy; to counter it, Dominic set up his order there and the school was made a *studium generale*. Both organizations used Aristotle's physical works extensively and explicitly against the Cathars. The earliest use of these works against the heretics is found in writings of Peter Martyr and Moneta of Cremona, which are rather late (about 1235 and 1241, respectively) but refer back to the early years of the thirteenth century, when the heretics were in open disputation with the Catholics and, like them, were using Aristotle's physical works. See Thomas Kaepelli, "Le somme contra la hérétiques de Pierre Martyr(?)," *Archivum Fratrum Predicatorum*, 1947, *17*:295–335; and Moneta of Cremona, *Adversos Catharos et Valdenses libri quinque* (Rome, 1743). The question is discussed at length in Roger French and Andrew Cunningham, *Before Science: The Invention of the Friars' Natural Philosophy* (London: Scolar, 1996). See also *Chartularium universitatis Parisiensis*, ed. Heinrich Denifle, O.P. (Paris, 1889), Vol. 1, p. 83; René Gadave, *Les documents sur l'histoire de l'Université de Toulouse* (Toulouse: Edouard Privat, 1910); and Pearl Kibre, *Scholarly Privileges in the Middle Ages* (London: Mediaeval Academy of America, 1961), p. 93.

So medicine, Aristotle's physical works, and Greek and Arabic teaching on the stars and planets were of great interest to the men of the twelfth-century West who knew of them. We can see why they found these things interesting: they had practical applications.[3] Medical men were among the first to seek out the new knowledge. The *Centiloquium,* thought to have been written by Ptolemy, was addressed to medical men as much as to astrologers and astronomers and was seen as directly *useful* by the prognosticating doctor of the Middle Ages. In the twelfth century it was perhaps routine for a medical practitioner to make use of astrology in some way. The medical man had traditionally put his special interest—man's body, the microcosm—in its place in the macrocosm, so that nature, the Greek *physis,* became the root of *physician.*[4] Both the doctors and the astrologers practiced in a marketplace where competition was not limited by regulation or formal qualification. Both groups had patients (the astrologers' clients were usually suffering in some way). Both groups advertised themselves by means of an assumed rationality that depended on an analogy between macrocosm and microcosm, where the correspondences included elementary qualities.

The power to predict the future was clearly an ability that was attractive to many (Roger makes it plain that he thought so), but it was perhaps most useful to the medical men. Their business involved prognostication, for which they had both ancient authority and a highly visible technique, uroscopy. Prognostication was explicitly held to have a dual purpose: the exercise of this particular skill was to generate a favorable image of the physician and to be of medical use to the patient.[5] Uroscopy was the characteristic activity of the doctor; the image of him inspecting the flask of urine by holding it to the light is widespread in medieval manuscripts. In such actions the doctor is publicly showing his skill in a partly ritual way.

The new Arabic astrology offered a technical apparatus that could extend the doctor's powers of prognostication. Its technical difficulty, once overcome, offered the same double advantage as uroscopy. The doctor believed that he was increasing the certainty of his prognosis, and he was doing so with a learned apparatus that enhanced his image. Because the doctor had long been held to possess special knowledge of the microcosm and its relationship to the macrocosm, astrology seemed to be an extension of his knowledge. Indeed, it seemed to offer a superior kind of knowledge. The most precise form of astro-

[3] Traditionally historians of astronomy have represented it as becoming scientific precisely by throwing off unscientific astrology. In fact, what looks to us like astronomy in the past was often no more than the mathematical preparation for astrology. Twelfth- and thirteenth-century terminology was too variable to allow us to see a contemporary distinction between astrology and astronomy. See Roger French, "Astrology in Medical Practice," in *Practical Medicine from Salerno to the Black Death,* ed. Luis Garcia-Ballester, Roger French, Jon Arrizabalaga, and Andrew Cunningham (Cambridge: Cambridge Univ. Press, 1994), pp. 30–59, esp. pp. 33–34. Charles Burnett, "The Translating Activity in Medieval Spain," in *The Legacy of Muslim Spain,* ed. Salma Khadra Jayyusi (Leiden: Brill, 1995), pp. 1036–1058, also emphasizes divination as the primary motive for translation, in which astronomy played a supporting role.

[4] See Jerome J. Bylebyl, "The Medical Meaning of *Physica,*" *Osiris,* 2nd Ser., 1990, *6:*16–41. On early efforts by medical men to seek out the new knowledge see French, "Astrology in Medical Practice"; on the use of the *Centiloquium* see Charles Burnett, "Adelard, Ergaphalau, and the Science of the Stars," in *Adelard of Bath: An English Scientist and Arabist of the Early Twelfth Century,* ed. Burnett (London: Warburg Inst., Univ. London, 1987). The texts on diagnosis and prognostication from urine and the pulse by Theophilus and Philaretus were basic treatises in the medieval textbook of medicine, later known as the *Articella,* which in the twelfth century consisted of five works.

[5] The Hippocratic *Prognosis* mentions the "glory" that follows from successful prognostication. Maurus of Salerno wrote of the "praise and glory" that came to the doctor from prognostications; see M. H. Saffron, "Maurus of Salerno: Twelfth-Century 'Optimus Physicus' with His Commentary on the *Prognostics* of Hippocrates," *Transactions of the American Philosophical Society,* N.S., 1972, *62:*5–104, on p. 22.

logical prediction was judicial astrology, which offered "judgments" on questions asked by the astrologer's client, but its very claims to precision made it look dangerous to some on religious grounds. It was accordingly more popular in royal courts than in monastic or other religious houses.[6]

These were the circumstances in which Roger wrote a number of works on astrological prediction. He was almost certainly the first Englishman to give a systematic account of the kinds of astrological prediction and perhaps the first Westerner to make available to medical men a way of making a "judicial" prognosis. But despite the natural relationship between medicine and astrology, the technical complexity of judicial astrology may have prevented doctors from taking full advantage of it. What we know of medical astrology of the time suggests that it continued to be at a simpler level of prognosis, for example, predicting favorable moments for surgery from the phases of the moon. The exception is Roger's younger compatriot, William of England, who was one of the first to use such judgments in the traditional area of uroscopy. This essay accordingly argues that the early close relationship of medicine and astrology made its judicial form (as exemplified in the writings of Roger) of potential use to doctors and that one doctor—William—realized some of that potential.

ABŪ MAʿSHAR, ASTROLOGY, AND MEDICINE

Roger was a key figure in the dissemination of Arabic astrology in England because he was familiar with the *Introductorium* of the ninth-century Muslim Abū Maʿshar. This text, translated in 1133 and 1140, was influential in the West, and Abū Maʿshar came to be perhaps the most widely cited author in Latin astrologies. Roger does not name him but was an early agent in the spread of the doctrines of the *Introductorium.* The text of this work shows clearly how medicine was closely associated with astrology. Perhaps fearing that the reader might be skeptical, Abū Maʿshar leads him gently into the subject. He begins with undeniable correspondences between the planets and the earth, such as that between the moon and the tides and menstruation. The most obvious correspondence of all is that between the sun and the seasons; Abū Maʿshar makes this the fundamental link, presenting a physical world picture that is largely Aristotelian. It is the sun that, in the spring, gives the season its elementary qualities of warmth and moisture: this leads to generation in the Aristotelian sense, and for Abū Maʿshar it is effected by the *temperies,* the "temper" or particular balance of elementary qualities, characteristic of the compound body in question. (The medical doctrine of *complexio* was very similar.) Corruption follows in the autumn as the sun's power lessens and the season becomes cold and dry. Abū Maʿshar's argument is that the necessity of celestial cause and mundane effect can be developed into a doctrine that can be handled rationally and so lead to prediction. It can also be handled experientially, just as the experience of farmers and navigators improves their ability to prognosticate the best times for sowing and sailing. His chief example is the medical man: experience, of course, improves his prognostication abilities, but he has another advantage as well. Indeed, the medical man is held to be linked to the astrologer by their common distance from the vulgar: Abū Maʿshar says that shepherds, sailors,

[6] On the relationship of the terms *physica, natural philosophy,* and *physician* see Bylebyl, "Medical Meaning of *Physica*" (cit. n. 4). On the perceived dangers of judicial astrology see Hilary M. Carey, *Courting Disaster: Astrology at the English Court and University in the Later Middle Ages* (London: Macmillan, 1992), p. 29. Walter Map, a colleague of Roger, was "eloquent" in his disapproval of astrology (*ibid.,* p. 30).

farmers, and midwives all can make predictions well enough on the basis of experience, but the astrologer and the doctor also make use of reason.[7]

It was natural for Abū Maʿshar to focus on the links of astrology with medical theory. The principal influences from the heavens, he says at the beginning of the *Introductorium,* are the four elementary qualities, and the most important effects are upon natural bodies compounded from the four elements. Among the least complex and most important of the compound bodies are the humors of the body: blood, red and black bile, and phlegm. Each has a pair of elementary qualities and corresponds directly to celestial influence. The humors are Abū Maʿshar's principal example of the link between medicine and astrology. The art of the medical man, he says, is based on knowledge of the elements, of the climates of the world (which were astronomically determined), and indeed of nature and what is natural, nonnatural, and contranatural (the Galenic categories fundamental to the theory of medicine). The task of the physician is to maintain the balance of the qualities of the humors; according to Abū Maʿshar, the skilled physician approximated the astrologer in his knowledge of the elements and their celestial governors. Abū Maʿshar sees medicine almost as a specialized form of astrology, dealing with the accidents that happen to elementary matter, while astrology proper deals more generally with sublunar motion. Abū Maʿshar uses medical language in claiming that the principles of astrology are to do with the "naturals" of the heavenly bodies, that is, the heat of the sun and the moistness of the moon (just as the "naturals" of the human body, to the doctor, are the parts, humors, and moving powers). He also uses the language of natural philosophy when he says that all individual things consist of matter and form. But to matter and form he adds a third, the influence of the stars. It may be general, like the sun being the principle of animal life, or it may be particular, like Mercury being the planet of man.[8] This doctrine of influences is also the basis for the planets' specific attachments to particular organs of the body: Saturn to the spleen, Jove to the liver, Mars to the blood.

Of course, Abū Maʿshar rates astrology a higher form of knowledge than medicine because of the nobility of the study of the stars and of causes; indeed, it is clear that his high opinion of medicine derives from its closeness to astrology. Central to both medicine and astrology were the doctrines of growth and decrease—the physician's job being, in Abū Maʿshar's view, to supply deficiencies, remove excesses, block external influences, and preserve a tempered state. This intervention was not merely corrective, but preventative. For example, the prognosticating doctor knew that when the summer came there would be fevers; as Abū Maʿshar notes, he therefore let blood and used the cupping-glass to try to prevent putrefaction and apostemes, which were among the causes of fevers. Knowing that a disease was coming allowed a doctor and his patient to alleviate its effects. It was good for the doctor to know that if a patient took to his bed early in the lunar cycle, he would fight the disease better.[9] And Abū Maʿshar also recognized that it was extremely useful for the doctor to know if his patient was about to die.

[7] I have used *Introductorium in astronomiam Albumasaris abalachi octo continens libros partiales* (Venice, 1506) (hereafter cited as **Abū Maʿshar, *Introductorium***), which is unpaginated. The initial discussion of correspondences and predictions is in Bk. 1, Ch. 1. See also Abū Maʿshar, *The Abbreviation of the* Introduction to Astrology *Together with the Medieval Latin Translation of Adelard of Bath,* ed. and trans. Charles Burnett, Keijo Yamamoto, and Michio Yano (Islamic Philosophy, Theology, and Science: Texts and Studies, 15) (Leiden: Brill, 1994). That the medical aspects of astrology—particularly the relations of microcosm and macrocosm—were important in its Christianization has been pointed out in Valerie I. J. Flint, *The Rise of Magic in Early Medieval Europe* (Oxford: Clarendon, 1991), p. 130.

[8] Abū Maʿshar, *Introductorium* 1.3, 4.2.

[9] *Ibid.,* 1.5 (importance of medicine, physician's job), 3.9 (lunar cycle).

But medicine and astrology were not the same. The medical man prognosticated chiefly through the inspection of urines, with which he made a professional display that generated the enduring image of the medieval medical man. He also, less ostentatiously, took the pulse. The copious division-of-the-sciences literature of the twelfth century always separated the two disciplines, and medical men down to the fifteenth century disputed whether astrology was part of medicine.[10]

The relationship between medicine and astrology at Roger's time was critical. The most important centers of medical teaching were Montpellier, Salerno, and Bologna, where students were finding it advantageous to group together to advance their common interests, and Paris, where the teaching masters were beginning to act in concert for similar reasons. The growth of institutions was central to the major changes that were about to come over medicine. When taught within a corporation that, with the consent of the church, issued licences to teach and practice, it became a profession whose members could seek to monopolize the practice of internal medicine and to control unlicensed practitioners, offering in exchange the perceived benefit to the public of their kind of medicine. It took about a century from Roger's time for the university physicians to finalize this program in fully formed faculties of medicine, but signs of its implementation are visible in the earlier thirteenth century.[11] In the northern universities, inserting medicine into the universities meant making it rational and learned in an Aristotelian sense, for the arts course and particularly its natural philosophy, on which the theory of medicine depended, were almost wholly Aristotelian.

But when Roger was writing about astrology, none of this had happened, and the medical men had hardly begun their battle to make medicine a subject to be taught in the new schools. The medical use of Aristotle's physical works in Salerno did not suggest any wider use of the new translations. Nor was it yet clear that the physical doctrines expounded in the major new astrological text of Abū Maʿshar (the *Introductorium*) were in fact Aristotelian.[12] Roger's role was as an agent broadcasting new Arabic material, by sharing and transmitting his enthusiasm for the physical knowledge of the Arabs and by organizing what he read in a form suitable for his contemporaries.[13]

[10] Pictures of physicians examining the pulse and urine of patients were a favorite theme of illustrators of medieval medical manuscripts, such as the *Articella.* A good example is Cambridge, St. John's College, D24. It was in the interest of the university physicians to stress that diseases were unique to each patient and required much personal attention from the physician; but the experience of great epidemics, in which many people had the same disease, compelled many to see disease as an external entity. Major—and rare—astrological events like the great conjunctions could then be invoked to explain the universality of diseases like the Black Death and the French Disease. See Jon Arrizabalaga, John Henderson, and Roger French, *The Great Pox: The French Disease in Renaissance Europe* (New Haven, Conn.: Yale Univ. Press, forthcoming). For examples of the division-of-the-sciences literature see Dominicus Gundissalinus, "De divisione philosophiae," in *Beitrage zur Geschichte der Philosophie des Mittelalters,* ed. Klemens Baeumker and Georg von Hertling (Münster: Aschendorff, 1906), Vol. 4; and Charles Henry Buttimer, ed., *Hugonis de Sancto Victore Didascalicon: De studio legendi* (Washington, D.C.: Catholic Univ. Press, 1939).

[11] For example, Frederick II decreed in 1231 that royal licenses should be given to properly prepared medical men in Sicily. See Michael McVaugh, *Medicine before the Plague* (Cambridge: Cambridge Univ. Press, 1993), p. 69.

[12] See Richard Lemay, *Abu Mashar and Latin Aristotelianism in the Twelfth Century* (Beirut: American Univ. Beirut, 1962). Many of the doctrines dealt with by Lemay are recognizable to him as "Aristotelian" but would not have been recognized as such by contemporary Latin readers. Certainly Roger, who drew extensively on Abū Maʿshar, had no notion that what he was reading derived ultimately from Aristotle.

[13] Students at Oxford were taught that Roger was as complete an Aristotelian as Alfred of Shareshill, who

What seems to have happened in the case of medicine is that the doctors chose to base the theory of their subject on Aristotle's physical principles and its technical content on the interpretation of Hippocratic texts offered by Galen (who himself used Aristotelian principles freely). This choice meant that the old links between medicine and astrology were not developed. Mathematical predictive astrology was new and was inapplicable to Aristotle's physical cosmology. The church was in any case not wholly in favor of allowing a lucrative trade like medicine to be taught in the universities and viewed astrology with great suspicion because it was not only lucrative but impious.[14] Books used in the early medical courses contained no astrology, and the *Articella,* the medieval textbook of medicine used in all the schools of medicine across Europe, is equally innocent of predictive astrology.[15]

Outside the universities, the case was different. The practitioners whom the new university physicians claimed the right to control had no need to break their links with astrology. At all times they were more numerous than the university physicians, and except where the faculty was close by and powerful they generally practiced internal medicine without hindrance. But they undoubtedly suffered in status as the university physicians succeeded in making their kind of medicine attractive to the rich and the powerful and the lawmakers. Astrological medicine remained at the popular level. In the southern universities, which were more secular and vocational and had been formed around extant teaching of medicine and arts, astrology probably maintained its links with medicine and ultimately even entered the university statutes.

Thus Roger's astrology gives us some idea of what techniques and doctrines could be used in non- and preuniversity medicine. His mathematically predictive astrology is central. Traditional Western astronomical knowledge had been provided by authors like Macrobius, Chalcidius, and particularly Martianus Capella. Pliny's *Natural History* was mined for extracts, often characterized by diagrams showing the motions of the planets. The possibilities of general prediction were made clear by texts attributed to Ptolemy, particularly the *Centiloquium.* They were also clear in Julius Firmicus Maternus's *Mathesis,* written in the fourth century but popular again by the eleventh; but without tables of the planets, this text could not be used predictively. The possibility of prediction was exciting (and scandalous) enough to prompt the search for fresh material from the Arabic. It is this context that gives Roger's production of a planetary table for Hereford its importance. With the new Arabic mathematical astrology came the notion that celestial causes were

---

translated and commented on the pseudo-Aristotelian *De plantis* and part of the *Meteorologica,* but this was simply a compliment implied by Alfred's dedication of the former. Roger's own knowledge of Aristotle seems to have been slight, and his predictive and mathematical astrology was incompatible with Aristotle's physical, nonmathematical, and nonpredictive cosmology. The teacher whose lectures were the source of the notes in the margins of British Library, Harleian 3487, fol. 224v, and Durham, CIII 17, fol. 313v, said of Alfred's compliment to Roger, "per hoc commendat hoc negotium et etiam personam cui inscripsit significando ipsam esse copiosam et provectam in philosophiam."

[14] When Gerard, the bishop of Hereford who was translated to York in 1101, died, a book "of curious arts" was found under his pillow. It may have been the astrology of Julius Firmicus Maternus; Gerard is said to have been denied a Christian burial as a result. See Burnett, "Mathematics and Astronomy in Hereford" (cit. n. 1). See also C. W. Clark, "The Zodiac Man in Medieval Medical Astrology" (Ph.D. diss., Univ. Colorado at Boulder, 1979), p. 178. Daniel of Morley, returning home from Toledo full of Arabic astrology, found it prudent to explain carefully what he was up to when he happened to meet the bishop of Norwich. See French, "Astrology in Medical Practice" (cit. n. 3).

[15] Of course, traditional notions of the effects of astral influences on the body were often repeated, and medieval hindsight made even Hippocrates an astrologer; but with Roger of Hereford we are at a point where the focus of astrology was changing from celestially determined mundane dispositions and nativities to mathematical and predictive elections.

linked to mundane effects in a necessary way, which implied that once the rules were known prediction was guaranteed. It was probably some such interest that made Adelard of Bath search out Abū Maʿshar's *Isagoge Minor* in Arabic-speaking countries, and certainly prediction fascinated the translator of the *Almagest,* Gerard of Cremona, and one of his visitors in Toledo, Daniel of Morley.[16]

THE MAN

Not much is known for certain about Roger of Hereford. He is addressed by Alfred of Shareshill at the beginning of the latter's translation of the pseudo-Aristotelian *De plantis,* made at about the beginning of the thirteenth century. Alfred calls him "dilectissimi mi Rogere" and presents his work to him as one would offer mature shoots of the vine to Bacchus or a golden stem of wheat to Ceres.[17] These are perhaps words of friendship rather than expressions of hope for patronage, and there seems little doubt that the two men knew each other well. The words also imply that Roger was learned in the kind of thing that Alfred was interested in: not, narrowly, plants, but the new Arabic learning that was generating excitement among their contemporaries. This is abundantly confirmed by the Arabic astrology that Roger made use of. It is not known whether, like Daniel of Morley, Roger himself traveled abroad to learn astrology or if he translated Arabic texts himself.[18] That he became known as Roger "of Hereford" suggests that this attribution might have become attached to him when he was somewhere else, as Alfred was known as "of Shareshill" when away from home and as "the Englishman" probably when in Spain. Roger held lands in the parish of Mordiford, some four miles from Hereford, and perhaps it was only at some greater distance that "of Hereford" became appropriate.[19]

Roger was active in the 1170s. He saw the eclipse of 13 September 1178 that was visible in Hereford and compiled planetary tables. In a *Compotus* written in 1167 Roger describes himself as "iuvenis," though he says he has spent many years in the schools ("regimen scholarum"). "Iuvenis" has prompted speculation that his surname may have been Young, but this seems unlikely. The name "Roger" appears on a number of documents that can

[16] See Bruce Eastwood, "Plinian Astronomical Diagrams in the Early Middle Ages," in *Mathematics and Its Application to Science and Natural Philosophy in the Middle Ages,* ed. Edward Grant and John E. Murdoch (Cambridge: Cambridge Univ. Press, 1987); and French, "Astrology in Medical Practice" (cit. n. 3).

[17] For Alfred's words see the critical edition of the text: *Nicholas Damascenus, De plantis: Five Translations,* ed. H. J. Drossaart Lulofs and E. L. J. Poortman (Amsterdam: North-Holland, 1989), p. 516: "tibique hoc opus, dilectissime mi Rogere, velut maturas Baccho palmites vel aureos Cereri culmos."

[18] In introducing the Hereford tables, Roger mentions the difficulty of following the Arabic years and months, which suggests that he was very close to his Arabic sources: "Maluimus haec quam annos Arabum et eorum menses propter difficultatem sequi, eo quod inusitati sint apud nostrates." See Thomas Wright, *Biographica Britannica literaria* (London, 1846), p. 218. But this was probably not a difficulty of *translation,* which Alfred, in contrast, wrote about in addressing Roger: "ex Arabico in Latinum transferens, in nostri idiomatis angustias . . . ex tam fluido loquendo genere, quod apud Arabes est." See Damascenus, *De plantis,* ed. Drossaart Lulofs and Poortman, p. 516. When Alfred's text was taught in the universities in the next century, the teacher explained what Alfred meant by *angustias:* "*angustias* hoc dicit quia qui addit scienciam addit laborem et penam. vel dicit hoc quia ydioma arabicum est fluidum et prolixum ut dicet postea et imo non potest verbo ad verbum transferri usque in ydioma nostrum." British Library, Royal 12 G III, fol. 193v. Clearly, said this teacher, the ideal translator worked from word to word without changing the author's opinion: "scilicet sententie aristotelis nihil rei addendo sed solum aliud ydioma ut scilicet latinum."

[19] See John Duncomb, *Collections towards the History and Antiquities of the County of Hereford,* Vol. 1 (1804), Vol. 2, Pt. 1 (1812), Vol. 3 (London: Cook, 1882), p. 68. The present family of Hereford (until recently "de Hereford") live at Sufton Court and Old Sufton, Mordiford. Tradition holds that Walter of Hereford, sheriff of Hereford in 1155, and Robert de Hereford, fined in 1158 for homicide, are members of Roger's family. Major Robert Hereford recalls that the family once had court rolls of the twelfth century (personal communication).

be linked to our Roger with a greater or lesser degree of certainty. In the *Compotus* he addresses Gilbert Foliot, bishop of Hereford until 1163 and a patron of learning; one of Foliot's documents was witnessed in 1173 by Roger. He is also to be identified with the Roger who, along with Walter Map, was a clerk and itinerant justice in 1185–1186, and possibly with the vice dean Roger, of Hereford, who owned three manuscripts now in Jesus College, Oxford.[20]

Whether or not he made his own translations from the Arabic, it is clear from his writing and his own admission that Roger was an educated man. R. W. Southern suggests that Alfred's address to Roger is one that would be made to a master, and the university historians have claimed him as their own: Thomas Fuller asserts that Roger was in Cambridge in about 1170, and John Pits lists him among the members of Oxford University. Here his name appears as Roger Herefordiensis Cantabrigiensis, but perhaps (given the nature of paleographic contractions) the last word is a slip for "Cambrensis," "of Wales," rather than "of Cambridge." Hereford was sometimes referred to as if it were in Wales, and Pits himself says that Roger was born "apud Herefordium in confinibus Cambriae." Roger calls himself a master, and some of the references to a "master Roger" in contemporary Hereford documents probably indicate the astrologer.[21]

THE SCHOOL

What kind of school was at Hereford? Almost everything we know about it comes from a poem written by a canon of the cathedral, Simon du Fresne, extolling the virtues of the school to Gerald of Wales, whom he hoped to attract to Hereford. Simon mentions the *trivii quadriviique locus,* the *artis septene . . . honos,* the *grammatice doctrina,* and the *ars logice.* To these five groups of doctrines he adds the work of the rhetorician; he elaborates on the contents of the quadrivial group by saying that the *ars numerosa* deals with solid, plane, and cubic numbers. He mentions how the geometrician can determine the height of towers by using the astrolabe and how the music teacher studies proportions. These topics are dispatched in couplets in lines 33 to 48. Astronomy also has a couplet, explaining that it teaches the motions of the sun and moon and when eclipses will occur. Astrology is mentioned in the person of the astrologer—*astrologus*—to whom are devoted eight lines of the poem, four times as many as the doctrines and their teachers that are mentioned before. The topics that follow are also dispatched in couplets: *fisis,* which

[20] "Compositi a magistro Rogero super annos Domini ad mediam noctem Herefordiae anno ab incarnatione Domini, mºcºlxxºviiiº post eclipsim quae contingit Herefordiae eodem anno"; quoted in Wright, *Biographica Britannica literaria* (cit. n. 18), p. 218. For Roger's self-description as "iuvenis" see Haskins, "Reception of Arabic Science in England" (cit. n. 1), p. 65; on Roger "Infans" and "Puer," which appear in different manuscripts, see Russell, "Hereford and Arabic Science" (cit. n. 1). The most recent work on Roger's judicial astrology is Nicholas Whyte, "Roger of Hereford's *Liber de astronomice iudicandi:* A Twelfth-Century Astrologer's Manual" (M.Phil. diss., Univ. Cambridge, 1991).

[21] Richard William Southern, *Robert Grosseteste: The Growth of an English Mind in Medieval Europe* (Oxford: Oxford Univ. Press, 1986), p. 91; Thomas Fuller, *The History of the University of Cambridge from the Conquest to the Year 1635,* ed. Marmaduke Prickett (London/Cambridge, 1834); and *Ioannis Pitsei Angli S. Theologiae Doctoris . . . Relationum historicarum in rebus Anglicis tomus primus* (Paris, 1618), pp. 964, 237. He is called Rogerus Herefordiensis and a *philosophus* in John Bale, *Index Britanniae scriptorum,* ed. Reginald Lane Poole (Oxford: Clarendon, 1902), p. 401, where a *Theorica planetarum* (the incipit reads "Diversi astrologi secundum diversos") and a *De ortu et occasu signorum* (the incipit reads "Orizon rectus est circulus magnus transiens") are attributed to him. Roger calls himself a master, for example, in the introduction to the Hereford tables, in Wright, *Biographica Britannica literaria;* Russell, in "Hereford and Arabic Science," is rather speculative about the identity of other Hereford Rogers.

teaches about elements and "hyle" (*ile*) as causes of the world, and the "new" and "old" law.[22]

So the topics we would expect to meet in a *studium generale* were taught at Hereford, if we can believe Simon's perhaps somewhat inflated account. But the amount of space given to astrology is unusual. It is the astrologer, says Simon, who teaches about the difference of the length of the day in the summer and winter and about the progress of the planets through the houses (Aries and so on). If we assume that the *astrologus* also taught astronomy, then ten lines of the poem are given to him. It is surely a reasonable guess that the astrologer at the school of Hereford was Roger, already known as an author (who had dealt with eclipses) and a principal attraction in a period when schools often flourished or failed on the reputation of a central teacher.[23]

But there is more to Simon's poem than that. What Roger was actually concerned with, and what excited men like Daniel of Morley, was predicting the future. None of that is mentioned in the ten lines of the poem devoted to astronomy and astrology. But then Simon goes immediately on to the *geomanticus,* who does indeed make predictions. *Geomantia* is recorded in English usage in 1159 as "predictions from earth," in which prognostication was made from patterns. Like astrology, geomancy in its new form was a product of the translations from the Arabic; the translator Gerard of Cremona said it was derived "from the truth of astrology." It took its terminology from astrology: the twelve "houses," the judgment, signs, and the querent (the inquirer). Judgment was made on sixteen "figures" distributed through the houses: the fifteen that are calculated (Simon says that the *geomanticus* "makes three times five figures") and the first, obtained by divination. As in astrology, it was held that the powers of the celestial bodies determined the terrestrial effects; indeed, geomancy was generally seen as a branch of astrology that had the advantage of requiring no astrolabe or tables. By figures and calculations the *geomanticus* predicts "which pathway, which people, which prison": just what Roger the astrologer was doing.[24] The *geomanticus* receives six lines of the poem and so is comparatively important among the attractions that Simon offers to Gerald. It is tempting to think that in all sixteen lines Simon is maximizing the appeal of Roger's activity by giving different parts of it

[22] The relevant portion of the poem is given in R. W. Hunt, "English Learning in the Late Twelfth Century," in *Essays in Medieval History,* ed. Richard William Southern (London: Macmillan, 1968), pp. 106–128. Charles Burnett thinks that Simon took these natural-philosophical terms from the *Isagoge* of Johannitius; see Burnett, "Mathematics and Astronomy in Hereford" (cit. n. 1). This was the first work in the medieval textbook of medicine; it makes natural philosophy the basis of medicine. Was the higher faculty of medicine also taught at Hereford? This interesting suggestion is made in Brian Lawn, *The Prose Salernitan Questions* (London: Oxford Univ. Press for the British Academy, 1979), p. xv, which discusses a manuscript written by an English scribe of about 1200 that uses as examples the sexual capacities of five men, three of them associated with Hereford. The poem's reference to the "new" and "old" law presumably reflects the recent recovery of Roman law.

[23] Southern identifies a "de-institutionalised" phase in the history of the twelfth-century schools, after a period of tighter control by the church and before the rise of masters' corporations; see Richard William Southern, "The Schools of Paris and the School of Chartres," in *Renaissance and Renewal in the Twelfth Century,* ed. Robert L. Benson and Giles Constable (Oxford: Clarendon, 1982), pp. 113–137. Hereford was one of at least forty schools in twelfth-century England that served the need of government and trade for a learned laity as well as supplying the church; see Southern, "From Schools to University," in *The History of the University of Oxford,* ed. T. H. Ashton, Vol. 1: *The Early Oxford Schools,* ed. J. I. Catto (Oxford: Oxford Univ. Press, 1984).

[24] See Thérèse Charmasson, *Recherches sur une technique divinatoire: La géomancy dans l'Occident médiéval* (Paris: Champion, 1980), pp. 9 (quotation), 13. I am grateful to the anonymous referee who drew my attention to this work. "Pathway," "people," and "prison" are categories within geomantic technique and not personal predictions. See also the details given by Burnett, who says, "Geomancy is the lazy man's astrology": "Mathematics and Astronomy in Hereford" (cit. n. 1). According to Whyte, these terms are derived from Gerard of Cremona's treatise on geomancy and provide a link between Roger and the Toledan translators; see Whyte, "Roger of Hereford's *Liber de astronomice iudicandi*" (cit. n. 20), p. 7.

different labels. Certainly the poem suggests that descriptive and predictive study of the planets—what has been called *astronodia*—was strong in Hereford, whether or not it centered on the "heroic" figure of Roger. Conversely, when Roger speaks of *astronodia* fructifying the other arts, he must surely have had in mind those mentioned by Simon in his poem and by himself in his *Compotus.*[25]

Simon does not mention theology in his poem. We would expect theology to be at the summit of studies in a thoroughgoing school. Certainly there were theologians in Hereford, for Simon's name appears on a charter together with that of another Simon, whose surname was probably Melun, who is described as a theologian. A "continuously reading" master of theology was also a feature of the school sometime before 1250, when the clergy and chapter resisted a plantation of Dominicans. One theologian was enough, they said. Like other schools, that of Hereford was at first under the control of the bishop's chancellor, but this ended when the incumbent bishop was translated to another diocese in 1375. When the school was revived, it was as a grammar school.[26]

THE CIRCLE

Roger belonged to a circle of Anglo-Normans, most of them with connections with the West Midlands and some associated with Oxford; all were interested to some extent in the new physical learning.[27] Roger may have suggested to Alfred of Shareshill that he should translate *De plantis,* and as we have seen Alfred addressed his translation to Roger. He dedicated his *De motu cordis* to Alexander Neckam. Neckam taught in Oxford and Paris; *De motu cordis* became statutory in Paris, and Alfred's commentary on his translation of *De plantis* came to be used in teaching the statutory natural philosophy texts in Oxford.[28] To write a commentary implies teaching—and the teaching we know of was by commentary—but there is no evidence to suggest where any of Alfred's teaching may have taken place. Robert Grosseteste was in the bishop's service in the 1190s and probably, then, in Hereford in Roger's lifetime, and it has been claimed for him, as for Roger, that he was a master of Oxford; he may have returned there in 1199 after the death of his employer, William de Vere, bishop of Hereford. If so, he would have been at Oxford for a short time with Alexander Neckam. It is from Gerald of Wales that we know that Grosseteste was a master of some university before 1198; Gerald praises Grosseteste's abilities in terms that

[25] The text of the preface of Roger's *Compotus* is given in Russell, "Hereford and Arabic Science" (cit. n. 1). On *astronodia* see Burnett, "Adelard, Ergaphalau, and the Science of the Stars" (cit. n. 4).

[26] Gilbert Foliot, a relative of the earls of Hereford, was bishop of Hereford from 1146 to 1163 and succeeded in securing the bishopric for his cousin Robert Foliot in 1176. One of Gilbert's letters to Robert was witnessed by a Roger of Hereford. See Whyte, "Roger of Hereford's *Liber de astronomice iudicandi*" (cit. n. 20). For Simon the theologian see Russell, "Hereford and Arabic Science." On the revival of the school at Hereford see Edward Dew, ed., *Extracts from the Cathedral Registers AD 1275–1535* (Hereford, 1932).

[27] In some ways this circle of men is comparable to the one that, in the same part of the country but slightly earlier, made a distinct English contribution to the renewal of Roman verse; see R. M. Thomson, "England and the Twelfth-Century Renaissance," *Past and Present*, 1983, *101*:1–21.

[28] There is a note in a manuscript of *De plantis*—Naples, Bib. Nat. VIII F 12—in Naples saying that the translation was made at the instance of Roger; see Georges Lacombe *et al., Aristoteles Latinus pars posterior* (Cambridge: Cambridge Univ. Press, 1955). Neckham taught in Oxford in the last decade of the twelfth century; see Hunt, "English Learning in the Late Twelfth Century" (cit. n. 22), p. 107. On the use of *De motu cordis* in Paris see D. A. Callus, "Introduction of Aristotelian Learning to Oxford," *Proceedings of the British Academy,* 1943, pp. 229–281, on p. 238. Alfred's text was adopted by midcentury for the last part of the *scientia naturalis inferior.* At Oxford, Alfred's commentary was used, for example, by the students who glossed the text in the British Library, Royal 12 G II, Royal 12 G III, and Royal 12 G V.

recall Simon du Fresne's description of the school of Hereford. Gerald himself was part of the circle, at least through correspondence. He read his *Topographia Hibernia* to the assembled scholars of Oxford in 1190, the year in which William de Vere gave him a Hereford prebend. But Gerald was not in favor of the Aristotle being newly translated in Toledo, fearing that it would lead to heresy if widely known.[29]

To some extent this circle of scholars was held together by patronage. Walter Map, Roger's fellow justice (and correspondent of Gerald of Wales) was a protégé of the bishop Gilbert Foliot, as perhaps Roger was too. Not only was the church able to offer positions to some of the men of this circle, but the king could choose to patronize them as well. Henry II made the innovation of appointing educated clerks rather than local magnates as justices; he had been taught some astrology by Adelard of Bath when young, and perhaps this had some bearing on his choice of Roger as a justice. Roger seems to have cast the horoscope of Eleanor of Aquitaine, Henry II's wife, so clearly he had strong connections with the court. And while predicting the future was important to a doctor, it was hardly less so to a king; royal patronage may have been another motive for scholars to tackle new Arabic material that furthered the art of prognostication. Possibly Henry II in England in the middle of the twelfth century played a role analogous to that of Sicily's Frederick II—for whom Michael Scot translated astrological treatises—in the early thirteenth. There are even horoscopes surviving from the 1150s that were probably cast by Adelard himself, perhaps as he considered whether to stay in the king's service.[30] These have been criticized on technical grounds, and there was no doubt room for the improvement in English astrology that Roger would help to introduce some twenty-five years later.

The cultivation of learning in Hereford grew from a number of sources. One was computistic material within the church, with which Robert of Losinga, bishop of Hereford from 1079 to 1095, was concerned. Robert was also known as an astronomer, and his computistic work survives in manuscripts with another on the course of the moon, an important topic in establishing the church's calendar, that was written by Walcher, prior of Malvern. From Walcher, knowledge of the astrolabe spread to other towns of western England until, as we have seen, the geometers of Hereford were using it to measure the height of towers and Roger the astrologer could assume that his readers were familiar with the instrument. Royal patronage was involved here, too, for Robert had been invited to join the court of William the Conqueror on the basis of his learning, which included knowledge of the abacus.[31]

BORDERLANDS

It is not easy to suggest specific reasons why a school that apparently had many of the features of a *studium* should have existed in Hereford and why such an impressive circle of men should have encompassed both it and the schools of Oxford. But there are features

[29] See James McEvoy, *The Philosophy of Robert Grosseteste* (Oxford: Clarendon, 1982), p. 6; and Whyte, "Roger of Hereford's *Liber de astronomice iudicandi*" (cit. n. 20), p. 7. Gerald was angling for a bishopric and could not, perhaps, afford to be seen as too "curious" about physical matters.

[30] On Roger's horoscope for Eleanor of Aquitaine see Whyte, "Roger of Hereford's *Liber de astronomice iudicandi,*" pp. 37–42. On what may be Adelard's horoscopes see Carey, *Courting Disaster* (cit. n. 6); and J. D. North, *Horoscopes and History* (London: Warburg Inst., Univ. London, 1986).

[31] See Burnett, "Mathematics and Astronomy in Hereford" (cit. n. 1); and Louise Cochrane, *Adelard of Bath: The First English Scientist* (London: British Museum Press, 1994), p. 7. Walcher (who died in 1135) had traveled to Italy and, like Roger, saw an eclipse and compiled planetary tables. See Haskins, "Reception of Arabic Science in England" (cit. n. 1).

of interest in the background to the story. Hereford was at the edge of a Norman kingdom and was one of a number of places fortified to secure the marches. It was so close to Wales that, as we have seen, it was sometimes thought to be in Wales. But Wales was not yet peaceful, and the last great Welsh revolt was still to come. In uncertain times borders are special places. The ruling ideologies have to be seen to be securely in place, for these are the spots where foreign—that is, dangerous—ideologies most threaten; borders, too, are often places where such ideologies are learned so that they can be counteracted. Another frontier of Norman expansion, Sicily, was a place where texts of the kind we have already met were translated. The other important border was the Christian-Muslim interface at Toledo, where Gerard of Cremona was at work and where Daniel of Morley went to learn Arabic astrology.

In all of these settings we can recognize not only the personal intellectual curiosity of the Latins of the West but, more widely, tactics intended to maintain an ideology in which military power and religious belief were fused. Many of the new translations were sponsored by churchmen, sometimes in efforts to improve their knowledge of their enemy.[32] One such translation was of the *De differentia spiritus et animae* of Qustā ibn Lūqa, which the bishop of Toledo wanted in Latin and which found its way into the collection of statutory texts of natural philosophy in the universities and was used by Alfred of Shareshill in his tract on the heart. Education was of course central to the maintenance of the ruling ideology. When there was a threat of heresy in Languedoc, the school of Toulouse was hastily upgraded to a *studium generale* expressly to contain the danger. The Dominicans established their own schools of natural philosophy and Eastern languages in order to defend and spread the faith. Crusades of the church were used to defeat heresy at home as well as to secure control of Greek Byzantium and the Muslim Holy Land; reeducation after military victory was essential. The Toulouse masters sent out a circular letter asking for more personnel; the new Latin Emperor of the East asked the Paris masters to come and set up a new school. When William de Vere, bishop of Hereford, visited the Holy Land sometime between 1170 and 1186, such issues must have been on his mind; at all events, he took the opportunity to bring home some Byzantine manuscripts.[33]

Two more topics suggested by the most recent publication on Roger speak to the geographical significance of the school at Hereford. In Roger's time the influence of the Celtic church was considerable.[34] At Deerhurst, close to Tewkesbury (just over twenty miles from Hereford), there had been unusually active engagement between the Celtic and Saxon

[32] The well-known translator Dominicus Gundissalinus worked under the patronage of the archbishop of Toledo, who must have been motivated more by a need to defend the faith than by intellectual curiosity. Peter of Cluny wanted Koranic materials translated from the Arabic because he believed knowledge of infidel belief to be the first stage in converting the Arabs. The papacy and the Dominicans supported Arabic studies for the same reason. See *Chartularium universitatis Parisiensis,* ed. Denifle (cit. n. 2), Vol. 1, p. 212; and David Lindberg, "The Transmission of Greek and Arabic Learning to the West," in *Science in the Middle Ages,* ed. Lindberg (Chicago: Univ. Chicago Press, 1987), p. 87. The Greek learning of the Byzantines had to be handled in the same way. Hugo Etherianus was urged by Hugh of Honau in Constantinople to translate Greek works to remove "dangerous doubts" that the Latins had adopted from Greek sources. At a theological disputation in Constantinople in 1136, with the translators James of Venice and Burgundio of Pisa, Moses of Bergamo stressed the usefulness, rather than the intellectual interest, of translations from the Greek. See Marie-Thérèse d'Alverny, "Translators and Translations," in *Renaissance and Renewal in the Twelfth Century,* ed. Benson and Constable (cit. n. 23), p. 432.

[33] On educational efforts to maintain the ruling ideology see *Chartularium universitatis Parisiensis,* Vol. 1, pp. 83, 131, 62. On the dual purpose of the Crusades see, e.g., W. L. Wakefield, *Heresy, Crusade, and Inquisition in Southern France* (Berkeley/London: Univ. California Press, 1974), p. 177. On de Vere see Julia Barrow, "A Twelfth-Century Bishop and Literary Patron: William de Vere," *Viator,* 1987, *18:*175–189, esp. p. 179.

[34] Moreton, "Before Grosseteste" (cit. n. 1), p. 564.

churches. A major point at issue was the church calendar, to which *compotus* techniques were central. (These figured, too, in the connection between the English West Country and Lotharingia after the Conquest: Robert Losinga, bishop of Hereford from 1079 to 1085, and Walcher, prior of Malvern, were both Lotharingian.)

The second topic is the presence of Jews in the area. By Roger's time the Jewish calendar had long been available in the West Country. It may be that Roger's knowledge of Arabic astrology came to him from Jewish sources. We have seen that there is no evidence to suggest that Roger, like Daniel of Morley, traveled abroad to obtain his Arabic knowledge. While Daniel discusses his adventures in Spain with apparent pride, Roger is reticent about his sources.[35] Perhaps he did not have to go farther than town on market day: the Jewish quarter of Hereford, about four miles distant from his land at Mordiford, was close to the southern gate of the city. Although the settlement is said to have been founded in 1179—slightly later than most of Roger's work—this does not preclude some contact with a Jewish community earlier or elsewhere. Private individuals like Daniel of Morley had Jewish help in making translations, and the translators of patrons in Spain like Alfonso X, "El Sabio," were mostly Jews. It is not unthinkable that a Jewish community, arriving in Hereford as its economic importance as a border staging post developed, carried with it traditional linguistic abilities.[36] We have little idea how learned such communities of Jews were, but their international connections provide a possible explanation for the dissemination of Arabic knowledge. When it became apparent that the new scholastic medicine was a profitable business, the Jews attained eminence in the field, despite being excluded from the universities and having no native tradition of this kind of medicine. Were they also the agents who carried the business of foretelling the future—as profitable as that of medicine—into the Norman borders of England? Their financial power made the king their friend, and their connections were international. Locally, in Herefordshire, their business was with the big families. Before the expulsion of the Jews in 1290, men with the surname Hereford—almost certainly from Roger's family at Mordiford—were involved in financial dealings with the Jews.[37]

ROGER'S ASTROLOGY

There are a number of works attributed to Roger in many manuscripts in British and European libraries. Their attribution and relationship have not been extensively studied, and the matter must contain many uncertainties.[38] But even erroneous attributions indicate

[35] *Ibid.*, p. 566. Roger does not even reveal the name of his major source, Abū Maʿshar. See *ibid.*, p. 581.

[36] On the founding of the Jewish settlement at Hereford see Joe Hillaby, "Hereford Gold: Irish, Welsh, and English Land, Pt. 2: The Clients of the Jewish Community at Hereford, 1179–1253: Four Case Studies," *Transactions of the Woolhope Naturalists' Field Club, Herefordshire,* 1985, *45*(1):193–270. The use of the West Country as a provisioning ground for Ireland seems to have been one reason for the establishment of a Jewish community. (I am grateful to an *Isis* referee for pointing this out.) On Jewish help with translations see French, "Astrology in Medical Practice" (cit. n. 3); and Burnett, "Translating Activity in Medieval Spain" (cit. n. 3).

[37] See Joe Hillaby, "The Hereford Jewry, 1179–1290, Pt. 3: Aaron le Blund and the Last Decades of the Hereford Jewry, 1253–90," *Trans. Woolhope Natur. Field Club, Herefordshire,* 1990, *46*(3):432–487. Robert de Hereford, probably from the family home at Mordiford, was on their books sometime between 1283 and 1290 as owing 40 marks. On Jewish success in scholastic medicine see, e.g., Joseph Shatzmiller, *Jews, Medicine, and Medieval Society* (Berkeley: Univ. California Press, 1994).

[38] Some of the attributions of manuscripts to Roger are mentioned in these notes. Perhaps one of the least likely is a *De rebus metallicis* said to be by Roger: Wright, *Biographica Britannica literaria* (cit. n. 18), p. 218 (where Roger is listed twice, under two different spellings). Any historical work on the manuscripts containing works attributed to Roger must begin with Whyte, "Roger of Hereford's *Liber de astronomice iudicandi*" (cit. n. 20).

that Roger's name was well known as a result of his astrological work, and it is worthwhile to take note of some of the texts attributed to him. There is a *Theorica planetarum* with the incipit "Diversi astrologi secundum diversos . . ." and a *De quatuor partibus astronomie* that begins "Quoniam principium huic arti dignum duximus de quatuor eius partibus agamus . . . ," part of which is similar to published work of John of Spain. Also attributed to Roger is a *De rebus metallicis* and a related *Expositiones Aelphidii,* which would seem to be a commentary on Alphidius's *De creationem metallorum.* There are as well at least five untitled tracts in Oxford manuscripts (they may be parts of Roger's two main texts, considered below) and four sets of tables—attributed to Roger, but without text—in manuscripts in London and Madrid. *De ortu et occasu signorum,* beginning "Orizon rectus est circulus magnus," is in an Oxford manuscript.[39] The so-called *Iudicia Herefordensis* may consist of abstracts of Roger's work, but in one manuscript it is actually the *De iudiciis* of Haly Rodoan (or Ridwan).[40]

It is well established that in 1178 Roger constructed astronomical tables based on the meridian of Hereford and that he used them in his local astrology.[41] The *Compotus* must also be genuine, for Roger's name appears in an acrostic in the table of chapters and in the work he addresses Gilbert Foliot (who had been bishop of Hereford until 1163; Roger wrote it in 1176). There seems no reason to doubt the attribution to him of the two works I wish to consider here, the *Liber de tribus generalibus judiciis astronomie* and the *De iudiciis astronomie.*[42]

In these works Roger is writing at a technical level. We can begin with the *De iudiciis astronomie,* which is the more general text. This is not a beginner's handbook but a work addressed to those who already knew the fundamentals of astronomy and astrology. Roger claims to be in a position to bring a number of sources together in a single work in a way not possible before.[43] This assertion agrees well enough with the idea that a theory of astrology was assembled gradually from a number of discrete Arabic sources.[44] It also indicates that there were enough astrologers in his intended readership to make it worth his while to write. He expects, for example, that his readers will be familiar with the use

[39] On *Theorica planetarum* see Thomas Tanner, *Bibliotheca Britannico-Hibernica sive de scriptoribus . . . Commentaria* (London, 1748); and Lynn Thorndike, *A History of Magic and Experimental Science,* Vol. 2 (New York: Macmillan, 1923). On the incipit see Bale, *Index Britanniae scriptorum,* ed. Poole (cit. n. 21), p. 401; and Haskins, "Reception of Arabic Science in England" (cit. n. 1), p. 3. On *De quatuor partibus astronomie* see Thorndike, *History of Magic and Experimental Science,* Vol. 2, p. 182. Haskins, "Reception of Arabic Science in England," p. 3, has a related title with a different incipit. For the attribution of *De rebus metallicis* see Wright, *Biographica Britannica literaria,* p. 218; however, as noted, this is probably erroneous. On *De ortu et occasu signorum* see Haskins, "Reception of Arabic Science in England."

[40] Thorndike differs somewhat from Haskins on the nature of this text and its manuscripts. We should also note a Magister Rogerus whose name appears on a text called *De eclipsi solis* and a *De divisione astronomiae* attributed to Roger of Hereford in manuscripts in Brussels and Paris. See C. A. McMenomy, "The Discipline of Astronomy in the Middle Ages" (Ph.D. diss., Univ. California, Los Angeles, 1984), pp. 509, 516. It has also been pointed out to me that there are tables attributed to Roger in manuscripts in Dublin and Brussels.

[41] They were based on the tables for Marseilles drawn up by Raymond of Marseilles in 1141, which were in turn based on the Toledan tables. See Burnett, "Mathematics and Astronomy in Hereford" (cit. n. 1). Raymond's work of astrological judgments was an important source for Roger (*ibid.*), and so was the *Introductorium* of Abū Ma'shar (Whyte, "Roger of Hereford's *Liber de astronomice iudicandi*" [cit. n. 20]).

[42] I have used Cambridge University Library (CUL), Ii.1.1, fols. 40r–51r, 51v–59r, checked in detail against CUL Gg vi 3; Oxford, Bodleian, Selden supra 76; and Oxford, Digby 149. The two texts may in fact be parts of a single work. See Whyte, "Roger of Hereford's *Liber de astronomice iudicandi.*"

[43] CUL Ii.1.1, fol. 40r: "Quoniam regulas artis astronomice iudicandi non nisi per diversa opera dispersas invenimus utili astrologorum desiderio satisfacere cupientes eisque ubi necesse fuerit explanacionem sive supplemencionem apponentes in unum breviter colligemus." Fol. 40v, col. 2: "cuius regulas universales nullus philosophorum huc usque simul collegisse invenimus."

[44] CUL Ii.1.1, fol. 40r, col. 1: "per diversas opera dispersas."

of an astrolabe. No doubt the Crusades and trading had made the astrolabe (which was also a navigational instrument) familiar to a number of Roger's readers, especially those who used it to measure angles in the school at Hereford. So from sources like Adelard, Walcher, and Daniel, there was enough knowledge of astrology in England to explain the level at which Roger pitched his text.[45]

To explain *why* Roger wrote what he did relates to why his readers found it interesting enough, often, to be copied. The answer is plain: to be able to predict the future. This is what Roger means when he refers to the "useful desire" of astrologers that he hopes his book will satisfy. But above all, as Roger bluntly says, the excellence of the art that compelled him to write—"nos quasi huius artis incomparabilis compulit excellencia"—lies in putting the man who knows it in a position superior to those who do not by giving him knowledge of things hidden in the future. Superfluous, then, to discuss any other use of the art.[46] This, Roger knew, was what excited people about astrology. Roger himself was clearly excited, both by the promise of foretelling the future and by the beauty of the method. The excitement overcame the difficulties: if you were as interested as Daniel of Morley, you had to spend a great deal of time and money in traveling to strange places at the very edge of Christendom, learn a foreign language, and hire some help. Probably you also had to give up a career to do so. Roger is direct about it: astrology gives man power over other men. True, it also reveals the hidden things of nature, but this is less an intellectual satisfaction than an extension of the argument for the certainty and thus the utility of astrology. So useful and powerful did Roger think astrology that in contrast all the other arts looked to him like the branches of a unfruitful tree.[47]

The image that Roger uses—the tree—calls to mind the division-of-the-sciences literature of the twelfth century, famously expounded by Hugh of St. Victor. It is a general feature of such schemes that they stress the unity of all knowledge, and philosophy is the knowledge of things divine, human, and natural. This is Roger's intellectual world, where Aristotle was known—outside the specialist circles of translators and medical teachers—only as a logician and accounts of the physical world were Platonic.[48] The "other arts" that seemed so unfruitful to Roger were essentially the whole range of knowledge; the claim for the superiority of astrology was therefore a major one. At the very least he means to assert its superiority to the seven liberal arts, as taught in the school at Hereford. He says something similar in the preface to his *Compotus*.[49] Roger argues that the superiority of astrology lies in the perfection of the planets and the signs through which they move. The contrast, of course, is with the corruptible and variable matter of the sublunary world, the physical world where things happen *physice*. While the other physical arts and sciences, says Roger, are concerned with an infinite range of subject matter, both individuals and kinds (and so are necessarily uncertain), astrology centers on the seven planets and twelve

[45] In 1185 astrologers disputed publicly about a coming eclipse. See Whyte, "Roger of Hereford's *Liber de astronomice iudicandi*" (cit. n. 20).

[46] CUL Ii.1.1, fol. 40r, col. 1: "utili astrologorum desiderio satisfacere." Fol. 40r, col. 2: "De huius utilitate autem superfluum esset agere cum ista hominem super hominem efferens futurorum ac omnium a natura absconditorum precium efficiat."

[47] *Ibid.*, fol. 40r, col. 1: "Sine hac et enim cetere artes quasi arboris infructuose rami extenduntur."

[48] See Buttimer, ed., *Hugonis de Sancto Victore Didascalicon* (cit. n. 10). Godfrey of St. Victor paints Aristotle as a fencing master who provides weapons and techniques for battle. As Alan Cobban points out, the "new logic" of Aristotle was exciting and was sought for its utility in social and intellectual life. See Edward A. Synan, trans., *The Fountain of Philosophy: A Translation of the Twelfth-Century* Fons philosophiae *of Godfrey of St. Victor* (Toronto: Pontifical Institute of Medieval Studies, 1972), p. 23; and Alan B. Cobban, *The Medieval English Universities: Oxford and Cambridge to c. 1500* (Aldershot: Scolar, 1988), p. 12.

[49] See Russell, "Hereford and Arabic Science" (cit. n. 1).

signs (and is accordingly more certain). A Platonic understanding underlies Roger's argument that if we can have certain knowledge of a thing like a rose, so variable in its matter in time and place, then how much more certain is our knowledge of astrology, which treats the incorruptible heavenly bodies.[50] Likewise, where he makes claims for the superiority of astrology because of the way it employs sense and reason, the "reason" at issue is largely mathematical in a Platonic way. It is, indeed, mostly the mathematical arts that he thinks are fructified by astrology: measures, proportions, divisions, and so on.[51] In the other arts, says Roger, each of the senses perceives individual effects, like seeing the whiteness of snow, tasting the sweetness of honey, and feeling the heat of wine. But in astrology *all* the senses are employed and perceive the effects of causes explained by certain reason: clearly Roger wanted astrology to explain all natural change in the physical world. He admitted that the other arts "have their fruit"; but the fruit of astrology is "universal judgment," pronounceable on everything except God's miracles, which are not subject to the natures of things.[52]

It was of course necessary to subjugate astrology to the highest kind of knowledge, that of God. Often enough in the twelfth century philosophy was called "knowledge of things human and divine," and it had to be clear that the purpose of practicing philosophy was to prepare the mind for higher knowledge. Roger says that astrology begins from knowledge of God.[53]

ASTROLOGICAL JUDGMENTS

We have to know something of the way in which astrology worked to understand both Roger's perception of astrology and how medicine became astrological. The basis of it was a set of correspondences between the heavens and corruptible things on earth, grounded in some form of similarity or sympathy. It drew strength from long-standing beliefs that the sources of things that happened on earth were to be found in the heavens. This sense was expressed, for example, in the ancient notion of the gods as direct causal agents. It could also be expressed in Aristotle's formulation of causes, where the ultimate cause was the heavenly unmoved mover. But the gods and Aristotle's causes were not features of Roger's astrology. He has some perfectly general remarks on earthly characteristics—like the sweetness, heat, and whiteness perceived by the senses—but these are not Aristotle's elementary causes and are not related to his causality. Their growth and decline follow only the rising and setting of the sun. He notes that each sign has an elementary quality, which to us (although not to Roger) might be evidence of an underlying Aristotelianism. Aries and Leo are fiery; Taurus, Virgo, and Capricorn earthy; Gemini,

[50] CUL Ii.1.1, fol. 40r, col. 2: "Certissima quidem, quia cum omnium aliarum aut sit materia variabilis ut physice e vel materie subiecta, ut patet in ceteris. In hac vero cum sit materia finita est et incorruptibilis et inalterabilis. Unde si rei variabilis et per locorum et temporum variaciones, ut rose possit haberi certitudo, quanto magis huius cuius plene tota materia invariabilis."

[51] Ibid.: "ad cuius comprehensionem non opinio tantum sensu commota, sed et ratio certissimis subnixa rationibus, et per numerorum et mensurarum tam in se quam motibus et quam temporibus, et per proporcionum certissimam doctrinam, et circa se et circa suos effectus sencire ascendit." Fol. 40r, col. 1: "subtiles eloquenciae, investigaciones numerorum innumerabiles divisiones mensurarum certissime distinctiones proporcionum aptissime copulaciones nisi ut hec velut satellites viam domine preparent, et quasi farinulas invenienda numeranda mecienda proporcionanda subministrarent."

[52] Ibid., fol. 40v, col. 1: "Cum igitur he sit fructus omnium aliarum arcium, habet et ista fructum sui iudicium universitatis, preterquam miraculorum dei, que natura rerum nequaquam subiacent."

[53] Ibid., fol. 40r, col. 2: "Est autem et hec finitissima, certissima, excellentissima, post creatoris cognicionem a qua ipsa incipit."

Sagittarius, and Aquarius airy; Cancer and Pisces watery. Leo is also choleric, Libra sanguine, Scorpio phlegmatic.[54]

Roger also points to general correspondences between the planets' elementary qualities and sublunar things. The elements of earth, air, fire, and water were common to Aristotelian doctrines and a number of others; Roger's use of them is not evidence for Aristotelianism. He notes, for example, that Mars is hot and dry and that Venus is characterized by cold and a sort of tempered wetness. Roger is not systematic here, but what he says could be of interest to the medical men. Not only might the qualities of the planets be medically interesting; the planets also produced particular effects, some of which were medical, some of which related to parts of the body, and some of which were expressed physiognomically. Again, Roger is not being systematic, and he may be drawing on a tradition other than that which gave him the more systematic "astrological anatomy" that is examined below. He links the nature of the planets to the personalities of people, again in a rather general way. For example, he says that Saturn is cold and dry, is responsible for pain in the body, and has sympathies with the right ear and spleen and that a Saturnine person has little hair, either on his chest or in his ugly beard, is gray-blue in color, and is sad. Mars is hot and dry, shares the liver with Jupiter and the nostrils with Venus, and is a bad indication for surgery, especially in significant astrological aspect with Saturn. The Martian man is short, with small eyes and red cheeks. Roger's descriptions here are brief and incomplete (that is, not all categories are dealt with in each case). He is eloquent only in the case of Mercury. Mercury, he says, relates to philosophy, teachers (*doctores*), pupils, eloquence, the highest of all wisdoms (especially mathematical divination), the use and exercise of all the sciences, and the discovery of new things through the intellect, especially by the man of Mercury, who is finely built, with graceful lips, nose and beard, and a "wise body." Perhaps the mention of mathematical divination made Roger identify with the man of Mercury, an image he adds to an account otherwise taken mostly unchanged from Abū Maʿshar.[55]

Beyond recognizing these general things, the astrologer's basic technique was to identify the client and his needs with a feature of the heavens. That feature then represented the client as it moved through the heavens. Its relationship with other features altered in a number of ways: the daily rotation of the heavens around the earth resulted in the differently positioned stars and planets rising and setting at different times; the planets also moved at different speeds across the background of fixed stars, some of them for a while moving backward. The astrologer not only divided the heavens into sections that were fixed in relation to the earth (so that all the heavenly bodies moved through them) but also divided the broad path along which the planets moved into parts. These parts were originally based on constellations of fixed stars, but it was found that the "map" or background

[54] *Ibid.*, fol. 42v: "Leo igneus colericus luxuriosus orientalis medie vocis calidus versutus multe audacie et angustie. habet mesopotamiam. ex locis valles cum amnibus rapidis loca metallorum." These qualities are traditional and can be found in Abū Maʿshar, *Introductorium* 2.4.

[55] CUL Ii.1.1, fol. 45v: "Mercurius promiscuus ad ascensus facilis. eius sunt puericia minores fratres. amor puerorum divinitatis fides philosophia eloquentia. doctores cum discipulis ingenium racio precepta eorum observacio. summa sapientia omnium studiorum precipue mathematice divinacionis scriptura. omnium scientarum usus et excertitacio cum eleganti novitatis invencione ac secretorum intellectu soli divinitati patencium. rarum gaudium et delicie rare providum consilium fama rumores ambicio causa glorie questores tribunarii. apotece. questus cum multo sumptu participaciones negotiaciones. furia fraudulencia malivolencia ignavia. timor. dubii affectus obedientia mitis. pius. amor fratrum mali propulsio. verax. cura. grata vox. aptitudo in omni artificium. iustorumque perfectio. cum fidenti omnium professione. suendi condendi pectendi manus apta. fontium scaturigines ampnium decursus. aquarum derivaciones. Eius est homo gracile habens corpus sapiens insistens lectioni completa persona multos adquirit amicos et in eis fortunam non habet. pulchram quoque barbam habens atque raram et parvam. labia subtilia et nasum subtilem." Cf. Abū Maʿshar, *Introductorium* 7 (sig. g4).

of fixed stars itself moved very slowly; as a result, as Roger knew, by his time the sections of the path no longer had a connection with the names of constellations and so were called "signs" of them: Aries, Taurus, and so forth.[56] Roger therefore had to explain the difference between the physical appearance of the heavens, as measured by the astrolabe, and tables that ignored the slow motion of the fixed stars.

Having identified the client and his needs with a feature of the heavens, normally a planet, the astrologer consulted his tables to see how that planet interacted with others as they moved through the houses. These relationships between the planets were "aspects," and their study was an important technique in astrology and one that invested it with an air of great mathematical precision. For example, planets in opposite positions in the zodiacal circle were "in opposition," or 180 degrees apart (generally an aspect would be given a range of 10 degrees or so, in order to extend its duration). Planets with different powers in opposition became weaker, while planets with similar powers and in conjunction became stronger. Planets 90 degrees apart were "at square"; "sextile" meant an angle of 60 degrees. Both aspects and planets were placed on a scale of benignancy and malignancy; for example, "trine" was not a favored aspect, and Mars and Saturn were regarded as evil. The manner in which the planets approached and left conjunction with each other was important; we shall see that Roger had a long list of technical terms describing this.

Each sign of the zodiac and each planet had its own particular relationship with the human body and its parts. This was of natural interest to the medical man and must have prompted his inquiry into the rest of astrological theory. Aries, the first sign of the zodiac, had the head and face; Taurus, the second, had the throat and neck; and so on down the body to the feet, of which Pisces, the final sign, was in charge. These are the relationships indicated on medieval "zodiac men." Those used by Roger are given in Appendix 1. While the planets had characteristics of their own, it was an important feature of astrology that the powers they exercised and the parts of the body they related to changed as they moved from one sign of the zodiac to another. Roger treats the planets systematically in each sign, always beginning with Saturn. Thus in Aries, the first sign, Saturn has the chest, Jupiter the belly, Mars the head, and so on through the seven planets. If we follow Saturn through the signs, we see that it rotates through the body in a similar way. In Taurus and Gemini Saturn has the belly and in Cancer the male genitalia. Saturn reaches the feet in the other signs and returns to the head and then the neck in Aquarius and Pisces, completing the circle prior to returning to the chest. Most of the other planets have part at least of such a cycle (see Appendix 2). While much of Roger's astrology is traceable to Abū Maʿshar, these correspondences are not, which suggests that Roger was drawing on a separate tradition of medical astrology. The result of all this was a systematic "astronomical anatomy" that was clearly useful to the medical men.[57] It gave them an additional technical apparatus with which to impress their patients, a celestial anatomy of their own proper business, the human body, in the period before they discovered the "new Galen" and insinuated themselves into the universities on the basis of a rationale of *physical* anatomy derived from him.

The more technical business of the astrologer began with the setting up of the houses

[56] He says that the motion of the fixed star "map" (i.e., the precession of the equinox) is 1 degree in one hundred years; it had now moved 8 degrees.

[57] The anatomical correspondences shown in Appendix 1 are conventional and are listed in both Abū Maʿshar's *Introductorium* and the abbreviation of it (Abū Maʿshar, *Abbreviation of the Introduction to Astrology*, ed. and trans. Burnett *et al.* [cit. n. 7]). On possible sources for the planetary correspondences see Whyte, "Roger of Hereford's *Liber de astronomice iudicandi*" (cit. n. 20), p. 23.

of the zodiac ("domification"), and this is a major concern for Roger in the *De iudiciis astronomie;* it is one of the few parts of Roger's text to have been read by a modern historian. An astrological "house" can be simply a sign of the zodiac regarded as the home of a particular planet, but it is probably better to use some other term for this and reserve *houses* for the divisions of the zodiac determined by the horizon at the moment of birth. In the simplest terms, the astrology available in the West before the twelfth century was a question of nativities, that is, the casting of horoscopes at the birth of a child to answer questions relating to matters like length of life, wealth, relatives, and illness. Such categories of things were to be found in the twelve houses: since the zodiac moves round the earth, a moment of time (for example, a birth) could be defined by a point on the circle (for example, rising above the horizon). This could be done with varying degrees of precision. The only surviving Roman horoscope is to be found in the *Mathesis* of Firmicus Maternus, and it is without the degrees into which the houses came to be divided. Much of Roger's interest is in this "judicial" astrology—which, like Ptolemy's, was more like prophecy than calculation—but he is very concerned to define the houses mathematically.[58] Roger's houses are subdivided, each division pertaining to some aspect of future life and each defined in degrees. Some of what Roger claims to be bringing together from different authors is expressed in his "table of hours," which enables the seasonally different daylight and night hours specific to the latitude of Hereford to be used to give precision to the houses. (He also here describes the use of the astrolabe.)

It was generally agreed that the twelve houses started at the ascendant and that the beginning of the tenth house was the point on the ecliptic directly south of the observer. But there was no general agreement about how to calculate the houses, particularly since, as Roger says (to look forward for a moment to the *Liber de tribus generalibus judiciis astronomie*), they differed at different latitudes.[59] Roger simplifies the matter by treating as his first house the whole sign in which the ascendant appeared, irrespective of its position in that sign. He then explains two methods for determining the remaining houses, one by using the astrolabe and the other by consulting tables giving the length of an "hour" at the appropriate latitude. A diurnal "hour" was one twelfth of the day and so was longer in the summer than in the winter, especially in the north. Roger's own tables for Hereford were probably the most northerly produced up to that time.[60]

The houses customarily related to many aspects of life, like personal relationships (concerning family, servants, friends), religion, inheritance, buildings, animals, career, and so on. Some of these were of particular interest to the medical man, and life span and its divisions were given prominence in the houses. The first house related to birth and the life of the body and soul (as well as to talking and reading) and the second to the completion of the youthful period of life. The middle of life was signified by the ninth house (as were

[58] Roger's houses of the zodiac have been considered in North, *Horoscopes and History* (cit. n. 30), p. 39. On astrology as prophecy rather than calculation see Cochrane, *Adelard of Bath* (cit. n. 31), p. 87.

[59] CUL Ii.1.1, fol. 51v, col. 1: "Notandum autem quod iste coniuncciones duobus modis fieri dicuntur, scilicet per celum vel per figuram. per celum, cum sit inter eos aut pars celi sexta aut quarta aut tertia aut media. per figuram vero cum secundum domorum disposicionem iunguntur. et hic diversificatur secundum diversitates climatum." On agreement with regard to starting at the ascendant and the beginning of the tenth house see Whyte, "Roger of Hereford's *Liber de astronomice iudicandi*" (cit. n. 20), p. 17.

[60] CUL Ii.1.1, fol. 41r, col. 2: "Compositionis autem hic est ratio tabulae subscripte maxima hora herfordie excedit minimam per 11 gradus et 40 minuta. Mediam vero per 5 gradus equales et 50 minutas. id est maxima excedit mediam 350 minutis, minimam vero 700 minutis horum autem quarta sunt 175 minuta sexta 116 minuta et 40 secunda."

philosophy and all branches of knowledge) and the end of this period by the eleventh.[61] The sixth house signified "the future before old age" and was the house of illness.[62] The third related to "life before death" and the fourth to death itself (and what happened afterward, that is, inheritance).[63] Likewise death was signaled by the twelfth house, and the "end of the years of life, after old age," by the eighth house, the house of death (which also related to fear of poisoning).[64]

Many a query to an astrologer must have been about the outcome of disease, whether life or death. The astrologer found answers by identifying his client with a heavenly body and his future with its journey across the heavens and the houses. Most often the client was represented by the "Lord of the Ascendant" (*Dominus Ascendentis*), the planet that ruled the sign of the ascendant, the point of the ecliptic rising over the eastern horizon when the query was made. Sometimes the moon was used instead, but Roger explains that in queries about life, the moon does not play the same part as in other queries and that judgment is taken from it only when it has significant aspects and the *Dominus Ascendentis* does not. The outcome in queries about life, says Roger, depends on the strength of the Lord of the House of the Ascendant and whether he is impeded by the Lord of the House of Death (i.e., whether his strength is diminished by unfortunate aspects with the latter). There is nothing to be feared, he adds, from the entry of the Lord of the Ascendant or the moon into the House of Death.[65]

The *De iudiciis astronomie* is, broadly speaking, judicial astrology in the sense used above, that is, relating to broad prophecies about the future based on the moment of the client's birth and employing greater or lesser sophistication in the construction of houses and their subdivisions, "the natures of the signs and the motion of the planets, the properties of the houses and of the planets and the quantity of these powers," as Roger puts it.[66] This judicial astrology, reflected in the title of Roger's work, also corresponds to the first of the four parts of astrology that he lists near its beginning. It is "simple judgment." But the new material that Roger had collected from the philosophers enabled him not only to construct a table of hours but to engage in different kinds of prediction. In such cases the

[61] *Ibid.*, fol. 46r, col. 1: "prima domus vite corporis animi et omnis originis et motus oracionis leccionis locutionis rumorum et inicium vite." See also fol. 46v.

[62] *Ibid.*, fol. 46r, col. 2: "et signat futura ante senectutem." Roger's dense style of writing may have led copyists astray: of the seventh house it is said "signat medietatem finis vite ante senectute. . . . Sexta domus egritudinis et esse eius status et habitudinis servorum ancillarum nequicie in iusticie cum participacione localis motus et animalium superviencium non equorum et signat futura ante senectutem."

[63] *Ibid.*, fol. 46r, col. 1: "Quarta domus patrum parentum generis radicis aquositatis campi agrorum civitatum castrorum edificiorum secretorum loci subterranei thesauri finis rerum mortis et reliquiarum mortui ac consequencium et signat finem carcerem et hereditatem et quid sequatur post mortem."

[64] *Ibid.*, fol. 46r, col. 2: "Octava domus mortis venenorum metus et perditi irrecuperabilis otii pigritie desidie fraudulencie interne vecordie desperacionis ire et hereditatum mortuorum laboris et tristicie bellorum et signat supervientes et auxiliatores adversariorum et signat finem annorum vite post senectutem." Fol. 46r, col. 1: "Nona domus itinerum exiliorum honestatis iusticie veritatis virtutum religionis legum templorum cerumoniarum philosophie omnis scientie scripture nunciorum visionum rumorum narracionum fidei preteritorum et viri degradati et signat dimidium vite."

[65] *Ibid.*, fol. 51v, cols. 1–2: "Et notandum est quod in omnibus luna participat cum domino ascendentis nisi in iudicio de vita, quantecumque fortitudinis sit domus ascendentis. Intelligendum quod si fortis fuerit dominus ascendentis et tamen non coniunctus domino rei et luna debilis et tamen iuncta figura accepcionem licet debiliorem. Si autem de vita queritur et dominus ascendentis fuerit fortis et in nullo impeditus a domino domus mortis, non impedit vitam. Sed si fuerit dominus ascendentis non aspiciens ascendens et luna aspexerit tunc a luna iudicium vite ut in ceteris sumetur. Sed et hoc valde notandum est si domus mortis receperit dominum ascendentis vel lunam non est timendum."

[66] *Ibid.*, fol. 40va: "et naturis signorum et temporibus planetarum . . . et quantitus virtutem." (Here and elsewhere, translations are my own unless otherwise noted.)

astrologer was consulted by a client with a particular question, just as a person with worrying symptoms went to see a doctor. In both cases the practitioner listened to the client, told him that the case was understood, reminded him of the grand principles on which the art was founded, told him that there was a good chance of success, wrote something on a piece of paper, and charged a fee. Part of the attraction of the new astrology must have been that it extended the practice of the astrologer in this way.

We can follow some of the details of an astrological consultation by looking at Roger's other text, the *Liber de tribus generalibus judiciis astronomie.* These "three judgments" seem to be the remaining items on Roger's list of the parts of astrology in his first text; and although the *Liber de tribus generalibus judiciis astronomie* begins as a separate book, it can be treated as a continuation of *De iudiciis astronomie.* At all events, the client, consulting the astrologer, told him what his problem was: perhaps he wanted to locate stolen goods or wondered when to embark on a new enterprise and whether it would be successful.[67] In general, such questions were "interrogations" when they were about specific items (like lost property) or "elections" when the client was seeking a propitious moment to begin something. The first of Roger's three judgments is about elections (the term he uses). Second, his "cogitation" (also called "intention") corresponds to a reply to an "interrogation" (he uses the term *interrogans* for the client).[68] The third judgment is another kind of interrogation; in the text we are now looking at he calls it the "pursuit of the Good."

In judicial astrology, the astrologer made a note of the time when the query was put to him and determined which planet should represent the client. He might also provide an astrological "history" of the client by drawing up a retrospective horoscope (as Roger did in his horoscope for Eleanor of Aquitaine), much as a medical man looked at the patient's medical history for help in making a prognostication. In both cases the practitioner wanted to discover the natural dispositions and characteristics of the client or patient, the better to predict how he would react in future circumstances. Thus Roger's first "judgment" (concerning the good or evil outcome of the case in hand) was made in various ways. In the simplest cases the client was usually represented by the moon. More often in complex cases it was the Lord of the Ascendant. Then the astrologer selected a "Lord of the Matter" (*Dominus Rei*), which signified the matter of the query. At its simplest, the prediction was that if the *Dominus Ascendentis* or the moon was moving to conjunction with the *Dominus Rei,* the outcome would be successful. The opportunities for making a prediction were increased by choosing which of the two—the *Dominus Ascendentis* or the moon—had significant aspects (conjunction was the most notable of them) with the *Dominus Rei.*[69] This simple prediction was hedged about with a wide range of qualifying conditions, in which lay most of the complexity of astrology. In brief, these were the good or bad aspects of the two lords to the other planets (themselves good or bad), the modifying effects of the signs on the planets and lords, and the positions of the signs and planets in the houses.

[67] *Ibid.,* fol. 51va: "Incipit liber de tribus generalibus iudiciis astronomie." Roger groups astrological questions into three categories: "Quoniam circa tria fit omnis astronomica consideracio videlicet circa consecucionem bonorum vel vitaciorum malorum et circa intencionem vel meditacionem et circa comparacionem vel eleccionem." These are the "three general judgments" of his title.

[68] *Ibid.,* fol. 57v, col. 1: "Sed et in questione eleccionis mira habenda cautela . . ."

[69] *Ibid.,* fol. 51v, col. 2: "Dinoscitur autem rerum consecucio tribus modis. primo scilicet a coniunccione domini ascendentis vel lune cum domino rei vel econverso. Dominus autem ascendentis vel luna signat querentem. Dominus vero rei rem quesitum. Sed si dominus ascendentis vel luna petant coniunccionem adquirens propria adquisicione rem adquiret. Si autem dominus rei pecierit coniunccionem ultimo veniet res quesita querenti. . . . Si dominus ascendentis aspexerit ascendens et non luna a domino ascendentis sumetur iudicium. Si luna et non dominus ascendentis tunc a luna. Et si uterque tunc a superiori."

Roger answers elective questions by treating the enterprise asked about as a process, with a beginning and an end, that can be judged and compared to other processes. The basic technique is the same, that is, the astrologer assigns a feature of the heavens to the querent and another to the process. In some cases the beginning of a long change might be indicated by the sun and its ending by the moon. Note the similarity to medical cases, where the sun and moon controlled acute and chronic diseases by means of their cycles; Roger calls this simple relationship "natural," while the more common "accidental" beginning of a process was the ascendant and its accidental end the house assigned to the process. Elaborations on this basic astrological scheme include a list of conditions under which the moon and planets have lesser powers (such as an eclipse, in the case of the moon) and a long list of relationships between the planets (such as *applicacio* and *separacio,* when a planet approached and retired from another). In the *De judiciis astronomie* Roger had listed eighteen such relationships, governed by the planets' location in the zodiac, retrogression (of some planets), and their aspects, like quartile and trine.[70]

The second of Roger's "three general judgments" was *intentio et cogitatio;* here he presents refinements of the general rules of astrology, for example, by subdividing the signs into ninths and twelfths—*novenarii* and *duodenarii.* Even each degree of a sign could have individual characteristics. Another refinement was to supply a planetary ruler for the hour in which the query was put to the astrologer. The hour was divided into three, and Roger knew what the *intentio* relevant to each third would be. A client asks about himself or his fellows in the first part of the hour of the sun; in the second, questions concern plans, wars, sieges, and so on.[71] The first part of the hour of the moon related to diseases of the eyes. Questions proper to the second part of the hour of Saturn related to the sex of unborn children, and those of the last part were about illness or pain experienced by the querent or his friends and about war or discord.[72] *Intentio* thus seems to be the astrologer's study of his clients (and of related "hidden things") and is apparently related to the astrological technique of providing retrospective horoscopes of clients in order to give weight to prediction. Since the horoscope was retrospective, the astrologer could readily demonstrate the cogency and potency of astrological arguments and procedures, and no doubt he used such things as advertisements for his practice. In a sense Roger was showing how to make a diagnosis of the client's complaint before the client complained. Doctors did the same sort of thing to impress their patients, and we shall see that William of England took the process a step further.

The third of Roger's judgments was "comparison or election." "Election" was normally a prediction based on using the birth chart, or nativity, of the querent in the new celestial circumstances of the present or future, and this before-and-after treatment seems to be what Roger means by "comparison." Many querents asked about length of life, but Roger is too busy with technical details to give an example. An election from the *Centiloquium*

[70] *Ibid.,* fol. 46v, col. 2: "Sunt 18 planetarum adinvicem habitus. Respectus. applicacio. separacio. parilitas. solitudo. alienacio. translatio. collacio. collocacio. prohibitio. redicio. contradiccio. impedicio. evasio. intercepcio. compassio. renunciacio. recepcio." Roger explains each of these in the text that follows.

[71] *Ibid.,* fol. 56r, col. 2: "Sed et per dominum hore aliter iudicatur de intencione et re abscondita ut cum sint planete 7 omnibus horis dominantes, quelibet hora in 3a dividitur. si autem amota fuerit quomodo in prima parte hore solis, querit de se vel socio. Res clausa erit annona vel herba. si in secunda querit consilium de bello vel obsidione, municione pavore potestate."

[72] *Ibid.,* fol. 56v, col. 2: "Si in prima parte hore lune de infirmitate oculorum. Res clausa herba odorifera. . . . Si in secunda, utrum pregnans masculum vel feminam pariat, et si fuerit planeta in die erit masculus si in nocte erit femina. Res clausa ferrum vel aliquid metallum vel aliud quod in ignem solet mitti. si in ultima de infirmitate sui vel amicorum vel de bello vel discordia vel dolore aliquod. Res clausa caput vespertilionis aut bicoloris avis."

will serve as an example: "When a sickness begins when the moon is in a sign in which at birth there was a malevolent planet, or in one in square with it or in opposition, it will be very hard to bear; if a malevolent planet is in a bad aspect, it will be dangerous; if the moon is in a house where at birth there was a beneficent planet, it will not be dangerous."[73]

PREDICTION AND PROGNOSIS

As we have seen, the medical man was already in the business of prediction. He had the ancient authority of Hippocrates that some fevers moved through a series of crises on certain—and therefore predictable—days. His examination of the pulse and of urine were both diagnostic and prognostic. The rationale was that the doctor was investigating the outward signs of fundamental bodily processes: the activity of the vital faculty in the heart and the generation of blood (the food of the body) by the natural faculty in the liver. Urine charts, volvelles, and posters he displayed were visible signs of the power of these rationales, designed to impress patients.[74] Signs of weakness and eventual collapse of the faculties were a regular part of pulse and urine lore. Hippocrates himself was supposed to have written an astrological text,[75] and it was a widely accepted fact that the phases of the moon were linked to growth and decay and to menstruation, all open to prediction. Some similarities between medical men and the astrologers have already been pointed out, and it is clear that on the most liberal reading the doctors wanted astrological techniques to make themselves better doctors in terms of prognostication. But probably more widespread was the recognition that an elaborate and technical apparatus that linked the patient to the celestial bodies themselves—the causes of everything—was sound advertising.[76] Roger said that astrology was second only to the study of the Creator and indeed sprang from it. There could scarcely be a greater endorsement.

It was suggested earlier that the learned medicine of the universities did not develop its links with astrology, but that practitioners outside the schools suffered no such constraints. We can now take as a case in point William of England, one of the first men to use astrology in the practical business of uroscopy. He is essentially unknown to historians: born in England in the late twelfth century, he was a generation or so younger than Roger (and there is no evidence that he knew of Roger's works). William calls himself a *medicus* but does not say whether what he learned (in Marseille) was the arts, medicine, or astrology. When he says that he was also an astrologer "by merit of knowledge," his words imply that he had learned his astrology informally. There was no new university in Marseille with a faculty seeking to control medicine, and it was perhaps a good place to learn astrology; certainly it was from here that Roger had taken the basis for his own tables. William settled there, becoming a citizen. The story of medicine at the hands of men like William runs parallel to its history in the universities, but the image should not be taken

[73] See S. J. Tester, *A History of Western Astrology* (Woodbridge, Suffolk: Boydell, 1987), p. 92.

[74] See, e.g., Clark, "Zodiac Man in Medieval Medical Astrology" (cit. n. 14). Belief in a natural spirit in the liver was medieval, not Galenic. A third spirit matched the three faculties and encouraged medieval doctors to see the liver as an important organ.

[75] The *Astronomia Ypocratis* was well known before the time of Maurus of Salerno; it is not mathematically predictive. A printed version is included with the *Regimen sanitatis* of Magninus Mediolensis (Lyons, 1505[?]).

[76] "Philosophy" in the twelfth century was knowledge of everything, human and divine. Because God was seen as omnipotent, "nature" was simply a collection of secondary causes used by God, not an autonomous principle. All causality flowed from God, and the motions of the heavenly bodies were readily seen as his secondary causes. Astrology on the Arabic model was dangerous because it seemed to establish autonomous causes.

literally. There was some convergence of the two traditions when medicine within the universities began to grow more astrological: William's *De urina non visa* was adopted as statutory by Italian schools.[77] Let us examine it.

William's claim to fame—and he does claim it, asserting that his work should be a memorial to himself because none of the ancients had attempted such a thing—was that he took the medical man's traditional means of prognostication, uroscopy, and added astrology to it. The result is his *De urina non visa* [*On unseen urine*], written about 1215.[78] That is, he claims to be able to make judgments about the urine and the patient it came from *without seeing either.* To us, since we believe in neither uroscopy nor astrology, it looks as if William is simply adding one dubious practice to another and so removing himself further from medical reality. But William and the Italian masters thought otherwise. One advantage of his system was certainly its advertising potential, the power of which in the medical marketplace we have already noted. To diagnose and prognosticate from a sample of urine without seeing the patient was already a technique designed to impress, and William is going one stage further, divining the nature of the urine and the disease and foretelling its outcome.

Like many who announce novelties, William finds it necessary to construct a little history for his new discipline, showing that its parts had the dignity and authority of age (even though none of the ancients had assembled them as William had). Thus William goes back to the classical use of augury to determine the proper time to begin an enterprise, drawing a parallel to the astrological determination of the best time for giving medicines, for example. He also alludes to Ptolemy's account of how the Egyptians used medical and astrological techniques in combination in order to be more certain of the result.

To make his point William has to do more than give his new idea a history; he must show the superiority of the method. Seeking to justify astrology rather than uroscopy, he turns to an argument from the schools: the upper causes of things are like universals, he says, while the effects on earth are like particulars. This is not an Aristotelian causal and physical relationship; William is closer to the twelfth-century debate on universals. In William's view, the universals order their particulars because they contain them. The universals are things like conjunctions and are, like celestial things in general, perfect. But the outcome on earth is not always perfect. The argument is similar to that of Roger, who stressed the perfection of heavenly motions and bodies in contrast to their earthly effects. Much more than Roger, however, William has the medical man's caution about making his prognosis too confidently—it was an unprofessional thing to do. William makes the neat point that the effects on earth of the celestial universal, being particulars of observation, are subject to errors of interpretation. As particulars expressed in mutable matter, they are also subject to accidents. It is the fault of matter, then, that the effects of the perfect cause are distorted and not regular; perhaps, for example, a thing destined to happen is delayed. With this apparatus William can argue further for the superiority of his new method. He notes that the medical man, in the course of his business, is concerned almost

[77] See McMenomy, "Discipline of Astronomy in the Middle Ages" (cit. n. 40). William's text was specified in the Bologna statutes of 1404 as a text for the fourth year. The statutes relate to astronomy and astrology, but the text is often found in collections of medical manuscripts. Although the statutory texts of medical education in the northern universities did not include works on astrology, it is very striking that university physicians almost universally held the causes of pestilences to be astrological. The Parisian faculty reported to the monarch about the Black Death in such terms, and later hardly anyone denied the celestial origin of the French Disease. See Arrizabalaga, Henderson, and French, *Great Pox* (cit. n. 10).

[78] William's text is widely distributed. I have used Vienna, National-Bibliothek 5207 (fols. 205–211); London, British Library (BL) Add 54543 (fols. 78v–79r); and Cambridge, Trinity College 0.8.31 (fols. 173–176).

entirely with particulars of sensory observation and derives from them primarily the "middle causes" that lie between the heavenly universals and the material particulars. The middle causes are things like the physicians' "complexion," the qualitative balance of the patient, which was important to the medical man who understood disease as an imbalance of qualities. The ordinary doctor, then, did not rise far above the notoriously imperfect material particulars. But the astrologizing doctor, William says, begins with the powers and positions (*status* and *disposicio*) of the planets and signs and descends in the light of knowledge so gained to specific complexions of things at certain times.

Thus William is claiming that astrological medicine is a higher study because it is closer to the upper, perfect, universals. This would have been an impressive story to anyone who held the priorities we would expect of the time, including a preference for rational understanding of natural principles over craft knowledge. Here is William on the difference:

> The medical man, whose judgment is largely bound by sense . . . finds certain causes for himself, such as time, complexion, and composition. The astrologer gives his attention to less familiar and more proper agents and by the state and disposition of the stars and signs he investigates the complexions of things in any hour, just as the medical man recognizes the cause and prognosticates about effect through his signs, which are sputum, urine, and sweat. So in a similar way the astrologer naturally anticipates the effect of a moving cause by a rational foresight; thus his deliberations are of a far higher order because they do not need matter.[79]

William's view of astrology as a higher study is what Roger had offered to medicine in setting it above all the arts, which were branches of an unfruitful tree in comparison. No doubt William believed that the astrologizing doctor was a better doctor; but he was also aware of the reputation to be gained from the use of astrology, and he quotes Abū Maʿshar's promise that, having astrologically determined the nature of the disease, the doctor can better tell when and if a medicine should be given, "and he will earn praise for his work." The medical man who adopts William's new method, he says, will investigate the color and substance of unseen urine according to the upper powers, "and the good medical astrologer will achieve glory."[80]

William adopts for medical purposes the basic technique of the astrologer in finding a lord for what is under investigation. As astrologers like Roger found the Lord of the Ascendant from what was rising above the horizon, so William has a "Lord of the Urine" and an appropriate house. Fundamental to his argument is the astrological "place of the liver." Doctors held the liver to be the organ where blood was generated from digested food. The blood itself was the food of the body and so was very important to its health. The generation of blood was the work of the natural faculty and involved the separation and removal of impurities, the black and red bile. The thick and fatty blood generated in this manner was too thick to flow through the small vessels of the liver and needed water to dilute and transport it. Once out of the liver, this water was collected by the kidneys

[79] Vienna 5207, fol. 206 (with modifications as noted): "Sed medicus cuius iudicii maxima pars circa sensum subiecta consistit quasdam causas de istis mediis ponit sibi [following BL 54543] proprias velut [following BL 54543] compositiones complexiones tempus et [following BL 54543] id genus. Astrologus vero minus usitatas et magis proprias utpote agentes attendit velud est presens tam signorum quam stellarum status et disposicio complexiones rerum in qualibet hora proprias [following BL 54543] investigat tunc sicut medicus per sua signa que sunt sputum et urina et humidum [BL 54543: humiditas] exterior et id genus de causa cognoscit [following BL 54543] et de effectum pronosticat. Similiter astrologus per causam moventem in previsione conjecturali effectum naturaliter antecedit. Unde et eius consideracio longe dignior cum subiecte materie non indiget."

[80] Vienna 5207, fol. 205v: "Cum enim ut ait albumazar previsa fuerit natura egritudinis et an prosit medicacio et quo tempore. nunc demum utiliter accedet medicus et laudem ex opere merebitur."

and excreted as urine. The consistency and color of the urine were held to reflect the processes occurring in the liver, so that, for example, the normal color of urine was the result of the blood becoming red. Abnormal colors and substances were produced when something went wrong and some qualities became attached to the urine.

In explaining how these abnormalities happen, William develops the astrological doctrine, found for example in Roger's work, of the qualitative nature of the planets and signs. These were the same elementary qualities that characterized things on earth, and the doctrine of "like affects like" accounted for many of the relationships between the upper and lower things. William, of course, believed that this happened at a level higher than the medical. He says that in investigating the urine we should have in mind, rather than the four humors with their pairs of elementary qualities, the celestial "triplicities." He means again that the humors, being material, share the mutability of all matter and that prediction is accordingly more difficult. The signs are not mutable and so are better for prediction; the triplicities are four groups of three signs, determined by their sharing common qualities. These are the same elementary qualities that the humors have, and they work their effects on the blood and elsewhere in the same way; but we can see why William thought he was being more precise. The planets have a similar effect on the humors, so that, according to William, the sun and Mars affect red bile (because all three are hot) and the moon and Venus affect phlegm (because they are cold).

The nature of the urine accordingly follows astrological rules that we have met, this time worked out in medical theory. For example, if the "place of the liver" is in Aries, and Mars is there too, or in significant aspect, then the heat of Mars weakens the power of the liver to separate superfluities from healthy matter and the patient will suffer from fever. The weakened power of the liver affects the substance of the urine by admitting gross substances, and the urine will also have a red color because of the adustion (burning) of the red bile. If instead both Saturn and the "place of the liver" are in Capricorn, then the urine will take on a black color, from mortification caused by Saturn's baleful effect.

William was looking to determine the nature of disease as well as the appearance of the urine, and again he uses apparatus put together by the ancient astrologers. William has a list of parts of the body controlled by the planets as they pass through different houses. It is very close to the list given by Roger (see Appendix 2), and William uses it for a sort of celestial pathological anatomy. Should the hot and dry Mars be causing a disturbance of the blood, then when Mars moves into a house that has a relationship to the chest (i.e., Cancer) the patient will spit blood. As we might expect of a medical man, William also lists the anatomical relationships of the signs to the parts of the body, top to toe; his list has much of what Roger's has but is more extensive. The same can be said of his list of the planets and their relationships to the body, which—although agreeing in part with Roger's—is more extensive, particularly in point of the diseases associated with each planet and generally caused by the elementary qualities of the planet in question.

A final feature of traditional astrology that the medical man found useful was the relationship between the signs and regions and features of the earth. In Roger's account, for example, Aries pertains to Palestine and Babylon, while Taurus has relationships with fields, mountains, and caves. Similarly, the planets had special connections with kinds of people and their activities. Saturn looked after carpenters and agriculture; Jupiter, princes, laws, and temples. Such categories helped the medical men to explain the local and general appearances of disease (and were still doing so at the time of the Black Death of 1348 and the French Disease in 1494). William uses the same language for regions and cities, changes of kings, disasters and plagues, famine, and corruption of the air and water.

Roger does not give his sources, even though his intention in writing was to bring them all together in a single work. William, in contrast, derives strength for his arguments and his new method by citing Ptolemy's *Quadripartitum* and the *Centiloquium.* He also cites Māshā'allāh and "Herman," no doubt Herman of Carinthia, the translator of Abū Ma'shar's *Introductorium.* William also relies on Alcabitius for the list of correspondences of the planets in the houses with the parts of the body, which is so close to that of Roger.

Finally, then, we can see that for both Roger, who was eager to assemble the rules of astrology from the Arabs in order to be able to practice it properly, and William, who more confidently wanted to extend the rules into medical practice, what was important was the ability to foretell the future. As we have seen, it was the interest and utility that they found in the new Arabic material that sent people like Daniel of Morley and Alfred of Shareshill scrambling off to secure fragments of Arabic star lore. Something similar was surely true for the pursuit of most Greek natural philosophy. It was not possible to discover the future with Aristotle's *Physics,* but it too had its uses: it was a suitable intellectual weapon to still the turmoil of the Cathar heresy and to set up schools of politically correct ideology to keep it still, and it was useful to the Paris masters in securing the arts a place in their university. But this knowledge was available to be used in these ways because it had been fetched for such purposes, not because it had diffused or been transmitted to the West.

APPENDIX 1
THE CONNECTIONS BETWEEN THE SIGNS OF THE ZODIAC AND THE PARTS OF THE BODY AS USED BY ROGER OF HEREFORD

Aries "has the head and face of man."
Taurus has the neck and throat.
Gemini has upper arms, lower arms, and hands.
Cancer has the chest, heart, stomach, ribs, spleen, and lungs.
Leo has the stomach, heart, sides, and back.
Virgo has the belly, intestines, and *tela*—literally, a web.
Libra has the loins, the back, the lower belly, the umbilicus, the *pecten* (probably the lower edge of the ribs), the genitalia, the *hancas* or *hanchos* ("haunches"), the *ilia* (intestines), and the nostrils.
Scorpio has the genitalia (especially male), bladder, anus, and upper legs.
Sagittarius has the upper legs.
Capricorn has the knees.
Aquarius has the lower legs down to the toes.
Pisces has the feet.

APPENDIX 2
ROGER'S ASTROLOGICAL ANATOMY

	Saturn	Jupiter	Mars	Sun	Venus	Mercury	Moon
Aries	pectus	venter	caput	femora	pedes	crura	genua
Taurus	venter	dorsum	collum	genua	caput	pedes	crura
Gemini	venter	verenda et inferiora	pectus	crura, cavilla	collum	caput	femora
Cancer	virilia et inferiora	femora	pectus	pedes	brachia, humeri	oculi	caput
Leo	verenda	femora, genua	venter	caput	cor	humeri, guttur	collum
Virgo	pedes	genua	venter	collum	venter	cor	humeri
Libra	genua	oculi	verenda	humeri	caput	venter	cor
Scorpio	cavilla	pedes	caput, brachia, femora	cor	verenda	dorsum	venter
Sagittarius	pedes	crura, caput	pedes, manus	venter	femora, brachia	verenda, cor	dorsum
Capricorn	caput, pedes	genua, oculi	crura, humeri	dorsum	femora, cor	verenda	dorsum
Aquarius	caput, collum	humeri, pectus, pedes	cavilla, cor	verenda	genua	femora, cor	verenda
Pisces	humeri, brachia, collum	cor, caput	cavilla, venter	femora	collum, dorsum	crura, verenda	femora

This table has been compiled from Roger's words. Expressed diagrammatically, it shows clearly the signs of an earlier systematic rotation of the body's parts as the planets pass through the signs. The column for Mercury is one step ahead of that for the moon and one step behind that for the sun. The sequence of organs for the sun is followed by that of Jupiter from Leo to Cancer. There are seven cases in which the column for Jupiter is one sign ahead of that for Saturn and nine where Venus is three signs ahead of the sun. It seems clear that *oculus* has been confused with *collum* at some stage in the transmission of these details; *collum* seems required in the sequences Venus–Mercury–Moon and Saturn–Jupiter–Sun.

VI

Astrology in medical practice

INTRODUCTION: A PARABLE

Daniel of Morley's journey to Toledo is something of a parable for the topic of this chapter and perhaps for the book as a whole. It has lessons for us. Let us first hear the story and then draw the moral from it.[1]

As Daniel told the Bishop of Norwich (probably in the early 1170s) there was little about the state of learning in the West that he found exciting. Paris was full of lawyers, arrogant and with closed minds, marking minute changes in their texts with asterisks and obeli. He was more interested in the *doctrina Arabum* being taught by the wiser philosophers of the world (as he called them) and so he took himself off to Toledo, where Gerard of Cremona was expounding the *Almagest* to a class of pupils, apparently during the course of its translation.[2]

What was exciting about the Arabic doctrine of the heavens was the belief that events on earth, day-to-day or momentous, were caused by the motions of the celestial bodies. This causal relation was *necessary*, which meant that, if the motions of the superior bodies were known, events on earth could be *predicted*. Daniel was partly horrified and partly fascinated. Did not prediction deny free will, he asked of Gerard, quoting some homilies of St Gregory. Moreover, how could a man born under Aquarius in a Spanish town miles from the sea or a river *necessarily* become a fisherman? Gerard, smiling at the young man's presumption, answered that

[1] The moral of a story was its higher meaning. See B. Smalley, *The study of the Bible in the Middle Ages* (3rd edn, Oxford, 1983).

[2] Daniel's text is given in K. Sudhoff, 'Daniels von Morley Liber de Naturis Inferiorum et Superiorum', *Archiv für die Geschichte der Naturwissenschaften und der Technik*, 8 (1918), 1–40. See also R. W. Hunt, 'English learning in the late twelfth century', in R. W. Southern (ed.), *Essays in medieval history* (London and New York, 1968), pp. 106–28, who identifies Daniel's sources as twelfth-century Paris masters and the pseudo-Avicennan *De celo et mundo*. See also the classic paper by A. Birkenmajer, 'Le rôle joué par les médecins et les naturistes dans la réception d'Aristote au xiie et xiiie siècles', in his *Etudes d'histoire des sciences et de la philosophie du moyen âge* (Warsaw, 1970). This edition includes an assessment of Birkenmajer's work by D'Alverny. B. Stock, *Myth and science in the twelfth century. A study of Bernard Sylvester* (Princeton, 1972), dates Daniel's book at about 1175.

the man would necessarily be disposed to be a better fisherman, which would appear should he ever have the opportunity to fish. Very well then, said Daniel, what about the son of a king and the son of a peasant, both born under a royal sign. It would surely be the case that only the son of a king would grow up to be a king. Ah, said Gerard, but the young peasant would be a king among the peasants. Indeed, he added, I was born under a royal sign myself, and I am a king. Oh, said Daniel, somewhat nettled, and where do you reign? In my mind, said Gerard coldly.[3]

The lessons for us are firstly that the exciting thing about such translations was that they seemed to supply powerful and useful knowledge about the world. It was almost a question of forbidden fruit tasting sweeter, for predictive knowledge of this kind hovered on the denial of free will and even of God's providence. Moreover, it was clearly pagan knowledge. Daniel had to explain to the bishop in his book how it was that pagan knowledge could be used by a Christian. It was, he said, like the gold the Jews borrowed from the Egyptians before the exodus: it was not holy, but it was useful. The same image of Egyptian gold was used by many in the twelfth and thirteenth centuries to excuse the use of pagan philosophy. The most significant use of the image is that of Gregory IX, who in 1231 set up a commission to remove what was offensive to faith from Aristotle's physical works in order to render them useful – to find their gold – in education. This event is essentially the formal acceptance of Aristotle's physical works in the *studium* of Paris and shortly predates the masters' construction of natural philosophy[4] – and as we saw in the introduction to this book, the importance of the reception of Aristotle's works for medicine was immense.

The second lesson from the story of Daniel is that this knowledge was fetched and did not come of its own accord. The twelfth-century Western Latin translator was a man who left home, spent a great deal of time and money on difficult journeys to uncomfortably hot places on the very fringes of Christendom, and learned a difficult language in order to read a highly technical book with the help of a Jew.[5] For all that, he surely had a

[3] Sudhoff, 'Daniels von Morley Liber de Naturis Inferiorum et Superiorum', pp. 40ff.

[4] This topic will be dealt with at length in Roger French and Andrew Cunningham, *Before science. The invention of the friars' natural philosophy*, forthcoming. For Gregory IX's bowdlerizing committee, see *Chartularium Universitatis Parisiensis*, ed. Henri S. Denifle and Aemilio Chatelain, 4 vols. (Paris, 1889–97), vol. I, p. 143.

[5] Adelard of Bath, a generation before Daniel, was another Englishman who travelled into countries where Arabic was spoken, and he translated some tables and some Euclid, as well as Albumasar's short *Isagoge minor* (an introduction to the *Introductorium*: see R. Lemay, *Abu Mashar and Latin Aristotelianism in the twelfth century* (Beirut, 1962), p. xxx). He was tutor to the future Henry II. See D. Lindberg, 'The transmission of Greek and Arabic learning to the West', in D. Lindberg (ed.), *Science in the Middle Ages* (Chicago, 1978), pp. 52–90; see p. 62. The material brought back by Adelard, Daniel and others was used by men like Roger of Hereford, on whom see N. Whyte, 'Roger of Hereford's *Liber de astronomia iudicandi*: a twelfth-century astrologer's manual', M.Phil. diss. (University of Cambridge, 1991).

motivation greater than the intellectual curiosity that we are sometimes left with as a motive in the diffusion of an '-ism'. Indeed, the motives of the twelfth-century translators are rarely touched on in the extensive scholarship that has gone into this question. This gap leaves unanswered the question of the *kind* of enterprise the translators were engaged on.[6] It is clear that much of the ecclesiastical patronage of translation was concerned with getting to grips with Koranic materials for the purposes of refutation. It was also necessary to work out how the newly discovered philosophical Christianity of the Greek Fathers could be reconciled with Latin theology. Some Arabic star-lore was desirable for the construction of calendars. It is very likely too that the astronomical, mathematical and medical works had a direct utility that explains the eagerness which had made Adelard of Bath travel to Arabic-speaking countries and translate Albumasar's *Isagoge minor*, which drove Gerard to pursue the *Almagest*, and which lay behind the travel-and-translate activities of Alfred of Shareshill.[7] To the early part of this list of Northerners we can add Walcher of Malvern and to the end, Michael Scot. With the exception of Gerard, they happen to be all Britons, for whom any knowledge of Arabic was an exotic quality; Walcher, Alfred and Michael all needed the assistance of Jews to help them translate from the Arabic. The existence of Hebrew versions of Arabic works is not so much evidence of a stage in some process of 'diffusion' as of the practical utility of the translated works to the Jews as much as to the Christians.

The third lesson is that little distinction was made between what we call astrology and what we call astronomy. We shall return to this below.

The fourth is that the person most likely to put predictive knowledge to some use was the medical man. He had a commercial use for prognosis, and had already developed uroscopy as a highly visible prognostic device in the business of securing a reputation. What sold learned medicine to the patient was the display of knowledge, on the part of the doctor, that impressed and comforted the patient. The doctor whose prognostications came true *proved* his learning. Here in knowledge of the causal relationship between upper and lower worlds was a field of learning that took medical prognostication back to the very fundamentals of the world picture.

This was very important. Medicine, as a service that could be bought and sold, existed in the market place. A medical teacher not only had to satisfy his patients but needed to attract pupils. He could attempt both by

[6] Much material which could be used to answer this question has been provided by historians of translation. See the work of M.-T. d'Alverny, for example 'Translations and translators', in R. L. Benson, G. Constable and G. D. Lanham (eds.), *Renaissance and renewal in the twelfth century* (Oxford, 1982), pp. 421–62. See also Lindberg, 'Transmission of Greek and Arabic learning to the West', pp. 52–90.

[7] On Alfred, see J. K. Otte, 'The life and writings of Alfredus Anglicus', *Viator*, 3 (1972), 275–91.

his authority,[8] by his learning and by his rationality: he could, as indeed Galen himself had done,[9] not only persuade the patient and pupil that he knew by experience and reading about this or that disease, but that he could *explain* it on the basis of a chain of argument that reached from the patient's symptoms back to the very fundamentals of the world picture. An important part of what follows in this chapter is the claim that the medical man's need for a rationalist prediction provided an important motive for the study of the upper world. It was a medical student who first attempted a translation of the *Almagest*. The medical men found that Ptolemy's *Centiloquium* was addressed to them as much as to anyone.[10] Daniel treats *medicina* as one of the eight parts, indeed, of astronomy. The others are equally predictive. For him *medicina* and astrology are indissolubly linked; he who attacks astrology destroys medicine. For Daniel, by contrast, *physica* was a study of the physical world, upper and lower. The process whose beginning we are looking at here is the taking over of *physica* by the medical man, who thus became the *physician*.[11] At the end of the process will be the physician who has been formed by adopting the new Aristotle and the 'new Galen'.

In the relations of theory and practice of medicine in the Middle Ages there was more than one role for medical learning. We shall see in later chapters to what extent it reached the surgeon and the other categories of practitioner and how it was put to use. Here we are concerned with how medical knowledge could also be used to organize the academic profession of medicine and to attract patients and students.

'ASTRONODIA' IN THE WEST

In the 'high' Middle Ages authors did not have our distinction between astrology and astronomy. (It is a distinction made by post-Renaissance astronomers and post-Enlightenment historians.) Sometimes these terms were used in approximately our sense, sometimes in the reverse.[12] Some-

8 The authority of the doctor, gained from his learning and rationality, was guarded by the ethics of the professional group for the often overt purpose of gaining advantage in the doctor–patient relationship.

9 An interesting introduction to Galen's use of rational chains of argument to secure a reputation for himself is found in P. Brain, *Galen on bloodletting* (Cambridge, 1986). V. Nutton, *Galen on prognosis* (Berlin, 1979, *Corpus medicorum graecorum*) is also very useful.

10 See C. Burnett, 'Adelard, Ergaphalau and the science of the stars', in C. Burnett (ed.), *Adelard of Bath. An English scientist and arabist of the early twelfth century* (London, 1987). Likewise the unpublished tract, *The reduction of the knowledge of astronomy to the faculties of medicine* (see pp. 53–5 below) freely quotes the *Centiloquium* for its medical content.

11 For Adelard, *physica* consisted of two equal partners, *medicina* and *naturalis scientia*. See Saffron, note 33 below. See also J. J. Bylebyl, 'The medical meaning of *physica*', in McVaugh and Siraisi (eds.), *Renaissance medical learning*, pp. 16–41.

12 Thus for Bartholomew of Bruges, discussing medical prognostication, it is the *astrologi* who agree with Galen on the influence of the moon, and *astronomi* who prognosticate on

times other terms were used for those who made predictive calculations, such as *mathematici*.[13] Sometimes the only distinction made was that the whole subject had practical and theoretical parts, like medicine.[14] Where judicial astrology was marked out for criticism it was *on moral or religious grounds*, not because it did not work, or was superstitious or fanciful. Indeed, almost everyone believed in 'astrology', and it can even be argued that our 'astronomy' was simply the necessary theoretical background to being able to practise 'astrology'.[15] The contemporary term 'astronodia' will be used here to cover all parts of the topic.[16]

These different terms were being used throughout the period we are concerned with. But the subject itself changed rapidly, from being qualitative and cosmological to mathematical and predictive. Before people like Daniel of Morley were seeking out Arabic works on the natural world, the West of the early twelfth century had some astronodial knowledge from authors like Macrobius, Chalcidius and especially Martianus Capella. It was largely Platonic, for the *Timaeus* was being used as a sort of secular and natural *Genesis*. In addition there were exerpts from Pliny's *Natural History* accompanied by characteristic diagrams expressing the order and periods of the planets, the harmonic intervals between their circular orbits and their ascent and descent across the latitude of the ecliptic.[17] Interest in astronodia in the West stirred before the first translations were made from the Arabic. Julius Firmicus' *Mathesis*, dating from the fourth century, is found in manuscripts in the West in the eleventh century. It was a work that made clear the possibilities of predictions, but on its own, without tables, it could

this basis. I am very grateful to Dr C. O'Boyle for providing me with a transcript of Bartholomew's as then unpublished commentary: see note 55 below.

13 Hugh of St Victor said it was the mathematicians who regarded the superlunar world as 'nature' and the sublunar as 'the works of nature' – a common twelfth-century view and one which would accommodate well the later predictive *astronomia*. Taken together these two halves of a single philosophy of nature are *physica* or *physiologia*. Quoted by L. Thorndike, *A history of magic and experimental science*, vol. II (London, 1923), p. 10. See also J. Tester, *A history of western astrology* (Woodbridge, Suffolk, 1987), esp. chapter 5.

14 The *Ergaphalau* text says that 'astronomy' is practical, being based on the use of instruments, and 'astrology' is theoretical (intellectual and mathematical). Raymond of Marseilles has an *astronomia contemplativa* and *activa*, the latter the making of talismans and images. See Burnett, 'Adelard, Ergaphalau and the science of the stars', pp. 133–45.

15 Thus the Italian commentators on Sacrobosco were primarily interested in astronomy as an introduction to judicial astrology. In general 'astrology' seems to have been a greater reason for studying 'astronomy' than was the need to construct a calendar and determine the date of Easter. See C. A. McMenomy, *The discipline of astronomy in the Middle Ages*, Ph.D. thesis (University of California, Los Angeles, 1984) (University Microfilms International), pp. 182, 522. On the widespread belief in astrology, Thorndike's famous survey, *A history of magic and experimental science*, is still very valuable.

16 The term is used in the text beginning 'Ut testatur Ergaphalau'. See Burnett, 'Adelard, Ergaphalau and the science of the stars'.

17 See B. Eastwood, 'Plinian astronomical diagrams in the early Middle Ages', in Edward Grant and John E. Murdoch (eds.), *Mathematics and its applications to science and natural philosophy in the middle ages* (Cambridge, 1987), pp. 141–72; and the same author's chapter on this topic in R. French and F. Greenaway (eds.), *Science in the early Roman Empire: Pliny the Elder, his sources and his influence* (Beckenham, 1986), pp. 207–12.

not be used to make them. But the very possibility of prediction was scandalous enough. Both Daniel and Gerard had read it and had perhaps been enthused by it to look further; John of Salisbury thought that 'mathesis' with a short 'e' was the equivalent of 'doctrine', and with a long 'e' was vanity and superstition; most scandalous of all was the Archbishop of York who died with the book under his pillow.[18]

The well-known 'nature poets' of twelfth-century Chartres also provided a picture of the celestial world. Their prosimetrons incorporated the device of allegory, which enabled nature and figures from the pagan pantheon to exist and act within a Christian world. The device was necessary, for the planets were called by the names of and often identified with the gods of the ancient world: Jove was not only the planet Jupiter, but the principal god of the Romans. Of the Chartrians we need only mention Bernard Sylvestris, for whom astronodia and medicine were the chief parts of philosophy, dealing with the macrocosm and the microcosm.[19]

Twelfth-century discussions of the kinds of knowledge, such as that of Bernard, are very much to the point here. They are not classifications of types of knowledge, but rather divisions of a single philosophy. The purpose of this philosophy was the religious one of repairing the damage done to the soul of man by the Fall. Gundissalinus, Hugh of St Victor, Robert Kilwardby in the next century are clear that 'perfection of the soul' and preparation for eternal life are the purposes of philosophy.[20] Astronodia and medicine – whether *medicina* or *physica* – are part of this philosophy. So were the quadrivial arts. Part of the quadrivium was *astronomia*, a knowledge of the heavens and their parts (just as geometry, at least in part, was a knowledge of the sphere of the earth and its parts). But *astronomia* – qualitative and cosmological – was neither physical, in the Aristotelian sense, nor mathematical and predictive in the sense that was to become clear from Arabic sources. Indeed, the nature of the quadrivium in general in the twelfth century is not entirely clear. There is a presumed prehistory in classical culture, particularly in late antique Roman civilization with

[18] For Bernard see Stock, *Myth and science*, esp. p. 26. The pre-Aristotelian nature of these views appears particularly in the belief that the heavenly bodies are animated and that they are composed of the four elements (views shared to a greater or lesser degree by Adelard, William of Conches and Raymond of Marseilles). See Lemay, *Abu Mashar*, and Thorndike, *A history of magic and experimental science*, vol. II, pp. 40, 56. Also useful, particularly on the relationship between the idea of nature and of law, is B. Stock, 'Science, technology and economic progress in the early Middle Ages', in D. Lindberg (ed.), *Science in the Middle Ages*, pp. 1–51.

[19] For Bernard Sylvester (more correctly Sylvestris) see P. Dronke (ed.), *Bernardus Sylvestris Cosmographia* (Leiden, 1978).

[20] D. Gundissalinus, *De divisione philosophiae*, in C. Baeumker and G. F. von Hertling (eds.), *Beiträge der Philosophie des Mittelalters* (Münster, 1906), vol. IV; C. H. Buttimer (ed.), *Hugonis de Sancto Victore Didascalicon. De studio legendi*, Studies in Medieval and Renaissance Latin, 10 (Washington DC, 1939); R. Kilwardby, *De ortu scientiarum*, ed. A. G. Judy (Toronto, 1976).

Boethius and Cassiodorus. There seems to be continuation with Isidore. But all this may be a construction of the newly vigorous schools of the twelfth century. The twelfth-century division-of-the-sciences literature, associated with and sometimes emanating from the schools, has an air of unreality. Gundissalinus gives an idealized system. Hugh of St Victor may well have been promoting the school at St Victor. All may have been involved with finding a formula with a Church that needed to control teaching, for which a history of the subject could have functioned as a partial justification. There is evidence[21] that some form of the quadrivium was taught in the early University of Paris and examined by the chancellor, but it is unlikely to have been in any thoroughgoing sense, either physical in the Aristotelian sense or mathematical and predictive in the Arabic sense.[22] No doubt some Capellan-Platonic or Chartrian alternative would have been acceptable, and so would a Sacroboscan one before mid century.

So prediction was not part of earlier twelfth-century astronodia. Arabic prediction relied on tables carrying the positions of the planets. These ultimately relied on observation, and had to be changed by calculation to adapt to places distant from where the observations were made. The astronodia sought by Daniel of Morley in the 1170s was being changed in this way by his countryman Roger of Hereford, who observed an eclipse and calculated tables for the meridian of Hereford in 1178.[23] Roger was among the first generation of Englishmen to be able to cast nativities and answer elective questions.[24] He certainly taught some form of astronodia in the cathedral school of Hereford; but, as the English schools came to be overshadowed by the two *studia generalia*, Oxford and Cambridge, astronodia seems to have been temporarily pushed to one side by the early thirteenth-century introduction of Aristotle's natural works, including his physical, non-mathematical treatment of the heavenly spheres.[25]

21 C. Lafleur, *Quatre introductions à la philosophie au xiie siècle* (Montreal and Paris, 1988). The introductions discussed by Lafleur are partly examination guides.

22 It is unlikely that the Church would have encouraged predictive astronodia, and the physical works of Aristotle were banned in Paris in 1210 and 1215.

23 See for instance the MSS in Cambridge University Library I.11.1 and Gg.6.3; Oxford, Bodley, Selden supra 76. For a preliminary interpretation of Roger see Whyte, 'Roger of Hereford's *Liber de astronomia iudicandi*'. It is hoped that a further treatment of Roger will appear in a joint publication by Nicholas Whyte and Roger French.

24 A nativity was the act of describing the astronodial circumstances at the moment of birth with a view to prediction; elections were answers to questions posed to the astrologer by his client.

25 Some of the material discussed by Lafleur, *Quatre introductions*, was composed of guides to the examination held by the chancellor. The chancellor was the bishop's representative and granted the licence to teach. He did not need to issue statutes and favoured an education that included the old liberal arts. The university statutes, in contrast, were drawn up by the masters, and concern the procedures necessary for inception into the masters' *consortium* and rely almost entirely on Aristotle. The masters also taught what was necessary for the chancellor's examination, but did so less formally, often in their own houses or colleges and on feast days and vacations. This included astronomy. See G. Beaujouan, 'Motives and

The physician at the time of the schools and the early *studia* thus had available to him two ways of developing his subject, and in so doing no doubt made it more attractive. By the 1160s or 1170s commentators on the *Articella* in Salerno were using the physical works of Aristotle to expand the theory of their subject:[26] finding value in the physical works, the medical men made the effort to go and find and use them. At the same time they had the possibilities of prediction, being used in the same period by the astrologers. What seems to have happened is that those physicians who guided their subject into the universities chose Aristotle as their vehicle. But the close ties between astronodia and medicine did not dissolve and university medicine was to become increasingly astronodial in the fourteenth century. Further evidence of this is provided by manuscript illustrations of the zodiac man, rarely found before the twelfth century and only incidentally concerned with medicine. However, after the translations from the Arabic, the figure took on its familiar form of showing relationships between the parts of the body and of the heavens. It is then clearly a medical illustration and served no doubt not only to prompt the memory of the doctor but to impress the patient. The coloured diagrams, the astrological volvelles carried by the visiting physician and the zodiac men that were used as posters in bath houses were all good advertising for the newly astrological medical man.[27]

The two ways open to the medical man to enrich and lend authority to his subject interacted to a certain degree. It was Aristotle's physical doctrines that persuaded the doctor that the planets, once thought animated and elementary, were quintessential and so not subject to decay. Their effect on earth was now not so much the sympathy exerted by their elements or souls but was derived from their 'aspects' to each other and to the earthly 'houses', a highly mathematical argument that could be deployed in an impressive way.

DANIEL ON THE UPPER AND LOWER THINGS

Having given the bishop a brief answer to his question on the relationship between upper causes and lower effects, Daniel extended it into a small book. This is essentially the translation of Arabic astronodia for a Christian context.[28] The Muslim emphasis on the unreachability of God enabled Arabic astronodia to be very deterministic. Avicenna, for example, had

opportunities for science in the medieval university', in A. Crombie (ed.), *Scientific change* (London, 1963), pp. 219–36.

26 Birkenmajer, 'Le rôle joué par les médecins'.

27 For details see C. W. Clark, *The zodiac man in medieval medical astrology*, Ph.D. diss. (University of Colorado, 1979).

28 Raymond of Marseilles similarly used Albumasar's texts and adapted them to Christian purposes, claiming, for example, that the sun stopped at the birth of Christ. Lemay, *Abu Mashar*, p. 141; Clark, *The zodiac man*, p. 239.

taught that God created only the outermost sphere or intelligence, which then created all below it, in a necessary fashion: God was not concerned with the particulars of creation.[29] Such a view could not be sustained in the Christian West, and Daniel, whose hesitations over determinism we have already met, found it necessary to establish the proper creational framework for his account. First defending his use of pagan philosophy with the story of the Egyptian gold, he sets out the Christian view of the world as created directly by God as the habitation of man. God's wisdom and bounty to man, says Daniel, are evident everywhere. The world, the *aula mundi*, is the image of God's will. That is, God uses the mechanisms of upper to lower causality to achieve what he wishes: nothing could be more directly opposed to deterministic Arabic astronodia.[30]

It is in this way that Daniel's astronodia is a complete account of the heavens and earth. It is introduced as a complete philosophy of God and his works, like the philosophy of other twelfth-century writers mentioned above, and like theirs has the overall purpose of remedying the natural defect of man's condition (in this case that he is partly corporeal). It also becomes a point of doctrine for Daniel that the world is not eternal (which would have been the Aristotelian position of some of his Arabic sources) and that God created it not by rearranging pre-existing matter (the Platonic position within surviving Western astronodial sources) but by creation *ex nihilo*. Daniel's knowledge of Aristotle's physical works is mostly second-hand,[31] and we would not agree with his analysis of Aristotelian causality; but it is important for his account that God created upper and lower realms together, so that the flowing down of causes from the higher has been the mode of God expressing his will from the start. The law that God gave for the continuation of the process is Nature.

Daniel frequently refers to the *physici*, whose concern with the physical world dealt with this point where the attractions of the old Western Platonic explanation of the world were being rivalled by the attractions of Arabic astronodia and its still largely hidden Aristotelian component.[32] As observed above, it seems that it was the business of the *physici* that the medical men took up when turning themselves into physicians. The important connection between the concerns of the *physici* and the *medici* that Daniel makes, following Albumasar, is to establish that the moon is not only an important celestial body for the *physici*, but the signifier of the

[29] See, for example, J. Weisheipl, 'Aristotle's concept of nature: Avicenna and Aquinas', in L. D. Roberts (ed.), *Approaches to nature in the Middle Ages* (New York, 1972).

[30] Islamic astronodia also had to be recalculated in terms of the Christian calendar; and the starting point for the Great Conjunctions was calculated back to the moment of Creation.

[31] Birkenmajer, 'Le rôle joué par les médecins', p. 3.

[32] Daniel quotes Albumasar freely, and it is likely that his knowledge of Aristotelian doctrines comes from the almost wholly unacknowledged use of them by Albumasar and others. Despite Lemay's emphasis on Albumasar as a vehicle of Aristotelianism into the West, very few western readers would have identified the Greek source of the doctrines. See Lemay, *Abu Mashar*.

querent (the client) in judicial astrology, and in addition the signifier of the acutely ill patient. This enabled the medical man to bring into the equation the Galenic rationale and calculation of the Hippocratic critical days. As Daniel sees, it is in the calculation of critical days that astronodia and medicine were indissolubly linked. It is here that he says that to attack the one is to destroy the other.

Daniel's astronodia moves without distinction from the physical description of the heavens (in which the ultimately Aristotelian spheres are combined with mathematical epicycles) and the great terrestrial circles to the medically important correlation between the signs of the zodiac and the parts of the body and between the planets and bodily functions. He does not enlarge upon the list of correlations he supplies, but it is clear the interest is in the *necessary* connection, giving the possessor of such knowledge the practical power of prediction.

THE 'ASTRONOMY OF HIPPOCRATES'

In treating the moon in this way Daniel was partly depending on an earlier and non-predictive medical planet-lore. Twelfth-century medical men like Maurus, in Salerno,[33] believed that Hippocrates had not only recommended that medical men should know astronodia, but that he had himself written a text on the subject. That Hippocrates himself should be seen to endorse astronodia was no doubt an additional reason for the medical man to be interested in acquiring further astronodial knowledge. This *Astronomia Ypocratis*,[34] apparently well known before Maurus, is not, therefore, predictive in the way that later medical astrology is. It is not concerned with the planets, their aspects and positions, but with the position of the moon in cases of illness. The reasoning here is that the moon clearly causes the sea to swell up – an effect taken to be greater at the full moon – and that there is a monthly periodicity in the growth of blood, leading to superfluity. As a cardinal humour the blood has a direct effect on the other three. Since the moon is held to be the cause of these things, then the celestial circumstances in which the moon finds itself reflect also upon the effect of which it is the cause, that is, the behaviour of the humours in illness.

Thus, should a disease begin when the moon is in Aries, together with the sun or Mars, then the patient's condition reflects the fact. His disease will be in his head, since – as the medieval zodiac figures demonstrate – Aries has control of the head (see Figures 1 and 2). It will be a hot disease because of

[33] M. H. Saffron, 'Maurus of Salerno. Twelfth-century "Optimus physicus", with his Commentary on the *Prognostics* of Hippocrates', *Transactions of the American Philosophical Society*, new series, 62: 1 (1972), 5–104, at 55.

[34] Included in the *Regimen sanitatis* of Magninus Mediolanensis (Lyons, ?1505), unpaginated. Maurus refers to other commentators who said that Hippocrates encouraged the use of astrology. The text has an editorial beginning which suggests that it was written round a remark by Hippocrates that the physician should look at the moon when it is full because the blood and the medulla increase and all things grow on earth and the sea increases.

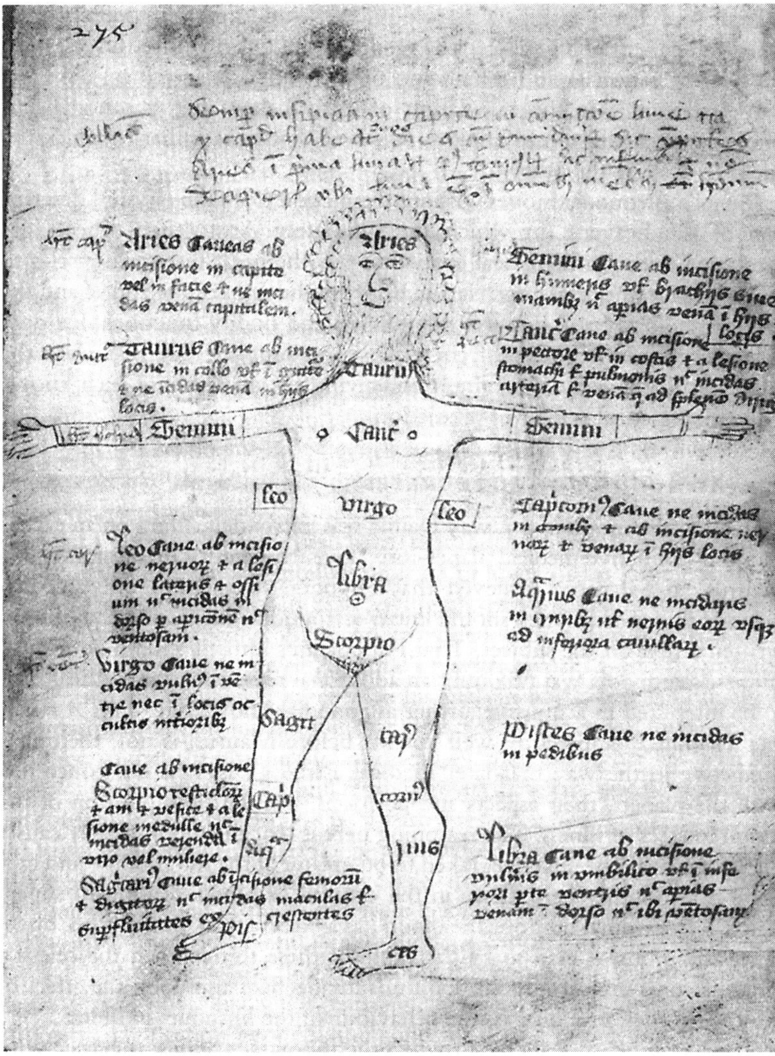

Figure 1 Zodiac man from a French *Miscellanea Medica* of the early fourteenth century.

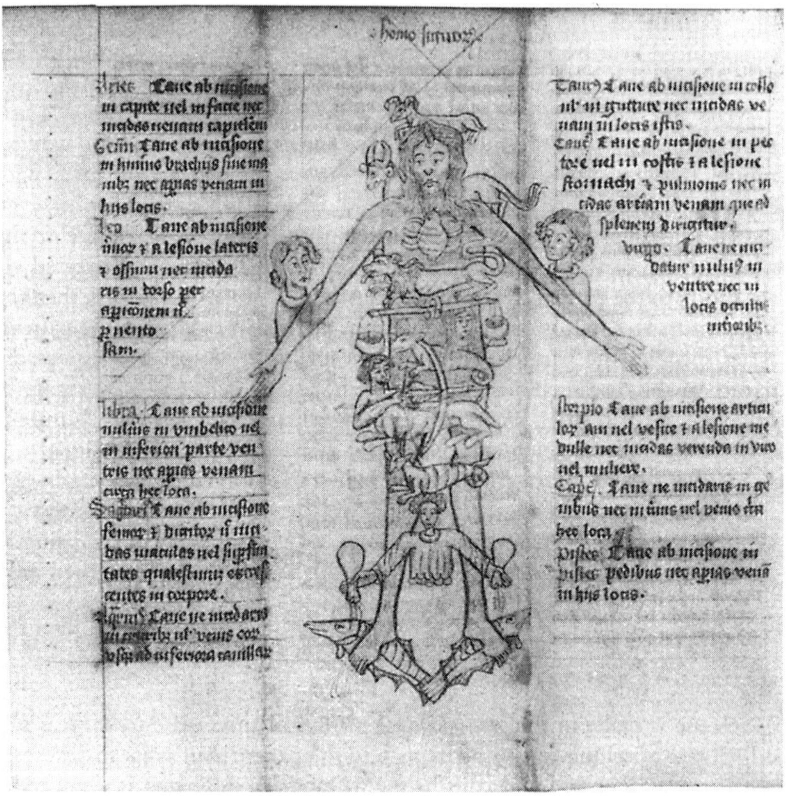

Figure 2 Zodiac man from a fifteenth-century calendar.

As in the case of the 'blood-letting men' (see figs. 4, 5 and 6 of Chapter 4 below) there was a standard 'zodiac man' illustration with a traditional text. The names (or pictures) of the signs of the zodiac are written on the human figure and the figure is surrounded by twelve sentences each headed by the name of a sign. These sentences offer surgical advice, that is, not to incise a part of the body when its corresponding sign was astrologically significant.

These figures are closely related to the phlebotomy figures, not only in the characteristics of the human figure, but because the astrological impediments to surgery applied also to blood-letting. These captions routinely advise when not to let blood. Like the phlebotomy figures, these do not represent the learned medicine of the early universities but an older and alternative tradition.

the warmth of the sun or of Mars. The treatment is to reduce the sun-induced heat by reducing the more readily available hot humour, the blood, and by the use of a 'cold' diet.

Mars and Saturn were regarded as evil planets – the Infortunes. Their position in regard to the moon was therefore critical. Should the waxing moon, drawing the disbalance of humours with her, be in Aries with Saturn and Mars, then the patient would die in seven days. That is, seven days is a quarter of a month and the moon is at 45 degrees or 'square' to the sun. This is a bad aspect and the full power of the Infortunes is exerted via the moon to the patient. If the moon in Aries is at square to Saturn, then the patient survives, but is driven mad: again the moon represents the patient, Aries specifies the part of the body, the planet in aspect determines the nature of the disease and the nature of the aspect determines its strength. Likewise the terrestrial, secondary cause, the excess of a particular humour, is determined by the elementary qualities of the planets and the signs.

In other words, the 'astrology of Hippocrates' is medical astronodia at a fairly simple and early level: the planets have their effect by elementary sympathies and by virtue of only the simplest relational positions: being in the same sign or at square. Such calculations as it uses are concerned only with critical days.

MAURUS ON THE *PROGNOSTICS*

Much use is made in the *Astronomia Ypocratis* of the future tense. It is not only a case of telling what will happen to the patient, but what the cause of the disease will be and what the disease will look like. That is, it seems to be a device for dealing with the patient unseen. Just as the doctor was expected to be able to say everything about a distant patient from a sample of his urine, so here what is on display and on trial is the doctor's use of technical knowledge. What we are seeing here is the sale of *rational* medicine: the doctor impresses his patient with a display of erudition that links the patient to the very workings of the world; the doctor proves his knowledge by the outcome of his prediction. Maurus, discussing prognostication, expressly says that one of its benefits is that the doctor collects 'praise and glory'.[35]

Maurus' commentary on the Hippocratic *Prognostics* is related in some ways to the *Astronomia Ypocratis*. Both texts are based on the motion of the moon; but Maurus does not describe the qualities of the planets, their aspects or relationship to parts of the body. He is in fact writing a tract on critical days. The Hippocratic authors had written that crisis in a fever happens most often at fixed times, such as the seventh, fourteenth or twentieth days, but had studiously avoided giving any reason for it. Any *rationalist* doctor, explaining and impressing his patient with natural

[35] Saffron, 'Maurus of Salerno', p. 22: *laus* and *gloria*.

reasoning, had to have an explanation for this fixed periodicity. The great rationalist himself, Galen, was clearly exercised to find a rationale, and so were our twelfth-century doctors.

Maurus' problem is to explain how in fever the twentieth day is critical, since a periodicity of a week would suggest the twenty-first. (He also wants to include an explanation of why sanguineous and phlegmatic apostemes erupt on the twentieth day, bilious on the fortieth and melancholic on the sixtieth.) His explanation consists of a brief introduction to astronomical calculation. He distinguishes between a solar week (one fifty-second of 365¼) and a lunar week (one quarter of the 29½ days it takes the moon to move across the zodiac). The first calculation gives him a week of six days and sixteen hours, three of which weeks are short enough to approximate to three weeks of normal speech each consisting of seven whole days. (It also comes close enough to explain the periodicity of the rupture of apostemes, allowing for some Hippocratic inconsistency.)

Maurus also had a doctrine of daily dominance of the humours which was his own invention.[36] Maurus divided the day into four six-hourly parts, during each of which a different humour became dominant in the body in accordance with the dominating elementary qualities of the ambient air. The doctrine was significant for his practice of bleeding, purging and so on, but it is not directly astronodial.

JUDICIAL ASTROLOGY

A man who was ill at the time of Maurus and later might well not have had the opportunity to seek Salernitan help. If there was no medical help available he might go instead to a practising astrologer. Such a man had a number of ways of predicting what would happen, even if he did not, in his own trade, have remedies to suggest. His predictions, later adopted by medicine, were now more mathematical and planetary than the early medical astrology based on the moon and the calculations for critical days.

The astrologer depended on a system of Houses of the heavens. This was essentially a grid that divided the sky up into twelve parts. The grid was fixed in relation to the earth by the points at which the ecliptic joined the horizon – broadly speaking where the sun rose and set, the east and west – and the top and bottom of the sky – that is, above and below the observer.[37] So the visible sky occupied half the Houses, and all the heavenly bodies passed in twenty-four hours through the twelve Houses. Each House, being terrestrial, related to aspects of life on earth. Family, fortune, friends all belonged to their proper Houses. This grid of Houses was the

[36] At least according to Gentile da Foligno, whom we shall meet below.

[37] The seasonal variation in the length of the day and the midday height of the sun led to many attempts to specify the extent of the earthly Houses more precisely. No single account became predominant.

astrological fine-tuning device that could locate celestial and terrestrial events down to a second or even trice of time. What the astrologer did when consulted was to see where the moon was at that time. He also made a note of what sign of the zodiac was rising in the east. This told him which was the important planet in the sky, because each sign had a special relationship to a planet. That planet was then the Lord of the Ascendant, which had a role similar to that of the moon in the *Astronomia Ypocratis*, that is, it signified the patient. The astrologer might find that the moon or Lord of the Ascendant was in the House of Life, or of Death. The outcome also depended on how far through the House the Lord of the Ascendant had proceeded; on what sign of the zodiac he was in; on aspects he had with Fortunes or Infortunes and so on. The astrologer depended utterly on ephemeris tables calculated for his degree of latitude, and the energetic ones, like Roger of Hereford, modified extant tables of Toledo or Marseilles for their home town.[38]

Astrological doctrine, used by such non-medical authors as Roger of Hereford, contained much material that related to health and disease. Each planet exerted its influence over a part of the body, so that, for example, Mars controlled the head, Saturn the chest, Jupiter the abdomen and so on to Venus, who had charge of the feet. The correlations between the planets and the parts of the body shifted as the planets moved through the different Houses, so that, for example, in Taurus Venus' connection was with the head, while in Cancer it was with the arms. These connections are the subject of many medieval figures in which the signs of the zodiac are imposed on parts of the body (see Figure 1) which indicated when surgery or blood-letting should be avoided.[39]

WILLIAM OF ENGLAND IN MARSEILLES

Marseilles in fact seems to have been a not unimportant centre of astronodial activity.[40] Here we have to locate the story a little more closely in time and space. We are in the Latin Mediterranean. We shall find in fact that the relationships between astronodia and medicine are different here from those further north. We are also at that time when the *studia* are emerging as formal and legal structures, in Italy and Montpellier as well as in the

[38] Roger of Hereford was a contemporary of Daniel of Morley and seems have been gripped by the same excitement about the predictive power of the new Arabic learning. Nothing he wrote has been published, but a number of MSS survive. I have not included a discussion of them here because Roger remained to the north of the Mediterranean, perhaps at the school in Hereford. Nor did he use his judicial astronodia in a medical context. I hope to publish something on Roger in the future.

[39] Roger of Hereford, 'De astronomia iudicandi', Cambridge University Library, MS I.1.1, fols. 42v, 43r.

[40] Thorndike describes a MS from Marseilles that claims to make the first use of Arabic astronodia (in either 1111 or 1139): *A history of magic and experimental science*, vol. II, p. 92.

north, and this also had its effect on the relationship between astronodia and medicine.

Marseilles was not only the place from which Roger of Hereford took his tables, but was home too, a few years later perhaps, to his countryman, known to us as William of England.[41] 'English by nation, medical by profession and astrologer in opinion', William wrote in 1219 a little book called *De urina non visa*, 'On unseen urine'. It is a predictive text, clearly designed to exploit the reputation-building potential of rationalized prognostication of both astrology and uroscopy. As William says, the medical man who can foresee the nature of the disease, devise a remedy and stipulate a suitable future moment for its consumption will deserve the praise he will receive. Glory (*gloria*) follows both astronodial and medical predictions.[42] His text became so useful in this respect that it came to be prescribed by statute to be read in the *studium* of Bologna.[43]

William emphasizes the links between medicine and astronodia. Did not Ptolemy record that the Egyptians practised the two arts in conjunction, to be more certain of their predictions? William of course is particularly interested in the links between the medical man's prognostication from urine and astronodial prediction. Both activities are parts of a range of natural operations: William stresses that the upper 'root' or ultimate cause is the motion of the heavenly bodies. Because they are perfect, their causation is perfect; but their effects, the lower root or secondary cause, operate in the realm of imperfect, corruptible matter. It follows that prediction can never be perfect since lower, terrestrial, corruptible things are subject to accident. Like Gerard of Cremona, and other writers, William has here a mechanism that will explain how prediction cannot in practice be perfect. It is also a mechanism that saves free will and providence: the planets provide invariant *dispositions* towards action in matter, but both accidents and determination in our material circumstances can overcome this disposition.

The corruptibility of matter was not only a reason for a lack of total precision in astronodial prediction, but it was also of course central to medical theory. Corruption of the air and of water, of which William writes, was a recognized cause of disease, leading to a corruption of the humours of the body. William has adopted the doctrine of the Great Conjunctions from Albumasar, a doctrine that lays down that the rare conjunctions of the Infortunes cause major political and natural disasters,

41 There was a school at Marseilles, where William and a close relative were educated. Perhaps it was here too that Raymond of Marseilles wrote his astronodial text in about 1139–40. It is based on Albumasar's *Introductorium* and the *De magnis conjunctionibus* in an emphasized Christian framework. See Lemay, *Abu Mashar*, p. 141.

42 Manuscripts of the work exist in astronodial collections from Rome to Cracow. I have used Vienna, National-Bibliothek, 5207; Cambridge, Trinity College, o.8.31.

43 McMenomy, *The discipline of astronomy*, pp. 452ff.

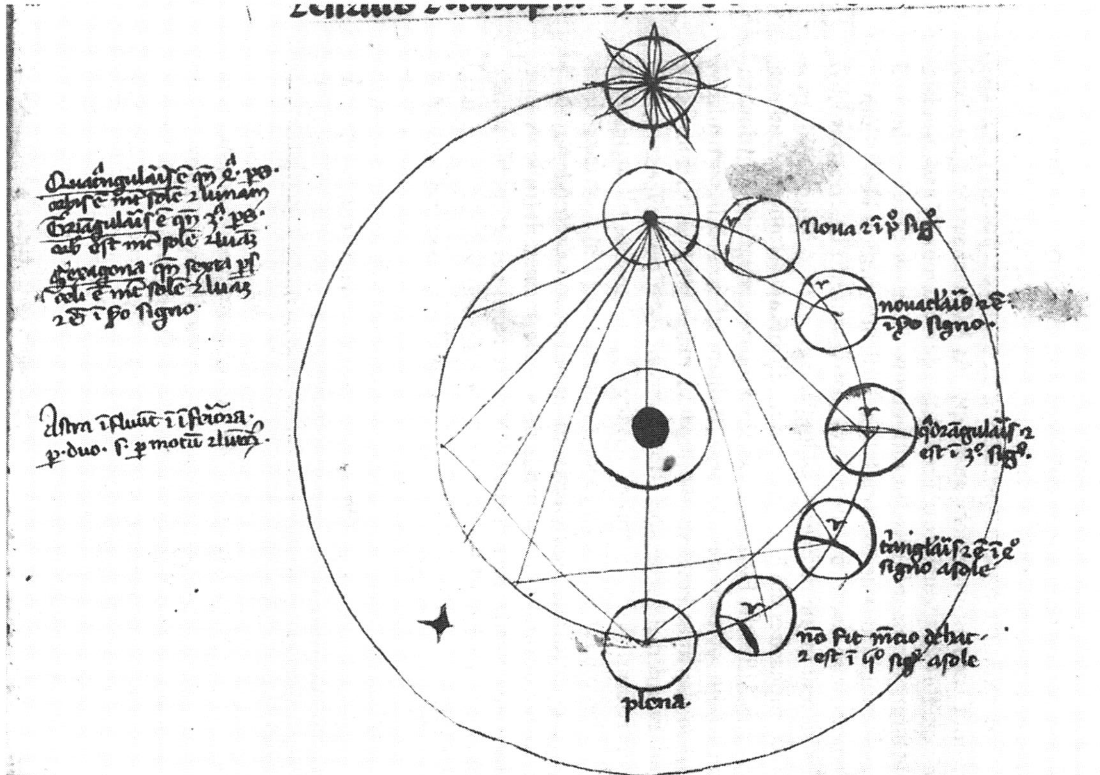

Figure 3 The medical week: the phases of the moon. From a collection of various works of Galen, mid fourteenth century. For explanation see foot of next page.

and particularly, by corruption of the air, plagues.[44] A related doctrine used by William is that lunar eclipses have similiar effects. The moon was, after all, the signifier of the patient and the cause of terrestrial growth. Its sudden and unusual loss of virtue was seen as a cause of evil.

A large part of William's text is taken up, as are many such texts, with a systematic exposition of the linkages between macrocosm and microcosm. Each planet (chapter 3) has particular influence on a part of the body, its function and its characteristic diseases. This link allows the macrocosmic system of aspects and the circumstances of the Lord of the Ascendant to relate to the anatomy of man. In a similar way each part of the body and its illnesses are distributed among the Houses (chapter 4), which provides an hourly guide for prediction. A third link is the special relationships each of the planets have with the parts of the body while the planets are passing through the signs of the zodiac in turn. After discussing the Lord of the Ascendant, William finishes indeed with an account of how to predict, astronodially, the nature of urine. It is 'unseen' urine because it is not yet in the jordan for inspection. But William knows what it will be like, because he can tell the qualitative nature of the heavens at some future time. He is bringing his astronodia to bear in particular upon the liver, of which he is concerned to find the macrocosmic place. It was in the liver that the production of urine was held to take place, as a superfluity from the fundamental process of the generation of blood. In normal uroscopy the colour, substance and contents of the urine told the doctor what was going on in the liver, where the natural faculty was making blood; William has reversed the process and is predicting both the state of the liver and the nature of the urine.[45]

In short, then, William's book represents the adoption of mathematical

[44] The doctrine of the Great Conjunctions became an important medical topic after the Black Death of 1348, right at the end of our period. Thereafter it became a common explanation of *epidemics*, that is, where normal horary, judicial and individual-centred astronodia could supply no explanation. It was concerned with cycles of very long duration (for example 960 years) between the conjunctions of the Infortunes and Jupiter at various positions in the zodiac.

[45] The text by Theophilus on urines was a standard part of the medieval textbook of medicine, the *Articella*. Occasionally it was replaced by a text by Gilles de Corbeil.

The earth is in the centre of the diagram and the sun at the top and its increasing light on the moon is shown in the descending positions of the moon as it moves from new to full. The new moon is the first of the five intermediate positions. The moon between its two extremes is 'quadrangular' because a square can be drawn (and has been) with its corners on the dark moon, the full moon and the two positions of the half moon; in other words, the half moon is a 'square' to the earth. In a similar way the other aspects of the moon are represented by triangles. The full and dark moons may be omitted in calculating the medical week.

prediction into medical astronodia. William would have needed ephemeris tables to know when planets were in conjunction. He would also have needed tables to tell what sign was rising at what particular moment and thereby to identify the Lord of the Ascendant. Marseilles was one of the few places with local tables.

MEDICINE AND ASTRONODIA IN THE *STUDIA*

When medicine became a university subject in northern universities like that of Paris, it does not seem to have been very astronodial. The picture we have of medicine in the early northern universities is one of a common curriculum, the *Articella*, expounded by commentary and disputed questions. Nothing in the *Articella* is astronodial. Since astrology could arouse as much criticism as medicine itself, perhaps the medical men took care not to encounter a double criticism by making their medicine astrological.[46] The picture we have of northern medicine being largely innocent of astronodia has perhaps also been rather cultivated by historians anxious to see medicine shaking off so unscientific a business. But we should remember that right at the end of our period the Paris medical faculty proclaimed that the plague was due to Great Conjunctions. How much and what kind of astronodia was taught in the liberal arts in the northern universities before the mid thirteenth century is not clear.

In contrast, some of the southern *studia* had started life as separate academic incorporations of law and of medicine combined with arts, and it was not a question of medicine *entering* them. Such medicine may have been more closely associated with astronodia than that of the north, perhaps because it found a natural place in the associated arts course. Evidence for what was taught in the early Italian *studia* is very scanty[47] but by the mid 1260s predictive astrology in Italy was of concern to the Dominicans. The order was spread throughout Europe and so in a position to make comparisons: it is significant that it is Italy and not the towns of the north that attracted their censure. The new master of the order in 1264 instigated a new Dominican astronodia, designed to replace the mathematical, predictive, deterministic and noxious *scientia* of the 'enemies of Christianity' with something more suitable.[48] Bologna had a full astrological course by 1405 – including the text of William of England – and the evidence points to growth of medical astronodia only in the later thirteenth and the fourteenth centuries. McMenomy found few manuscripts of

46 For the attacks on medicine and astronodial/physical branches of knowledge, see S. C. Ferruolo, *The origins of the university: the schools of Paris and their critics, 1100–1215* (Stanford, 1985).

47 See N. Siraisi, *Arts and sciences at Padua. The studium of Padua before 1350* (Toronto, 1973).

48 M. Grabmann, 'Die "Summa de Astris" des Gerardo da Feltra OP', *Archivum Fratrum Praedicatorum*, 11 (1941), 58–82; see also R. Creytens, 'Hugues de Castello astronome Dominicain du xive siècle', *Archivum Fratrum Praedicatorum*, 11 (1941), 95–108.

'medical astrology' in the thirteenth century. Perhaps, then, medicine became astronodial only after the faculties had become well established; and this was in the later thirteenth century, later than hitherto thought.[49] The standard teaching texts of *studia* astronodia are also comparatively late; at least they postdate the origin of the Paris and Italian *studia*. Sacrobosco's *Sphere* was written sometime between 1215 and 1235, and the other main source of medieval astronodia within the *studia*, the anonymous *Theorica planetarum*, dates from between 1260 and 1280.[50]

This mathematical astronodia was matched within the *studia* by the more physical accounts of the heavens, based on Aristotle's *De caelo*. This text was part of the natural philosophy of the later part of the arts course in Paris, specified in the mid 1250s and soon copied in many European universities. Natural philosophy came to Padua in Taddeo's time[51] when, perhaps, *De caelo* was added to the astronodial works of the medicine-and-arts course. All in all then, it looks as if the southern pattern may have been that the twelfth-century interest of the medical man in the single *philosophia* of the world and in Arabic prediction persisted in the *studia* and was supplemented by the addition of Aristotelian physical works in the later thirteenth century. In contrast, the natural philosophy of the later arts course in the north was astronodial only in so far as commentaries on *De caelo* became predictive rather than physical. Even this preceded and was not part of the medical course. It seems general that the development of astronodia in medicine was the product of the fourteenth and fifteenth centuries.

To dwell for a moment on commentaries on *De caelo*, there are several manuscript examples of a regent master's commentary being written down, to say nothing of the exceptional and famous commentaries by people like Aquinas. These commentaries are 'physical' in the Aristotelian sense, rather than mathematical and predictive. The manuscripts are examples of the physical *corpus* of Aristotelian nature books that formed the textbook of natural philosophy of the Middle Ages. In the generous margins of these volumes, and sometimes on the flyleaves, is found material that is distinctly unAristotelian but which represents the efforts of thirteenth-century teachers to place Aristotle in a context that is both Christian and astronodial. Sometimes the *Sphere* of Sacrobosco appears. The front leaves of such a volume annotated in Oxford fill out Aristotle's creatorless world with a discussion, based on Plato, of the divinity of natural things.[52] It proceeds to an astronodial description of the upper and perfect causes and

49 See C. O'Boyle, 'The founding of the French university faculties of medicine. The life and work of Bartholomew of Bruges', Ph.D. diss. (University of Cambridge, 1987).

50 McMenomy, *The discipline of astronomy*, pp. 16, 127.

51 N. Siraisi, 'Pietro d'Abano and Taddeo Alderotti: two models of medical culture', *Medioevo*, 11 (1986), 139–62: 147.

52 London, British Library MS Royal 12 G v; 12 G II and III contain postils and glosses also derived from lectures.

of their effects among lower corruptible matter, dealing in particular with the nature of the planets and of the people who are influenced by them. As time went on this process of adding different material to the simple list of Aristotle's nature books specified in the mid thirteenth century was institutionalized. The Oxford statutes of 1350 add Sacrobosco's *Sphere*, a compotus and Euclid's geometry to the traditional thirteenth-century list of the nature books (reflected in the *statuta antiqua* of 1340). The statutes of Paris of 1366 have something similar.[53]

Montpellier in some respects followed the northern pattern, and the statutory medical course in 1340[54] contained no astronodia. Masters are said to have used the subject in discussing critical days and bleeding and we would expect extensive use of it when the new Galenism arrived and the masters had to comment on Galen's *Critical days*. Bartholomew of Bruges provides a detailed mathematical analysis of the Hippocratic-Galenic problem of calculating critical days, but this is in a commentary on the *Prognostics*, and he is not concerned with planetary aspects and qualities. In the south, Gentile da Foligno has a similar treatment of critical days.

THE CALCULATION OF CRITICAL DAYS

Bartholomew of Bruges[55] provides a worthwhile example of the medical use of astronodia.[56] He was an exponent of high scholastic medicine at the end of our period, having taught arts in Paris and medicine in Montpellier. He taught the new Galenism, which transformed the old curriculum based on the *Articella*. He was heir, then, to rational medicine in the sense used in this chapter, that is, medicine whose intellectual connections to other branches of knowledge made it attractive to patient and students, justified it institutionally and laid the basis of common professional belief and practice. We can emphasize again the importance of prognosis in a medicine of this kind, and that no kind of prognosis in medicine was much more important than the prediction of critical days, the days that dramatically sealed the fate of the patient.

It will be useful to compare what Bartholomew has to say on critical days with Gentile da Foligno's *quaestio extravagans* on the same topic.[57]

53 McMenomy, *The discipline of astronomy*, appendix.

54 L. Demaitre, 'Theory and practice in medical education at the university of Montpellier in the thirteenth and fourteenth centuries', *Journal of the History of Medicine*, 30: 2 (1975), 103–23, at 110.

55 See C. O'Boyle, *Medieval prognosis and astrology: a working edition of the* Aggregationes de crisi et creticis diebus: *with introduction and English summary* (Cambridge, 1991) (Cambridge Wellcome Texts and Documents, no. 2).

56 Bartholomew of Bruges, *Dicta super* Prognostica, Österreichische Nationalbibliothek, Vienna, MS Vind. Pal. 2520, 50v–68r.

57 Gentile da Foligno, *Quaestiones et tractatus extravaganates* (Venice, 1520). In this collection, Gentile's tract on critical days follows his commentary on chapter one, tract four of the 14th fen of the *Canon*.

Both were teachers at the end of our period, when medicine was firmly Galenic and its theory was firmly based on the natural part of Aristotle's philosophy. This made Gentile's handling of critical days different from that of Maurus, whose arguments about critical days Gentile dismisses as rhetorical and vulgar in not proceeding from propositions in a demonstrative way with proper use of logic. In fact he links Maurus with many other earlier writers whose explanations lay in the power and perfection of numbers, such as the superiority of odd numbers like 7 which consists of 4 and 3. Such numerology for Gentile is not only insufficiently based on Aristotelian demonstration, but has no connection with the physical world. This brings him, in the company of Bartholomew, to Galen. In Bartholomew's Montpellier, the bachelor of medicine becoming a master[58] had to have read Galen's *Critical days*, and we would therefore expect that it was the job of regent masters to comment on it. In fact Bartholomew's treatment of the Galenic text is part of a larger commentary on the Hippocratic *Prognostics*. Since much of Galen's own writing on crises is a Hippocratic commentary, Gentile and Bartholomew have a strongly Galenic style of rationalizing commentary.

It is with Galen that they base the calculation of critical days not on a numerology that Gentile attributes to most earlier writers, but on physical arguments. The centre of their attention is the moon. This is partly because of the normal astronodial use of the moon as the signifier of the patient and the controller of his humours, and partly because the periodicity of the moon can be mathematically related to the Hippocratic critical days. Bartholomew sets up the physical situation in astronodial language: the *radix superior* consists of the heavenly bodies, the *radix inferior* the generable and corruptible material things of earth; *all* motions, if controlled at all, are controlled from above.[59] As Gentile says, the relationship between the upper cause and the crisis is necessary, *ordinatus*. What happens on the non-critical, or intercadent days, says Bartholomew, has its (secondary) causes in the lower *radix* and so is variable and uncertain.

Of the celestial bodies, our authors say, the sun controls chronic diseases with its yearly cycle, while acute diseases follow the shorter lunar cycle. Since the phases of the moon depend on the sun, the sun is not without influence in critical days, both in this physical sense and in the mathematical techniques of calculating. Bartholomew and Gentile, like Maurus and Galen himself, are engaged in the exercise of rationalizing the Hippocratic critical days. What, they ask, is the physical reason that explains the crises of the seventh, fourteenth and twentieth day? If the number seven is important why is not the twenty-first day critical? (or why does Hippocrates say that three weeks are completed in twenty days?).

The physical answer they were seeking is the one we have already met,

[58] Demaitre, 'Theory and practice', pp. 108–12.

[59] Bartholomew of Bruges, *Dicta super* Prognostica, fol. 60r.

that the moon has a special relationship to the patient and his humours. The mathematical problems are solved by an elaborate analysis of the moon's periodicity. Apart from the calendar month, which Bartholomew calls 'artificial' because of its different lengths, and the 'month' of common speech that was thirty-two days, our authors have at least four different kinds of months. The first is what Gentile calls the month of conjunction, which is, as we can read in Bartholomew, the month in which the moon goes through all the astronodial aspects to the sun: conjunction, sextile, square, at triplicity and opposition. These are the phases of the moon as it goes through the angles of 45, 90, 135 and 180 degrees on the fourth, seventh, eleventh and fourteenth day. From this position, full moon, it returns in reverse order to conjunction.[60] The second kind was the 'month of peragration' in which the moon completed a circuit of the signs of the zodiac. (This was also called the month 'of proper impression'.) This, say our authors, is twenty-seven days and eight hours. The third kind was the 'month of common impression' or the 'manifest vision'; that is, while the moon's means of influencing us, its light, was apparent. This month did not include the period when the side of the moon facing us was not illuminated by the sun. This month was reckoned to be twenty-six days twelve hours.

In fourth place was the medical month. This was calculated by the medical man, says Bartholomew, from the second and third kind of natural month as follows: compare the length of both; divide the difference – twenty hours – into two and add ten hours to the month of common impression, making a month of twenty-six days twenty-two hours. So the medical month was ten hours longer than the month of common impression and ten hours shorter than the month of peragration. Since it was also shorter than a month of four weeks each of seven whole days, there were 'medical weeks' and 'medical days' each proportionally shorter than natural weeks and days. Thus medical days did not coincide with natural days, and so provided an alternative way of counting when calculating critical days. It was also possible to count 'continuously' or 'discretely', the second of which is what we would now call an 'inclusive' week ('from the first to the seventh inclusive') which meant in practice taking day seven as the last day of the first week and the first day of the second week. All in all these procedures enabled the rationalizing doctor of the first half of the fourteenth century to explain Hippocratic critical days, and particularly why three weeks added up to twenty days, on the basis of what we might want to call physical astronomy. The reason for doing so was, it can be argued, to enhance medicine by means of an attractive story about its macrocosmic 'fit'.

It is for this reason that Bartholomew and others do not make a distinction between astronomy and astrology in which historians of science

[60] Bartholomew of Bruges, *Dicta super* Prognostica, fol. 61r.

could look for signs of emancipation of science from superstition. Bartholomew's purpose is rather to strengthen medicine with knowledge about the natural world. The very sun and moon are vitally important in medical matters, as in the world at large. The sun makes the seasons and causes animals to generate, as Bartholomew read in Aristotle. The moon causes the tides, menstruation and swelling of the brain. The primary mechanism of this causation is the light of the moon, which varies as the moon passes through different aspects to the sun. In describing the moon's motion round the zodiac, Bartholomew passes without hesitation into what we would call astrology. He does not have this distinction, and indeed for him it is the *astronomi*[61] who predict and the *astrologi* who study the active influence of the moon. According to Bartholomew, it is not only the relative amount of light sent to us by the moon that determines the course of a disease, but whether the moon, when the disease began, was in a sign together with a Fortune – Jupiter, Mercury or Venus – or an Infortune, Mars or Saturn.[62] Bartholomew proceeds to nativities with the same confidence. If a man is born, he says, when there is a Fortune in Aries and an Infortune in Taurus, then his disposition will be good when the moon – as always, his signifier – moves into Aries or into one of the two signs having the good aspect of square to Aries. For similar reasons his disposition will be bad when the moon enters Taurus, and these reasons govern the course of a disease that starts at an identifiable moment.

Bartholomew claims that most of this can be found in Galen, and it is at this point, he says, that Galen becomes oblique in his language. Having given here, he says, what the good medical man needs, Bartholomew recommends that anyone who wishes to understand what Galen is being obscure about should study *astrologia*. But Bartholomew is not separating medical knowledge from superstition, but recognizing there are practitioners of prediction – he calls them again *astronomi* – who are not medical men. The medical man should be prepared, he says, to accept from the *astronomi* what is established in their field. The difference between the two kinds of prediction is that 'astronomical' prognostication concerns only the future influence of the planets – what Gerard of Cremona would have called the necessary forming of a disposition – while the medical man has to balance the strength of the disease against that of the influence of the planets.

THE *REDUCTION OF THE KNOWLEDGE OF ASTRONOMY TO THE MEDICAL FACULTIES*

This unpublished text represents a further degree of integration of the theory of medicine with that of astronodia.[63] It was written probably in the

[61] Bartholomew of Bruges, *Dicta super* Prognostica, fol. 61v.

[62] Bartholomew of Bruges, *Dicta super* Prognostica, fol. 62r.

[63] I have used Cambridge, Trinity College, MS o.8.31, fols. 132v–133v. L. Thorndike and P. Kibre, *A catalogue of incipits of mediaeval scientific writings in Latin*, 2nd edn (London,

early fourteenth century, and certainly after the time of Bernard of Gordon, whose book on prognostics it cites. It comes, that is, from the time when the 'new Galenism' of the fourteenth century had been developed, and its doctrines bind up the Galenic system of faculties with astronodial systems.

The author justifies his work by Hippocrates' recommendations of prognostication and on Bernard de Gordon's observation that the medical man is expected, whether he likes it or not, to know the nature and complexions of the signs and planets. As in the *Astronomia Ypocratis* and our other sources, the moon is the most important of the planets, not because of its size but because it is closer to us. 'Nature and complexions' of the signs and planets are the key to this marriage of medicine and astronodia, because the four Galenic faculties are also said to have qualitative causes. The faculty of attraction is in this way said to achieve its works by the hot and the dry, that of retention by cold and dry. The digestive is correspondingly warm and wet and the expulsive cold and wet. In this way the four faculties correspond to the four sets of 'trigons' or 'triplicities', each of which is a group of three signs having two elementary qualities in common. The hot and dry attractive virtue thus corresponds to Aries, Leo and Sagittarius, the hot and dry signs. In a similar fashion Taurus, Virgo and Capricorn control the retentive faculty, Gemini, Libra and Aquarius the digestive, while the expulsive is governed by Cancer, Scorpio and Pisces.

Naturally enough the hot and dry planet Mars relates to attraction, Saturn to retention, the sun, Jupiter and Venus to digestion and the moon to expulsion. These simple correspondences give shape to the practice of medicine recommended by the author. Despite the relation of the moon to expulsion it remains, as in other schemes, the signifier of the patient. So, when the doctor wants to strengthen the attractive virtue, he does so when the moon is in one of the three signs that favour attraction. If the Lord of the Ascendant is with the moon, so much the better, and better still if the sign ascending is one of the triplicity of the faculty in question. This formula is repeated for each of the three remaining faculties.

In addition the author's practice is shaped by the relationship between, on the one hand, the humours that are to be evacuated by his therapeutic techniques and, on the other, the planets. Blood, being hot and wet, is favoured by the sun (hot) and Venus (wet). When blood is in excess and has to be removed, then it should be done when the planets that favour it are weakened by reason of their celestial aspects. Jupiter is said to strengthen all natural things, including the faculties and humours, so any attempt to

1963), give the alternative title *Virtues and signs of the planets*. The work is found also in an Oxford MS: Bodley, Digby, B Ld 29, fifteenth century, fols. 179r–181. See also the short but learned article by C. Burnett, 'Astrology and medicine in the Middle Ages', *Bulletin of the Society for the Social History of Medicine*, 37 (Dec. 1985), 16–18.

remove a humour and restore a balance while the influence of Saturn is strong will not be successful. Not dissimilar arguments are used for the proper times of taking medicines: the watery triplicity will aid the dispersal of an ingested medicine, and the Lord of the Ascendant, if below the earth, will draw the medicine down. Should it be above the earth, vomiting will ensue. Lastly, astronodially suitable times should be selected for the preparation of medicines (which of course operate by reason of the elementary qualities).

PIETRO D'ABANO

The period covered by this book begins when the first translations from the Arabic were being added to the descriptive astronodia of the pre-*studia* West. It ends when the Black Death all but disrupted the universities, in which mathematical and predictive astronodia was an established and statutory study. We can gain some insight into this change by looking at Pietro d'Abano, because he defended the increasing use of astronodia within medicine.

We have seen that astrology may have been more a feature of the south than the north. Pietro taught astrology (and medicine and philosophy)[64] in Padua, in a country, that is, where astrology was already in demand in court circles.[65] He had also been to Paris, where we may suppose he became familiar with the northern style of university.[66] His *Conciliator* was finished in 1303, but he claimed to have been working on the material for ten years.[67]

Pietro announces his enterprise in terms that had been used by those who wrote in the twelfth century about the 'divisions of the sciences'. That is, he saw philosophy as single, knowledge-as-a-whole that had the purpose of perfecting man's nature or at least remedying the faults caused by the Fall. Its ultimate purpose was religious, both for the twelfth-century authors and for Pietro: 'All branches of knowledge agree in one purpose', he said, 'which is the acquisition of perfection of the human soul that prepares it for future happiness'.[68] But, unlike his twelfth-century predecessors, Pietro's apparatus for explaining and achieving this is Aristotelian. It is to the *Ethics* and *Politics* of the arts course that Pietro refers when explaining man's desire to 'live well and be happy'. 'To live' is the form of the living, says Pietro from *De Anima*, and 'to live' for the living means to strive for a more perfect and divine state: the ultimately religious nature of philosophy

64 See Siraisi, 'Pietro d'Abano and Taddeo Alderotti', p. 142.
65 Siraisi, *Arts and sciences*, p. 72.
66 Siraisi, *Arts and sciences*, p. 282.
67 *Conciliator*, prologue.
68 'Omnes scientiae communicant in una utilitate, quae est acquisitio perfectionis animae humanae praeparantis in effectu eam ad futuram foelicitatem', *Conciliator*, p. 4r.

is not far below the Aristotelian surface in Pietro. Indeed, while he thinks of happiness as an operation of the soul in terms of Aristotle's *De Anima*, and of man's desire to know in terms of the *Metaphysics*, yet the 'happy life' acquired through philosophy can culminate in beatitude of a religious kind, a perfect state of the aggregation of all that is good.

But, continues Pietro, man's basic desire for life and happiness is not enough. Things can go wrong. In a word, *differences* appear. It was his purpose in putting together his *Conciliator* to remove some of these differences, particularly those that arise in medicine between philosophers and physicians. The *Conciliator* consists of 210 'differences', each treated in a formal disputational way. For Pietro it is Aristotelian methods of argument and Aristotelian philosophy that provide the power – *potestas* – to bring the basic desire for life and happiness to actuality. Part of this discipline of living is the need to know the good and evil influences of the stars.[69] It is Pietro's view of the oneness of philosophy that directs his arguments for regarding astronodia as useful to, essential to, and indeed part of medicine. He represents medicine as that which, of all the *scientiae*, is the most devoted to particulars. It relies, then, upon more general *scientiae* that deal with universals, that is, upon natural philosophy and the seven liberal arts. Even the trivial arts, like logic, are for Pietro part of the philosophical enterprise: 'Logic is an organic part of the whole of philosophy, defending us from evil in practice and from the false in theory.'[70] The quadrivial arts, especially astronodia, are equally necessary, but it is plain from Pietro's treatment that his interest lay primarily in astronodia. Arithmetic is said to be useful simply for calculating critical days, and geometry for assessing the size and shape of wounds. As for music, Pietro simply refers to a separate *differentia*, and says nothing about its relation to medicine.

The formal principles on which Pietro constructed the *Conciliator* obliged him to lay out the most fundamental differences first. The first ten *differentiae* form a complete section of the book and are concerned with the nature and relationships of medicine; the doctor should be familiar with the other theoretical *scientiae*, including logic; his medicine is indeed such a *scientia*, theoretical as well as practical; at the same time it is the most excellent of the arts. Its subject is the human body, which is best committed to the care of a single doctor, who should be aware that, for philosophical and religious reasons, it is now more fragile than in ancient times. The final 'difference' of this first section is whether the doctor's astronodia can help cure his patients.[71]

69 Ibid., prologue.

70 'Logica est pars organica totius philosophiae defendens nos a malis in practicis et a falsis in speculativis', ibid., p. 3v. (*Differentia* 1: does the medical man need to know the other *scientiae*?).

71 Not included in the list of *differentiae* given here is Pietro's long discussion of that widely debated question on what Galen intended by the three 'orders' or 'doctrines' by which he began the *Tegni*: it is number eight.

Pietro's formal principles also oblige him to begin the discussion of each disputed question with an account of the arguments against the position he is defending. This is a device of the schools, but it is probable that some of these arguments in favour of a negative resolution of the question were those used by the opponents of Pietro's position. Thus the arguments *against* the doctor knowing other subjects are arguments against medicine being learned, that is, a university subject. They may well have been used by those who did not wish to see medicine taught in institutions that they felt served religious purposes.[72] According to Pietro, they centre on the empirical nature of medicine and its status as a manual craft. Had not the great Hippocrates avoided theory?

In answering such questions in the first section of the book, Pietro is leading up to the final treatment of astronodia. The other *scientiae* are the necessary preliminary steps for the medical man. He should be familiar with them but not study them for their own sake. 'Don't grow old in arts', was the cry of the ambitious teaching master in Paris, who wanted to proceed to higher studies. Pietro says the same – 'neque antiquandum est in aliis scientiis'[73] – for excessive concern with the subtleties of language or of universals discourages the attention to sensory observation and particulars that is so fundamental to medicine. While the other disciplines are preliminary for medicine, Pietro argues that astronodia is part of medicine. He was encouraged in this assertion by his belief that Hippocrates himself had written on astronomia: it is the text we have looked at above.

Having thus arrived at the medical uses of astronodia, what does Pietro say? How is this most particular of disciplines, this most excellent of arts informed in its practice by the *scientia* of the heavens and earth? The answer is: not very much. In general, says Pietro,[74] the astrologizing doctor can foretell the qualitative changes of the air and so adjust the regimen of his patients. Astrology also provides suitable times for providing medicines.[75] It shows when the moon is tempered by the Fortunes. It explains why the effect of purges (as we have seen) is diminished when the moon is with Jupiter. It supplies some rules for surgery (including phlebotomy),[76] for 'it is horrible to take the knife to any part when the moon is in the sign of that part'.[77] But this is not very much when compared, for example, with his enormous digression on the 'three doctrines' of Galen. It is clear that Pietro is concerned with the *principle* that astrology is part of medicine, and not with details of astrological practice of medicine.

Some of the reasons for adopting this principle were external to the

[72] For the opposition to medicine as a learned, university subject, see Ferruolo, *The origins of the university*.

[73] *Conciliator*, p. 4r.

[74] Ibid., p. 17v (*Differentia* 10).

[75] Ibid., p. 3v.

[76] Ibid., p. 17v.

[77] Ibid., p. 3v.

perceived technical superiority of astrological medicine. Some had to do with the expectations of the patient, for, as Pietro says,[78] the doctor must be able to deal with a patient who has already seen an astrologer. It was expected that the doctor knew his astrology, and many would have agreed with Pietro's advice that no one should put themselves in the hands of a doctor who was ignorant of astrology.[79] Indeed, Pietro makes it plain that part of the doctor's authority derived from his impressive knowledge of the stars.[80] His authority with the patient was an important part of the doctor's armoury: Pietro goes into some detail in giving what was probably a standard account of medical ethics, a great deal of which was concerned with the building and defence of the doctor's reputation. The doctor with authority was in control of the relationship between himself and the patient, particularly if he was in sole charge of the patient (as Pietro argues in the seventh *differentia*). He could influence the patient in the matter of fees. The very authority of the doctor generated a confidence in the patient which itself helped him to recover. For Pietro this authority – the doctor's reputation – could be increased in a number of ways. Treatment of the poor without a fee 'generates fame'.[81] His modest behaviour in civil life demonstrates that he is worthy of faith and confidence. And Pietro's preferred route to a reputation is through prognostication. Joy for the doctor and glory for his reputation are the results of successful prognosis.[82] Use of astrological signs not only reinforces the doctor's own confidence but enables him to convince the patient and the assistants, and to build his reputation, says Pietro explicitly.[83] But the hazards are considerable, and rules must be obeyed in order to avoid disaster. The doctor and the astrologer should never be absolute but always tie their predictions to conditional circumstances, says Pietro; the patient must be obedient, and the assistants skilful. Nothing is certain, especially in acute cases; but, if death looks certain, advises Pietro, then change your expression and say with an assumed grief to the assistants, 'Only a divine miracle can restore health'. The result is a prognostication that does not detract from God's freedom of action and which is good for the reputation of the doctor.

CONCLUSION

So what, ultimately, is the moral of the story of Daniel's journey to Toledo – what different message does this way of looking at the story give us? At

[78] Ibid., p. 4r.
[79] Ibid., p. 4r: 'Cuiusmodi est medicus, qui astrologiam ignorat, nullus debet se in eius manus ponere.'
[80] Ibid., p. 4r: Doctors, says Pietro, ought to know the *scientia* of the stars 'ut per eam sciant sui magisterii radices certissime'.
[81] Ibid., p. 5r.
[82] Ibid., p. 5r.
[83] Ibid., p. 17v.

his time, the *moral* reading of a story, perhaps a parable, was held to give a higher meaning than the *literal* reading.[84] To transfer this distinction to modern scholarship: a *literal* reading of the history of translations and translators gives us an event which is often called 'the reception of Greek and Arabic science'. Perhaps the *moral* reading shows us that there was a different kind of historical dynamics at work than some mysterious 'reception'. For, to be able to predict the future gives one power. This is the moral reading, this gives us the cause and reason why people translated Greek and Arabic works in the Middle Ages. If we are looking for causes of the medieval reception of someone else's 'science' then, in terms of excitement and practicality, the practical need to foretell the future comfortably beats as an explanation the desire just to curl up by the fire with Aristotle's *Physics*.

Finally, and to repeat an earlier point, this chapter has not sought to give a systematic account of medical astrology in the period. It points indeed to a gap at that particular spot in the literature and suggests that it might be plugged by a more detailed look at the manuscript sources, some of which are briefly examined here, and by a re-evaluation of the historical dynamics of translation, 'transmission' and 'assimilation'. In relation to the connections between learned and practical medicine from Salerno to the Black Death, it suggests an alternative view of the uses of medical learning in the medical market place.

[84] See Smalley, *Study of the Bible*, esp. pp. 26ff.

VII

THE USE OF ALFRED OF SHARESHILL'S COMMENTARY ON THE "DE PLANTIS" IN UNIVERSITY TEACHING IN THE THIRTEENTH CENTURY

The later twelfth century was a critical time in the intellectual history of the West. The introduction of Aristotle's texts into the new studia marked the formation of a body of doctrine that remained canonical down to the seventeenth century. With hindsight we can see that implications were great for Western rationality, and especially the dominance of northern logic in the thirteenth and fourteenth centuries. In natural philosophy the framework of "science" in the Middle Ages and even of the "scientific revolution" of the seventeenth century was set by the use of Aristotle's libri naturales in the universities.

It is therefore of great interest to see how these texts were used. How did thirteenth-century Christian clerks understand Greek natural philosophy? What resources did they use? What methods did they adopt in expounding their Latin versions of the physical works? Some answers to these questions can be found by examining Alfred of Shareshill's engagement with one such text, the pseudo-Aristotelian *De plantis*. Below we meet his problems with the intellectual content of his text, with the language in which he found his text, and with the resources he could draw on in explaining it. These problems and his answers were all constrained by, and illustrate, the difficulties of using Aristotle's physical works in a Christian society. That is the theme of this paper: while Aristotelian philosophy could be put to good use, it also contained things that looked offensive and dangerous to the devout. The issue ultimately at stake was the stability of Christendom and the uniformity of belief that was a necessary condition of that stability.[1]

These issues were of long standing, and now, at the end of the twelfth century, were brought into sharp focus by the new translations of philosophical works. The church did not need philosophy for internal purposes like the maintenance of faith and discipline. But it did need philosophy for the external purposes of proselytization, and attack and defense against the infidels and heretics.[2] The church used Plato's philosophy for these purposes in the early centuries, and Plato remained the church's philosopher down to the twelfth century. But when it became clear that the Aristotle whose logic had

[1]The Albigensian heresy, flourishing at the time when Alfred was writing, was crushed (by a newly strengthened papacy) only by a whole crusade complete with massacres and the end of a civilization, that of the troubadours. See R. K. French and A. R. Cunningham, *Before Science: The Invention of the Friars' Natural Philosophy* (Aldershot 1996).

[2]A considerable part of the industry of translating Arabic materials on physical philosophy was sponsored by the church to meet the Muslim threat. The Dominicans set up special schools for Eastern languages and natural philosophy to train the brothers for Christian campaigning. See French and Cunningham (n. 1 above).

already been used to construct a new dialectical theology had also written extensively on the natural world, dangers were seen. Aristotle's physical world was eternal, not created. He was accordingly criticized for giving too much attention to the world and not enough to its Maker. "What value is it, Aristotle, for you to be concerned with the summits of the heavens and the depths of the earth, when you do not know about your creator?" asked Peter of Poitiers in a rhetorical question that encapsulates the reaction of the religious to secular learning.[3] Further, Aristotle's metaphysics could be seen as ambivalent on the question of God's goodness,[4] and his work on the soul had little on its immortality in a Christian sense. There was a widely held belief that too much attention to the physical world was idle curiosity that stood in the way of the mind's turning to higher matters.[5] Yet Aristotle's doctrines were uncommonly useful for the special tasks of suppression of heresy and the education of the young in sensitive areas,[6] and the general task of constructing a world view that embraced the whole of Christendom.

A resolution was needed. Before the prohibitions of Aristotle's physical works in Paris in 1210 and 1215,[7] before Gregory IX's attempted emasculation of them in 1239,[8] and before the condemnations of natural propositions in 1277, Alfred of Shareshill and the first teachers of the *libri naturales*, especially in Oxford, had to work out their own reconciliation of Aristotle and Christianity. This paper argues that Alfred's very early solution of the problem was to treat Aristotle as a specialist who supplied information about the way in which the created world worked but who had lived before Christ and was ignorant of revealed knowledge.

ALFRED AND THE ENGLISH CIRCLE

Alfred of Shareshill,[9] in Staffordshire, was one of a circle of Englishmen interested in Arabic learning in the late twelfth and early thirteenth century. In the prologue of one

[3]Quoted by Stephen F. Ferruolo, *The Origins of the University* (Stanford 1985) 254.

[4]It was thought that the shortcomings of the *Metaphysics* could be met with the text *De causis,* or the "Book of Pure Goodness." See J. Kraye, W. Ryan, and C. Schmitt, *Pseudo-Aristotle in the Middle Ages: The Theology and Other Texts* (London 1986).

[5]Vincent of Beauvais, on becoming a bishop, felt rather guilty about his own earlier curiosity when writing his *Speculum naturale.* Vincentius Burgundus, *Speculum quadruplex, naturale, doctrinale, morale, historiale* (Douai 1624), *Speculum doctrinale* bk. 1 chap. 26.

[6]The heretics of course behaved in accordance with their beliefs, and this put them outside papal control. The new *studium* of Toulouse was explicitly designed to control the ideology of the area. The same may be said of the new Latin *studium* of Constantinople, after another crusade had been diverted from its original purpose. The main source of relevant documents is H. Denifle, O.P., *Chartularium Universitatis Parisiensis* (Paris 1889) vol. 1 (hereafter CUP).

[7]A. Birkenmajer, "Le rôle joué par les médecins et les naturalistes dans la réception d'Aristote au XIIe et XIIIe siècles," in his *Etudes d'histoire des sciences et de la philosophie du Moyen Age* (Wroclaw 1970) 8 argues that at least two of Alfred's commentaries, on the *Meteorology* and on *De plantis,* were among those included in the ban.

[8]Gregory IX set up a committee to remove from Aristotle's physical works anything offensive to the faith. See CUP 1.143.

[9]Alfred was also known as Alfredus Anglicus and "of Sarashel." Otte agrees with Russell that "Sarashel" is a corruption of the English "Shareshill" (I adopt its modern spelling). Shareshill, Staffs. is near Lichfield, of which Alfred became a canon. See James K. Otte, "The Life and Writings of Alfredus Anglicus," *Viator* 3 (1972) 275–291 at 283. See also (with caution) J. C. Russell, "Hereford and Arabic Science in England about 1175–1200," *Isis* 18 (1932) 14–25. "Shareshill" is accepted by R. W. Southern, *Robert Grosseteste: The Growth of an English Mind in Medieval Europe* (Oxford 1986) 91.

of his works he addressed another member of the circle, Roger of Hereford, who was active in the 1170s. Roger's interest, like that of Daniel of Morley,[10] was in Arabic astrology,[11] and he probably taught some form of astronomy at the school in Hereford. We know about the school at Hereford mostly from the poem of Simon du Fresne (ca. 1195–1197) addressed to Gerald of Wales.[12] Simon, a canon of Hereford, mentions the liberal arts, the trivium and quadrivium, law, natural philosophy and he emphasizes astrology and astronomy: his purpose was to persuade Gerald to come to Hereford. Simon clearly had an interest in astronomy and astrology and we can count him as a member of the circle.[13] Possibly Daniel of Morley was associated with this school[14] (and if so he was a fourth member of the circle), and certainly the presence of Grosseteste in the city in the employment of its bishop was significant. When the bishop, William de Vere, died in 1198, it is "not unlikely"[15] that Grosseteste went to teach in Oxford, of which it has been claimed he was already a master. The "new Aristotle" was being taught in Oxford by 1209, and thus a circumstantial picture builds up of possible routes that linked scholars, masters, and their corporations. Another link is Alexander Neckham, to whom Alfred addressed his *De motu cordis.* Neckham taught in Oxford and would have been there when Grosseteste arrived; and he noted what appears to have been the clandestine way in which the texts of Aristotle were read,[16] which may be an indication of the problems of the texts in a Christian society. As we shall see, Alfred's commentary on *De plantis* was remembered in Oxford more than half a century later, and it may have reached there by some of these routes.

Although some of the evidence for the connections between the members of this "circle" is circumstantial rather than concrete, it is suggestive that many of them came from the West Midlands. If we care to begin with Walcher of Malvern, the first Englishman to own an astrolabe (by 1092),[17] we can pass on to Adelard of Bath,[18] and the

[10]See Roger French, "Astrology in Medical Practice," in Luis Garcia-Ballester, Roger French, Jon Arrizabalaga, and Andrew Cunningham, *Practical Medicine from Salerno to the Black Death* (Cambridge 1994) 30–59.

[11]The most important of Roger's astrological works are the *De tribus generalibus iudiciis astronomiae* and *De iudiciis astronomiae.* Manuscripts containing Roger's astrological works are widespread. Convenient for British scholars are Oxford, Bodleian Library Selden supra 76, Cambridge CUL Gg.6.3 and Ii.1.1.

[12]The relevant part of the poem is reproduced by R. W. Hunt, "English Learning in the Late Twelfth Century," in R. W. Southern, ed., *Essays in Medieval History, Selected from the Transactions of the Royal Historical Society on the Occasion of Its Centenary* (London 1968) 106–128.

[13]He gives a disproportionate amount of space to the topic *astronomia* and the persons of the *astrologus* and *geomanticus.* The descriptions he gives, combined, of all three, agree with what Roger actually did.

[14]See James McEvoy, *The Philosophy of Robert Grosseteste* (Oxford 1982) 6.

[15]Ibid.

[16]Although he was familiar with medical works and with some of the physical writings of Aristotle, Alexander's purpose was the moral one of drawing the reader's mind from nature to the creator. He says he will leave to others (and it would apply to Alfred and Roger) "the golden chain of Homer" which rises physically or philosophically from nature to universals and down again to particulars. See his *De naturis rerum,* ed. Thomas Wright (London 1863) 2. For the secret reading of Aristotle, see R. W. Hunt, *The School and the Cloister: The Life and Writings of Alexander Nequam (1157–1217),* ed. and rev. Margaret T. Gibson (Oxford 1984) 68.

[17]Southern (n. 9 above) 103.

[18]See Charles Burnett, "The Introduction of Arabic Learning into British Schools," in Charles H. Butterworth and Blake Andrée Kessel, eds., *The Introduction of Arabic Philosophy into Europe* (Leiden 1994) 40–57 at 43.

western astrolabe users, including Roger and the geometers at Hereford.[19] Shareshill is arguably in the West Midlands and it was largely from the west that the University of Oxford drew its members. It has been argued[20] that the men of this circle gave up good careers to pursue their intellectual interests, perhaps traveling, like Daniel and Alfred, to centers of translation and returning perhaps to a minor position in the church.[21] Alfred's interest in Arabic learning led him to translate from the Arabic the text *De plantis* (or *De vegetabilibus*).[22] This was at that time thought to have been written by Aristotle, and it received Alfred's attention just when Aristotle's physical works were becoming known.

Rival doctrines of soul

We have seen that there were grave dangers in using a pagan, ancient, and Greek philosophy in a European, Christian, and thirteenth-century society. This is illustrated by one of Alfred's admirers, David of Dinant,[23] who proved to his own satisfaction and with Aristotle's help that the soul, God, and matter were the same substance. In the resulting scandal David's works, along with the physical books of Aristotle, were banned and burned in the early thirteenth century in Paris.[24] Significantly, the physical books continued to be taught in Oxford, and when natural philosophy was reintroduced to Paris, it may have been from English sources.

A central issue in the battle for and against the Aristotelian texts was Aristotle's doctrine of the soul as the form of the body, a doctrine that had to be reconciled with the Christian teaching that the soul was the means of personal immortality. There is a sense in which the whole Aristotelian physical program centers on the natures of things (not on a transcendent 'nature')[25] and culminates in a study of the most complex nature-of-a-thing, the human soul as the principle of life and form of the body. There is no need to spell out the centrality of the immortal soul in Christian doctrine

[19]Simon says that the geometers used the *alkidade*—part of an astrolabe—to measure the height of towers.

[20]Southern (n. 9 above) 90.

[21]Alfred was almost certainly a canon of Lichfield, and Roger is said by Southern to have been a canon of Hereford. Neckham became a canon of Cirencester. There is also evidence that Roger was, like Daniel of Morley, a royal justice. Southern (n. 9 above) 90 thinks that Adelard had a local position in royal government.

[22]The text has been edited and attributed to Nicolaus Damascenus: H. J. Drossaart Lulofs and E. L. J. Poortman, eds., *Nicolaus Damascenus De plantis: Five Translations* (Amsterdam 1989) 465–561. This edition supplants that of E. H. F. Meyer, *Nicolai Damasceni De plantis libri duo Aristoteli vulgo adscripti* (Leipzig 1851).

[23]See R. James Long, "Alfred of Sarashel's Commentary on the Pseudo-Aristotelian *De plantis*: A Critical Edition," *Mediaeval Studies* 47 (1985) 125–167 at 167.

[24]In 1210 a group of bishops met in Paris on the matter of heresy. The heretics were to be burned, apparently, over a fire of the books of Aristotle. The works of David of Dinant were also to be burned, and no one, on pain of excommunication, was to read the *libri naturales* of Aristotle or the commentaries thereon. It is clear that the bishops were worried that Aristotle could be used to support heresy. Scholars have long wondered whose commentaries were banned. There is a possibility they were Alfred's. See CUP 1.70; G. Théry, *Autour du décret de 1210* 1: *David de Dinant: Etude sur son panthéisme matérialiste*, Bibliothèque Thomiste 6 (1925).

[25]See Roger French, *Ancient Natural History: Histories of Nature* (London 1994), esp. chap.1.

and discipline; clearly Aristotle's doctrines required special treatment if they were to prove acceptable. The question of the soul was a central issue, and Alfred took a particular interest in it.

His interest in *De plantis* was that it set out (he thought) Aristotle's teaching on the vegetative soul, the soul of plants that represented the vegetative faculties of the higher human soul. Alfred not only translated *De plantis*,[26] but wrote a commentary on it. It is the first commentary in the West on any of the *libri naturales*.[27] To write a commentary implies teaching, and whether or not Alfred himself ever taught at Oxford, his commentaries were later used there and in Paris in teaching.[28] Indeed, it has been argued that his commentaries were those that were excluded from teaching in Paris by the ban of 1210 that covered the works of David of Dinant and the *libri naturales* of Aristotle.[29]

The Kinds of Knowledge

Before we look in detail at the particular nature of Alfred's interpretation of his sources in his treatment of the vegetative soul, we must look at the framework that supported the discussion. The validity of Alfred's opinions, for himself and his readers, depended on the soundness of their relationship with knowledge as a whole, and with special knowledge of a related kind. Twelfth-century formulations of philosophy as a knowledge of God-and-his-works provided a place and a justification for everything that could be called knowledge. Even Aristotle's philosophy, itself a regulating and justificatory system, had to be introduced into this framework.

Alfred's preface to his commentary on *De plantis* tells us something about how he saw specialized knowledge of plants fitting into knowledge as a whole. The preface is a dedication to Roger of Hereford and there is a sense in which it is a comment on the

[26]Alfred seems to have made the acquaintance of Arabic while in Spain. Birkenmajer (n. 7 above) asserts that Alfred was studying medicine in Spain when he was introduced to some of the *libri naturales* of Aristotle. Lindberg says that Alfred was there in search of Arabic learning; he was taught by the Jew Salomon Avenraza. See D. C. Lindberg, "The Transmission of Greek and Arabic Learning to the West," in idem, ed., *Science in the Middle Ages* (Chicago 1978) 52–90.

[27]Hunt (n. 12 above) 111. Alfred is said also to have corrected and divided up a version of *De generatione et corruptione* made by Henry Aristippus, and to have made glosses on it. See G. Lacombe, A. Birkenmajer, M. Dulong, and A. Franceschini, *Aristoteles latinus* 1 (Rome 1939) 464–465.

[28]That is, not only in the anonymous *glossa anglicana* but fragmentarily in the commentaries of Adam of Buckfield; Roger Bacon also used Alfred's commentaries. See D. A. Callus, "Introduction of Aristotelian Learning to Oxford," *Proceedings of the British Academy* (1943) 229–281 at 236–237. Apart from commenting on the whole of Aristotle's *Meteorologica*, Alfred also commented on what was thought to be part of it (which in fact was part [on minerals] of Avicenna's *Shifa*). This was used also by R. de Stanington; Grosseteste refers to the commentary on *De plantis*. See J. K. Otte, *Alfred of Sarashel's Commentary on the Metheora of Aristotle* (Leiden 1988) 6, 11. Outside Oxford Alfred's commentaries were known to Albertus Magnus and Moneta of Cremona, in his book against heresy. Bernard of Gordon, the Montpellier doctor, used only two recent authorities in natural philosophy, Albertus Magnus and Alfred (L. Demaitre, *Doctor Bernard de Gordon: Professor and Practitioner* [Toronto 1980] 24). At least 157 manuscript copies of Alfred's translation of *De plantis* are known. See G. Lacombe, "Alfredus Anglicus in Metheora," *Beiträge zur Geschichte und Theologie des Mittelalters, Supplementband 3.1: Aus der Geisteswelt des Mittelalters* (Münster 1935) 463–471 at 463.

[29]Birkenmajer (n. 7 above) 3, 8.

text, like the glosses that Alfred attached to his translation of the text.[30] Indeed, the dedication serves as an *accessus* to the subject matter of the text. An *accessus* was a device of Aristotelian scholarship which introduced a new text to an audience by asking a series of routine questions of it. The overall result was to locate the text's area of knowledge in relation to other areas, and so prepare the student. Alfred's dedication accordingly shows that the work on plants is a small but essential part of philosophical knowledge. Philosophy is also "located" in being described as a gift of God. This by implication put philosophy into relation with God's other gifts (such as other kinds of knowledge) but, more importantly, it justifies the use of Greek knowledge in a Christian society.

Alfred's justification of philosophy is based on a doctrine attributed to Empedocles that three things associated with the practice of philosophy demonstrate its munificence as a divine gift. These are contempt of affluence, a desire for future happiness, and an enlightenment of mind. These three things caught the attention of the later teachers, and comments on them form a part of the *glossa* common in the English universities (described below). But by then they had become standard parts of introductions to philosophy written by teaching masters for their students, perhaps to help them answer the chancellor's questions when he examined them for the license to teach. Such introductions are known, for example, in Paris,[31] and one of them, the *Accessus philosophorum VII artium liberalium,* has Alfred's three items as the third of its opening reasons for practicing philosophy (the first two are to improve the mind and to perceive the magnitude of the Creator). Alfred's remark that "nothing is more honest than the first, nothing happier than the second, and nothing more efficacious than the third" is also given. This text dates from between 1220 and 1230, and so is later than Alfred. Perhaps both took it from a common source, for it is a tag that would fit well the twelfth-century literature on the "divisions of philosophy." But it could well be the case that this piece of English natural philosophy had moved from Oxford to France, no great intellectual distance away: we have met the circumstantial connection between Alfred and David of Dinant; Alexander Neckham taught in both Oxford and Paris; Parisian philosophy students came to read Alfred's book on the motion of the heart.[32] The three items discussed by Alfred are discussed by at least three later French scholars writing on philosophy, and they also appear in two more introductions to philosophy.[33] The statutes that specify which of Aristotle's works were to be read for inception include *De plantis;* the manuscripts containing the work, no doubt many generated by the formalization of statutes, all seem to have the work in Alfred's translation.[34] If the three items with which Alfred introduced his address to

[30]Alfred did not find it necessary to gloss his own dedication, and so provided no material for selection by the thirteenth-century Oxford teaching masters.

[31]See Claude Lafleur, *Quatre introductions à la philosophie au XIIIe siècle* (Montreal 1988).

[32]The *libri naturales* were banned again in Paris in 1215 by the papal legate, but no such ban existed in Toulouse—expressly in order to allow the use of Aristotle against the heretics—nor in Oxford. If the ban remained in force until Gregory IX's commission to investigate the use of Aristotle in teaching had reported, then probably much more natural philosophy was being taught in Oxford than in Paris, and may have been reintroduced from England. For the statutory reading of Alfred's *De motu cordis,* see CUP 1.143.

[33]See Lafleur (n. 31 above).

[34]See Long (n. 23 above) 129.

Roger are the source of the later tradition, Alfred becomes more important in the story of medieval natural philosophy.

HEART AND SOUL

We have glanced at Alfred's use of the *accessus* and the three doctrines of "Empedocles" as devices to locate and justify Greek philosophical knowledge in the Christian system of knowledge in *general.* Because of the importance of the soul in this process, we must look briefly too at how Alfred related the topic of *De plantis* to a *specialized* area of knowledge, the soul of man.

Some time after finishing his commentary on *De plantis*, Alfred wrote a *De motu cordis.*[35] He was almost initiating a genre of literature. A certain Alexander wrote another, and so did Aquinas. The topic recurred in the universities frequently down to the time when William Harvey was writing his own (very different) work with the title. It provided much material for disputations within natural philosophy and medicine, and may owe its long career to the fact. But in Alfred's day there were no medical men in the universities, and natural philosophy was still being formed by men like himself. His resolution of the differences between Greeks and Christians was successful, for his text was adopted as part of the university curriculum in Paris.[36]

Another part of the curriculum dealing with the same issues was the *De differentia animae et spiritus* by Costa ben Luca. This was explicitly[37] written to report on the ancient opinions of Aristotle, Plato, Theophrastus, Galen, and Hippocrates on the topic of spirit and soul. Clearly these terms had to be related in some way to the same terms in the Bible and in the fathers; and in requesting a translation from Johannes Hispalensis, Raymond, archbishop of Toledo, evidently wanted to face this major issue. Alfred drew on the *De differentia animae et spiritus* for his own work on the heart and no doubt thought that he was superseding it. Perhaps he was, for his text on the motion of the heart was quoted as an authority in one of the later glosses of a manuscript containing Costa ben Luca's work.[38] (The biggest gloss deals directly with the question of the soul.)[39]

The central question, then, was what physical attributes of the soul described in Greek philosophy did the immortal soul of Christians have? Aristotle and the Greek doctors maintained that the soul of man had many directly physical attributes, from digestion to generation, which were not necessary to old Christian traditions about the nature of the soul. Were they even desirable in that tradition? Could they be accepted in the early thirteenth century? Alfred sets up the problem in a significant way. The soul, he says, is subject to physical inquiry only in that it is united to the body. It is *only* the physical attributes of the soul that are the concern of the philosophers. What we know about the soul from revealed knowledge is (by implication) a

[35]It has been edited: Carl Sigmund Barach, ed., *Excerpta e libro Alfredi Anglici De motu cordis, item Costa-ben-Lucae De differentia animae et spiritus* (Innsbruck 1878).

[36]See Callus (n. 28 above) 238: Alfred's text was adopted by mid-century for the last part of the *scientia naturalis inferior.*

[37]Barach (n. 35 above) 120.

[38]Ibid. 121.

[39]Ibid. 132.

higher truth, to which the specialist Greek philosophers could add supporting physical knowledge. As we have seen, it was precisely this supplementary knowledge that was regarded with some concern as mere "curiosity" by Christians at the beginning of the thirteenth century. One of the teachers who taught Alfred's translation of *De plantis* in the universities accordingly thought it advisable to begin with a quotation from Boethius to the effect that philosophy was not knowledge that should be held for its own sake, but merely for the removal of ignorance.[40] This quotation was a part of the common *glossa* that elaborated on what Alfred himself had said about philosophy being justified only as a divine gift. Only when mundane knowledge prepared the mind for the (specifically Christian) knowledge of eternal things and a future life was it justified.

Thus Alfred is dealing with a central topic when discussing the corporated soul. In being corporated, he says, the soul offers signs of itself that are visible to the senses; and since the senses are powers of the soul, it is investigating itself. It was the soul that gave man his power of intellection, the reason that was generally seen as man's distinguishing characteristic and God's gift to man. The soul was also the immortal part of man and belonged to God.

It is with these thoughts in mind that we must read what Alfred has to say on the soul. He tells the reader that what he has to say is unknown to the philosophers. He calls them the *physici*[41] and clearly thinks that he is going beyond them; what he in fact does is to show that philosophical accounts of the soul and its action in the heart can be explained in Christian terms, an attempt that lies behind the whole enterprise of using Greek philosophy of nature. Alfred is familiar with a wide range of Aristotle's work and here takes his notion of soul first from the *Metaphysics*. He also uses the *Celestial Hierarchy* of Pseudo-Dionysius the Areopagite, where Platonic doctrines of soul had already been reformulated in terms appropriate to Christianity. Alfred is here addressing Alexander Neckham, just as he had addressed Roger of Hereford in the prologue to *De plantis*. We have seen that Alexander was another of those who, like Alfred, had early knowledge of the physical works of Aristotle,[42] and Roger, like Alfred again, was engaged in the enterprise of seeking new knowledge about the natural world from Arabic sources. All of them faced the problem of presenting what they had read or discovered to contemporary society. We have noticed that Alexander implied that Aristotle was first read secretly;[43] and Roger had to justify his astrology as (like Alfred's philosophy) a divine gift.[44]

Alfred begins with a discussion very similar to that in *De plantis* about life and sense in plants. He needs to do so in order to explain why in animals the more numerous faculties of the soul require numerous organs. He takes Aristotle's *De anima* as the

[40]Many thirteenth-century commentators regarded ancient philosophy as akin to the valuables that the Israelites took from the Egyptians: useful but not holy; to be used but not enjoyed. See French and Cunningham (n. 1 above) passim.

[41]Barach (n. 35 above) 83–84.

[42]Alexander taught in Oxford not long after 1190 and taught in Paris from about 1175 to about 1182. See Hunt (n. 16 above) 4.

[43]Hunt (n. 16 above) 68.

[44]"Est autem et hec finitissima, certissima, excellentissima, post creatoris cognicionem a qua ipsa incipit"; Roger of Hereford, *De iudiciis astronomie*, Cambridge, CUL Ii.1.1 fol. 40 col. 2.

source of doctrine about the soul's powers but is quick to assert that the *sapientissimus auctor* of the soul and its powers is God.[45]

Alfred also goes beyond the philosophers in his discussion of spirit, *spiritus.* The term was of course biblical, sometimes meaning God's agent. It was also medical and philosophical, for the body was said in a physical way to contain two or more spirits that had precise functions. Alfred's interest centers on the heart because it was there that philosophers said that air drawn in by respiration was turned into spirit that heated and vivified the body. The heart was the central organ of life: *Vita cor!* he says.[46] It was for this reason, he continues, that God arranged the arteries, veins and blood to take the spirit to the body from the heart. It was God too as *sapientissimus omnium artifex* who arranged that the heart has all it needs to maintain life.[47]

Alfred's tract is called "On the Motion of the Heart" because his main argument is that the heart is moved by the soul. The constant motion and heat of the heart for Alfred presupposed an immaterial first, moving cause, while the muscles and nerves of the heart are the efficient cause (and the spirits are the agents of the soul). Alfred wanted to go beyond not only the philosophers, but also the physicians. In Alfred's view they too did not include as much of the divine into their doctrines as they should have done, and Alfred does not rate their thinking highly. For him they were merely "mercenary treaters of disease," *mercenarii morborum curatores,*[48] opponents from whom it was easier to take medicine than it was to give them natural philosophy.[49] The problem was that the doctors wanted to prove that it was nature, not the soul, that moved the heart. They argued that the soul, being tied to the body, could only produce effects with the body's help, and that a rational soul would not be unaware of what it was doing (i.e., that in fact we are not aware of making the heart move).

The thrust of Alfred's reply is that "nature" is not an autonomous principle. It is neither substance nor thought, he says, and its changes would tend to destroy rather than prolong life. To see nature as an autonomous principle could easily be seen as detracting from the omnipotence of God, as natural philosophers in the twelfth century found to their cost.[50] It was just this "curiosity" that had be guarded against when teaching Aristotle's physical works to young men in the universities.[51] Alfred, like some theologians, saw medicine as a lucrative profession, and he looked down his nose at it. When he mentions Salerno and Montpellier he probably thought of them as vocational training grounds, and the *schola medicorum* does not mean a school in an institutional sense but is a rhetorical and rather disparaging term for "crowd." Alfred thought of himself as a philosopher, following Aristotle in a plane of thought higher than medicine. Some of

[45]Barach (n. 35 above) 85–86.

[46]Ibid. 87.

[47]Ibid. 89, 90.

[48]Ibid. 94. In his commentary on the *Meteorology* of Aristotle, Alfred speaks of "plebeian professors of medicine." See Otte (n. 28 above) 42.

[49]That at least is a possible meaning for Alfred's rather dense apothegm, "Sic igitur opponentibus facilius est, medicinam adimere, quam physicam concedere"; Otte (n. 28 above) 93.

[50]William of Conches, for example, was attacked for his "naturalism" by Abbot William of St-Thierry; PL 180.333–340 at 340.

[51]The Dominican Vincent of Beauvais also regretted his own early "curiosity." His prologue to the *Speculum* shows clearly how the works of Christians and "gentiles" (philosophers and poets) were to be used in the interests of the faith and to satisfy his own curiosity. But after he had become a bishop, he retracted this. See Vincentius (n. 5 above) general prologue chaps. 1 and 18.

the technical details he describes are accordingly Aristotelian rather than Galenic: the heart has three cavities, not two; there are two spirits, not three; the seat of the soul is the heart, governing the actions of the brain and liver through agents. This is the stuff of scholastic disputation and Alfred covers many of the points that were endlessly reworked in universities in later years. But this was not a university disputation. Alfred's *De motu cordis* was written not much later than the period when the universities were first recognized as corporations. There is no direct evidence that Alfred taught in a university, and Salerno never became a university. While the Salernitans were among the first to use the physical works of Aristotle in their medical theory, Alfred found their understanding of them to be defective in an important way. It was a defect—the autonomy of nature—that hovered dangerously around Aristotelian studies from the Dominican confrontation with the Cathars at the beginning of the century until the condemnations of 1277. Rather than seeing Alfred's contest with the medical men in terms of a scholastic disputation we should see it as part of the broader picture of using Greek natural philosophy in a Christian context. There is a strong implication in Alfred's words that while a *medicus* might claim special knowledge of the human body, it was the job of the *physicus* (a term he applied to himself) to explain the natural world down to first principles. They were of course principles consistent with Christian truths and Alfred's message is that only philosophers could achieve such consistency.

Medicine had an anomalous role in these matters. It was a late-comer to the universities and many, like Alfred, saw it as a lucrative trade and thought that it should not be in a university.[52] Yet the Salernitans' use of Aristotle in commentaries made possible a learned and rational medicine. Medicine was a route by which the new Aristotle could be drawn into discussions about the physical world by other scholars, like those we are examining. Alfred's time in Spain was partly spent studying medicine.[53] Alexander Neckham was familiar with the works of the Salernitan teacher Urso,[54] and had given some thought to the question of who had translated the standard medical texts.[55] Yet Alfred scorned the medical men and Alexander's work on the natures of things is a monastic contemplation of the divine, not a physical or philosophical treatment. While it has been argued[56] that *physica* became more medical in meaning through the twelfth century here we see that *physica* was held to be far superior to medicine, which, like Aristotle's physical works, could be useful but which could also lead to mere curiosity or error. Alfred's and Alexander's views and actions illustrate the fact that the process we are concerned with here is not the active arrival of Aristotelianism, like a sort of intellectual rising damp, but an activity on the part of people who had reason to search out texts, understand them, and solve the problems involved in that understanding, in that society. It was a process of construction, not reception.

Alfred's account of how each planet has a particular influence on the developing organs of the body[57] should also be seen in the context of pagan philosophy in a Christian context. This is an astrological doctrine that perhaps Alfred shared with his

[52]See Ferruolo (n. 3 above).

[53]Birkenmajer (n. 7 above) 6.

[54]Hunt (n. 16 above) 71.

[55]See Per-Gunnar Ottosson, *Scholastic Medicine and Philosophy: A Study of Commentaries on Galen's Tegni (c. 1300–1450)* (Uppsala 1982) 11.

[56]J. J. Bylebyl, "The Medical Meaning of Physica," *Osiris* ser. 2, 6 (1990) 16–41.

[57]Barach (n. 35 above) 101.

friend Roger of Hereford. Roger, taking astrology to be the queen of the arts, without which all the others would be like the branches of a barren tree, goes to some trouble to explain how the new Arabic astrology he has discovered fits into a Christian world.[58] It was not only a case of adjusting to a Christian calendar and Creation but of explaining that astrology was not determinist in any sense that detracted from God's omnipotence and was indeed a gift of God himself. Here Roger was at one with the views about philosophy of Alfred and the teachers who taught *De plantis* and used Alfred's commentary on it in their glosses, as we have seen. Alfred achieved his overall aim by seeing God as the omnipotent Creator who had chosen to make the world in a partly Aristotelian way. Aristotle's causes become God's laws. "Fixit in aeternam causas, quo cuncta cohaerent, se quoque lege tenens," says Alfred.[59] Even in the case of the effects of the planets on the growing body (not an Aristotelian doctrine) there are no autonomous powers of parts of nature (the planets), for Alfred's peers, the *physici*, assert (he says) that the effect of the planets on the parts of the body is God's direct command, as in the case of iron moving to the magnet.

Textbooks

In Oxford and almost certainly in Cambridge,[60] substantial parts of Alfred's commentary on *De plantis* were added to a standard commentary to be found in a number of English manuscripts. This *glossa ordinaria*, or at least *anglicana*,[61] is remarkably uniform in the different manuscripts; and one of the ways in which the different users of it vary most in their annotations is the extent to which they use Alfred's commentary.

These manuscripts were textbooks. Historians of Aristotelianism recognize two medieval collections of the physical works, the "older" and the "newer." The *corpus vetustius* is almost wholly confined to the second half of the thirteenth century and includes the works specified by statute in Paris in 1258 to be read by the prospective master of arts. The collection is generally housed in a single large manuscript in a format intended for the reception of marginal glosses. This textbook, then, represents the final acceptance into Western Christian society of the physical doctrines of Aristotle after earlier bans and purges. It is significant that the Aristotelian text itself occupied but a small area of every folio (a quarter or fifth): the textbook was incomplete until it had received the standard interpretation, which included instructions and examples of how to read Aristotle in a Christian context.

The *corpus recentius* volumes are later and smaller but contain more works; their margins are smaller and contain fewer notes. Clearly the mode of teaching had changed, perhaps from commentary to disputed question, but the texts remained statutory in many universities and the textbook was reproduced in some form down to the time of printed texts and often announced to the reader that it contained all that

[58]Roger of Hereford, *De iudiciis astronomie*: Cambridge, CUL Ii.1.1 fol. 40.

[59]Barach (n. 35 above) 104.

[60]Alfred's commentary appears in a manuscript now in Cambridge (Caius College 506), but it is not clear where it was annotated.

[61]I hope to publish shortly in *Physis* the version of this *glossa* to *De plantis* found in London, British Library (BL) Royal 12 G III.

was necessary for the MA.[62] The texts within the textbook were arranged in the thirteenth century in more or less the same sequence that had been established by Aristotle's ancient editors, that is, the *Physics* came first, because it set out in an abstract way the principles of natural motion, and it was followed by treatises dealing with natural motion, arranged on a scale of increasing complexity. The medieval student read about the natural motions of the heavens and on earth (*De celo et mundo),* those involved in the production and destruction of natural objects *(De generatione et corruptione)*, those of the natural events and objects, including living ones, of the air and earth *(Meteorologica)*, and those of the soul *(De anima)* and its particular powers *(De memoria et reminiscentia; De somno et vigilia; De sensu et sensato; De longitudine vitae* and *De differentia spiritus et animae).* The student had already read many of these before he got to *De plantis,* which he understood the better with the help of his teacher's reference back to the works earlier in the curriculum.[63]

The *corpus vetustius* manuscripts were notebooks as well as textbooks by virtue of the very large blank margins left by the manner of arranging Aristotle's text. This text is also written out to allow for the insertion of interlinear glosses. The routine marginal glosses are placed as close as possible to the relevant lemma in the text and follow the elaborate ruling of the big margins in two or more columns, consequently forming alternate squares in a checkerboard pattern down the margin. The upper and lower horizontal margins offered more space and were often reserved for extra material. Occasionally a whole different text is written out over many pages in one manuscript, and not represented at all in the others.[64] Large quotations from authorities like Alfred, Boethius, Isidore, and Aristotle are also often placed here. There is evidence that the *glossa* was written out as fair copy of notes taken during a lecture and placed close to the lemmata, while the quotations were copied from a written exemplar[65] and made to fit the large spaces distant from the text, that is, the top and bottom of the columns of text. Quite possibly the glosses taken from Alfred's commentary were added to the text later than the glosses of the *glossa anglicana.*[66] It may simply be that the larger size of some of the separate quotations from the authorities makes the top and bottom of the folios a natural place for them; but the prominence they have there seems to indicate that those locations were in some sense privileged. Some quotations from authorities are marked with a drawing of a face, as if to indicate a "voice." Sometimes the quotation is opened by a drawing of a head and closed by a drawing of something else, perhaps a tail, like illustrated quotation marks. (We shall see a number of examples.) Certainly introductory

[62]See note 22 above.

[63]The *corpus vetustius* also contained *De causis,* a work not by Aristotle, in which emphasis is put on the benign nature of natural causality.

[64]Caius Coll. 506 fols. 246–249 (in the gloss on the *Physics*) has a tract on perspective, incipit "Perspectiva cum sit una de scientiis doctrinalis..." and the gloss on the text *De differentia spiritus et animae* contains the *Algorismus* of Alexander de Villa Dei.

[65]See the comment to gloss 63.

[66]This is seen more clearly in Royal 12 G II, where Henry of Rainham used a wider nib for his quotations from Averroes and, according to Parkes, wrote more carefully. See M. B. Parkes, "Tachygraphy in the Middle Ages: Writing Techniques Employed for Reportationes of Lectures and Sermons," in his *Scribes, Scripts and Readers: Studies in the Communication, Presentation and Dissemination of Medieval Texts* (London 1991) 19–33 at 22.

glosses, which often act as an *accessus* stressing the subsidiary nature of secular knowledge, are given prominence by their positioning on the folio.

The lemmata are often repeated and underlined at the beginning of the gloss. Some glosses are linked to their lemmata by a form of asterisk or obelus. Each student scribe had a large repertoire of signs and used a few of them much more than the others, often beginning a new folio with his favorite. The glosses emend the text where necessary, explain technical terms and textual obscurities, give additional examples, and generally make the text intelligible at a literal level.

The Manuscripts

The British manuscripts that contain texts of *De plantis* annotated by students are Cambridge, Gonville and Caius College 384 (James 506); Durham, Cathedral C III 17 and C III 18; and London, British Library Harley 3487, Royal 12 G II, Royal 12 G III, and Royal 12 G V. Royal 12 G II, annotated by Henry of Rainham, has a *glossa* that is basically *anglicana* but differs in a proportion of its glosses; Durham C III 18 has fragments of the *glossa anglicana* in the dense annotation of the first three folios but is thereafter so sparsely annotated that it has to be grouped among those British manuscripts without annotations on this text.

Glosses Taken from Alfred

The *glossa* common to the English manuscripts contains a number of individual glosses taken from Alfred's commentary, which is at the same level of complexity. Both are essentially collections of enlarged glosses without the structural features of the commentaries of the great masters like Aquinas in Paris. But Aquinas may have been making his ultimate analysis for the benefit of fellow friars at the level of theology. In contrast, when Henry of Rainham, under the aegis of Rochester Abbey, went up to Oxford and completed his textbook of natural philosophy by means of notes taken from lectures,[67] it was the simple *glossa* that did the job.[68] Probably the form of a commentary was determined by the intended audience. The well-known master

[67]Ibid. 29 holds that Henry's glosses are a direct *reportatio* of lectures and so show simplified forms and abbreviated statements. Yet although Henry departs from the *glossa anglicana* more than the annotators of the other manuscripts, he uses it in a form very close to that used by the other annotators. Some the awkwardness of the *glossa* derived from the fact that the glosses are essentially continuations of the text and sometimes, for example, nouns are in unexpected cases. Study of the *glossa anglicana* in different manuscripts makes it difficult to believe that they are direct lecture-notes; they seem to have been copied out neatly at leisure from hasty notes made while listening.

[68]Henry of Rainham (de Renham) wrote the glosses of Royal 12 G II (he says so on a flyleaf). He seems to have been supported at Oxford either directly by the abbey at Rochester or by funds from Walter de Merton's will. Merton College offered a comparatively large number of Fellowships to men "de Renham": see A. B. Emden, *A Biographical Register of the University of Oxford to AD 1500* 2 (P–Z) (Oxford 1959). Caius Coll. 506 was "corrected" by "G. de [H]aspal" (Callus [n. 28 above] 272–275). Aspall was a fellow student of John Peckam and his commentaries on three of the *libri naturales* survive. In Caius Coll. 506 Aspall is described as *magister* and the inscription thus probably refers to his lectures or his corrections in his own text rather than to the glosses written on the text.

Adam of Buckfield in Oxford used fragments of Alfred's commentary in his own large and highly structured commentary,[69] but it is less easy than in the case of the common gloss to see its role in institutional terms—its audience and purpose.

The importance of Alfred's commentary on *De plantis* has been recognized, and it has appeared in a critical edition. But some quotations from the commentary in these manuscripts do not appear in the critical edition, and we must conclude that Alfred's work was originally larger. Sometimes the quotations from Alfred's commentary in the *glossa* are longer than those of the edition, but conceivably this is explained by the presence of interpolations by the teacher.[70] They are recorded here, however, for quotations from authorities are given special treatment by the annotator, as though to treat them as apart from the *glossa,* and they accordingly give us more information on classroom practice.

A large proportion of Alfred's commentary is used in one of the manuscripts, British Library Royal 12 G V. Of the 339 lines in the edition by Long, about 186 lines (over 60%) are quoted in conjunction with the *glossa*, generally in large paragraphs. But the commentary used in this way is only a small proportion of the *glossa* as a whole which, approximately, is ten to twelve thousand words in length, or about 1100 lines of the length of those in the printed commentary. In other words, the teaching course on plants in Oxford in the later thirteenth century was about three times as long as Alfred's commentary, which must date from close to the beginning of the century. It was also a little longer than the text of *De plantis* itself.

If we assume that the teacher who employed (or supplied) the glosses from Alfred's commentary for use in annotating the textbook of natural philosophy had a fuller text of it than represented by the fragments, then he was being selective, and we can form some notion of what it was in Alfred's commentary that he found especially interesting. Comparing the glosses he chose with those available in the critical edition, we can see that the teacher was interested in Alfred's introductory remarks on the nature of the physical world and its mixed bodies. He at once picks up the topic of the soul and its powers in the three groups of animated beings, plants, animals, and man. He passes in silence over Alfred's reference to the texts *Meteorologica* and *De congelatis* but picks up the reference to *De anima.* He prefers Alfred's discussion of sensation (as a power of the soul) to the discussion of the kinds of vapor, to a logical consideration of man as biped and mortal, and to some detailed differences between animals and plants. He has a sizable piece from Alfred that begins with the three kinds of soul, once more, and goes on to the birth and growth of plants in different environments and their edibility.

From this point Alfred's commentary is reproduced almost in its entirety, and the master had ceased to select from it. What his earlier selection tells us is that a consideration of the soul is central: it provides a link from plants to the better known sensitive and motive soul of animals and the rational and divine soul of man; it explains how the faculties of the vegetative soul empower the actions of the plant, such as nutrition, and it provides an explanation for vital action in a physical world of vapors,

[69]Callus (n. 28 above) 236.

[70]This may be the case for example where Alfred appears to refer to Aristotle's *De animalibus* by the number of the relevant book: Alfred does not do this elsewhere and we do not know of an earlier translation than that of Michael Scot.

humors, elements, qualities, and structure that is otherwise wholly materialist. Let us examine the selected glosses.

The Glosses: Text

The glosses edited below are taken primarily from Royal 12 G V, which has more quotations from Alfred's commentary than the other manuscripts. Glosses in pointed brackets < > come from other manuscripts, as indicated in the notes and comment. Material in italics is absent from the critical edition by Long. Lemmata given by the annotator are underlined; those in brackets are not given and have been supplied from the text.

The following sigla are employed:

A = Royal 12 G V
C = Cambridge, Caius 506
D = Durham C III 17
H = Harley 3487
L = Royal 12 G II
R = Royal 12 G III

It is especially the annotator of Royal 12 G V who often puts quotations from Alfred's commentary in noticeable positions, usually in the wide margins at the top or bottom of the two columns. He first quotes Alfred's opening words in a gloss at the foot of column 2 on folio 165v. The gloss is indicated as a quotation by a drawing of a grotesque animal with a dragon's and a man's head, its hand pointing to the initial *Alvredus.* The gloss is slightly abbreviated in comparison with the text of the critical edition.

fol. 165v:

1] Alvredus. corporum inferioris mundi quatuor sunt genera confusa congelata, plante et animalia. Sunt autem confusa que sola mixtione ab elementi extremitate extorta elementorum quam prope servant vestigia que vulgus dicit elementa. Congelata sunt que generationem tantum recipiunt. crementum vero et sensum repudiant. Sunt enim corpora inanimata terminata. planta autem que radice suffulta est generationem suscipit et crementum sensum quoque suscipiens. est enim substantia animata sensibilis. In duobus autem horum scilicet planta et animali dicunt vitam consistere. Vitam in animalibus et plantis. [lower margin]

2] Plato Alvredus Plato vim attractivam, retentivam, digestivam, desiderium vocat. Sic enim se habentia desiderare videntur. Aristoteles autem in disputatione ipsam veritatem elimat et ideo sic infert. Et dicit vehementem secundum alvredum *quia plante egent nutrimento non solum ut nutriantur sed ut multa ex se generent. Vel potest hoc dicere quia virtus nutritiva magis eget suo objecto quam sensitiva suo.*[71] [lower margin]

3] in animalibus manifesta Alvredus quia in animalibus multi apparent affectus anime *ut sensus motus localis et huiusmodi* in plantis vero pauci[72] <sunt anime effectus. Unde in ipsis est vita occulta. Vix enim dinoscitur in quo differat planta a congelatis.> [right margin]

[71] The text in italics is common to H, A, R (fol. 193v), and D.

[72] A ends here; the commentary is continued in A fol. 193v, here in brackets.

4] Alvredus desiderio scilicet florum frondium et fructuum. horum enim absentiam illis molestam esse dicebant.[73] [right margin]

fol. 166r:

5] (habere animam) idest eas esse animalia secundum alvredum.[74] [left margin]

6] (desiderio quoque affici) alvredus quod non est necesse ipse enim in libro de anima ostendit differentias inter partes anime scilicet vegetabilem etc.[75] [left margin]

7] (quicquid cibatur) Alvredus cibari cum delectatione sensibili convenit animali sine delectacione sensibili convenit plante.[76] [left margin]

8] (dispositiones nisi cum sensu Alvredus. est enim fames nutrimenti appetitus ex attraxione membrorum sensibilis fitque in solo stomacho. prius enim necesse est ut sentiat superius os stomachi attraxionem a membris huiusque appetitus molestia tristatur patiensque supervenientis cibi nutrimento exhylaratur. Utrumque ergo mediante sensu fit.[77] [lower margin]

9] mirabilis erat Vel secundum alvredum idest cum diceret eas desiderare et tristari innuebat eas sentire. huius ergo mirabilis erat sententia qui dicebat eas sentire. [left margin]

10] <desiderium non est Alvredus visus apprehendit delectabilem et tunc accipere eius species in anima et indicatur ex sensu et ratione species esse boni tunc incipit anima velle et tunc convertit forme voluntatis sue ad illum sensum et movet tunc ad desideratum per illud sensum a quo concepit rem desideratam.>[78]

11] (nostre voluptatis)[79] Et secundum alvredum dicit nostre *ad excludendum illud desiderium quod habet anima separata a corpore.* Alvredus membra enim singulis sensibus deputata ab aliis in aliis sibi similia sunt ut oculi irradiacio naris concavitas et similia.[80] [left margin]

12] (sensus est causa) Alvredus vita sine sensu mortis tenet ymaginem sensus autem vite prestat illustrationem.[81] [right margin]

13] (illustrationis vite) Alvredus *cognicionis et discretionis quia per sensum accipitur in anima species sensibilis vel intelligibilis que animam illustrat. Dicitur tamen quod hec illustratio consistit penes rerum comprehensionem et comprehensarum discretionem, et discretarum fugam vel electionem.*[82] [right margin]

14] (ponamus) Unde alvredus conchilia sentiunt. unde ad libitum conchas aperiunt vel claudunt. [right margin]

[73]Also in H and D (where the name of Alfred is omitted).

[74]This gloss is common to A, H and C. The dotted *habere* between *eas* and *esse* in A has been omitted.

[75]fol. 166. Not H. R (fol. 194r) has the fullest gloss, L the smallest (it omits the names of the three species of soul).

[76]The gloss is common to the other manuscripts of the group. (R fol. 194r).

[77]The annotator of A has placed the gloss at the bottom of fol. 166r col. 1. It is not shared with the other manuscripts.

[78]This gloss is not in A, and is here taken from R fol. 194r.

[79]Lulofs and Poortman (n. 22 above): *voluntatis.*

[80]The text in italics seems to be a report of Alfred's view rather than a quotation. See Long (n. 23 above) 150 line 72.

[81]Characteristically L has "commentator" in place of "alvredus." R has its "Alfred" face; D has a face and a pointing hand and a large Arabic 4 in the margin.

[82]While the whole gloss seems to be attributed to Alfred, what follows *Dicitur* may have been drawn from elsewhere. D marks the end of the quotation with a face. The gloss is also in R (fol. 194) and H.

15] (scimus) Alvredus. *Omnia generaliter animalia que sunt dure teste sunt media inter arbores et animalia. Ut in fine quinti decimi libri de animalibus dicitur et conveniunt cum animalibus quia tantum habent gustum et tactum. cum plantis quia non habent masculum divisum a femina.*[83] [lower margin]

16] (plante et animalia) Alvredus dicit quod tacuit hic de quibusdam serpentibus qui radicitus terre affixi sunt et hoc quia manifeste habent motum voluntarium et membra singulis sensibus deputata.[84] [lower margin]

fol. 166v :

17] (genera dant) Alvredus idest ex genere est diffinitio et nomen diffinitioni equale. est enim diffinitio et ratio nominis idem significans ut hec substantia animata sensibilis et hec appellatio animal.[85] [left margin]

18] (est sensus quia) Alvredus quem quia non habet planta non vivit. quia facit animal idest per sensum scitur an vivit animal. [left margin]

19] (ut animal perfectum) Alvredus. dicitur inperfectum aut quia non habet omnes sensus aut quia non potest generare sibi simile.[86] [lower margin]

20] aliquem sensum scilicet aliquo modo secundum tamen alvredum legatur litera affirmative sic et scilicet cum planta habuerit aliquem sensum idest aliquam virtutem attractivam alimenti que assimilatur gustui. Unde Alvredus per sensum intelligit virtutem attractivam retentivam et expulsivam.[87] [upper margin]

21] <planta indeterminata vel sic secundum Alvredum indeterminata scilicet ad operationes proprias ergo planta non habet sensuum.>[88]

22] indeterminata Alvredus[89] vegetativa in officio sibi deputato est infinita et interminata circa suum proprium subiectum quia numquam in alia arbore tot ramos vegetat quin plures in eadem possit vegetare. et similiter anima animalis in sensu et ymaginatione se habet. similiter etiam anima rationalis se habet in ratione et intellectu quia numquam intellectus tot comprehendit quin plura possit comprehendere. [upper margin, following 20 directly]

fol. 167r:

23] (quia vigilare) Alvredus cum sensus est in effectu tunc est vigilia. Item aristoteles in libro de sompno et vigilia. Sompnus est immobilitas sensuum velud vinculum vigilia vero est solutio et remissio eorundum. Item aristoteles sompnus est interceptio primi organi sentiendi ab actu sensus.[90] [left margin]

[83] *divisum* is taken from R (fol. 194r); the contraction is not clear in A. For the use of Aristotle's *De animalibus* here, see n. 116 below.

[84] This gloss is also in a privileged position at the foot of column 2 of fol. 166r. It is shared by D, H and A, but not R.

[85] Fol. 166v.

[86] This is at the foot of col.1, fol. 166v. The alternatives are bracketed graphically after *aut.*

[87] This and the previous two glosses are reports of Alfred's opinions, not direct quotations. Not H or R, but D has this part of the gloss, omitting, however, Alfred's name.

[88] This gloss is taken from R (fol. 194v) and is not in A, H, or C; D replaces Alfred's opinion with another.

[89] D has Al marked in the margin.

[90] R (fol. 195r) L and C omit *Alvredus* at the beginning. C does not quote the first Aristotelian opinion. D attributes the second opinion to *averoys;* not in R or L.

24] (et dormit) alvredus[91] scilicet cum vapor elevatus ibi infrigidatur ex frigiditate cerebri et condensatur et descendit obturans meatus spirituum et impedit ipsos ne possunt mīnistrare ipsis sensibus particularibus. [left margin]

25] <vigilat scilicet alvredus oportet in planta non est iste ascensus et descensus quare etc.>[92]

26] et ipsum indiget Alvredus. planta indiget hieme ad congregationem humoris seminarii sine emissione. et indiget vere temperato ad emissionem humoris seminarii. quia tunc nec est vehemens frigus congelans nec calor vehementer adurens, corrumpens semen. Indiget etiam sole resolvente partes ipsius constrictas a frigore precedente ut calor ingrediens segreget humorem seminarium a nutritivo et semen extrahatur. indiget etiam terra ex qua principium materiale sui nutrimenti et principium generationis factum est a sole sicut ab efficiente.[93] [upper margin]

27] <generationem fructuum Alvredus hic accipitur fructus pro omni eo quod excipiatur ex semine plante.>[94]

fol. 168r:

28] (cadunt de planta partes multe non terminate) scilicet non necessarie ad esse plante. secundum enim alvredum partes determinate tam in animali quam in planta sunt partes quas natura determinat ita quod nec planta nec animal possit esse sine hiis.[95] [right margin]

fol. 168v:

29] (hoc est radix stipites) Alvredus stipes plante nascitur super terram ad sustentationem corporis plante ad similitudinem corporis animalis sustinentis membra eius.[96] [right margin]

fol. 169r:

30] (sed rami sunt) Alvredus. et assimilantur manibus et pedibus animalis in hoc quod non inveniuntur rami nisi in plantis perfectis sicut nec manus nec pedes nisi in animalibus perfectis.[97] [left margin]

fol. 169v:

31] quedam nascuntur et vivunt. Alvredus coniungit nasci et vivere cum unum necessario sequatur ad aliud secundum locum bonum tamen contingit quod nascantur in uno loco in quo non vivant nisi pauco tempore.[98] [left margin]

[91]L characteristically omits the name Alfred, as do H, A, and D. R: fol. 195r.

[92]Not D, A, L, or H. R, fol. 195r.

[93]Also R fol. 195r. L characteristically omits Alfred's name and has simply *commentator.* A places the gloss in the privileged top right of the margin (and so balances a gloss derived from Aristotle in the top left) and marks it as a quotation with a crowned head and arm holding a club or sword (the Aristotle gloss is marked with a crowned or mitered grotesque). fol. 167r. Not H. This gloss is certainly attributed to Alfred by the annotator.

[94]Not A. R: 195v. It is the second half of the next gloss in D.

[95]Fol. 168r. In D this gloss is marked, unusually, with a large gibbet and a pointing hand. It is also in R fol. 196r.

[96]Also R fol. 196v.

[97]Fol. 169r. Again the lemma is in the part of the text apparently ignored by Alfred.

[98]Fol. 169v. The gloss is common to the other manuscripts of the group, although the wording is slightly different in L. Again from the "silent" part of Alfred's commentary. R: fol. 197v.

32] <habent nodos scilicet ad colligationem partium successive generatarum in planta secundum alvredum et ad calorem recipiendum per maiorem porositatem in nodis.>[99]

33] <maxime radicum Alvredus. a diversitate radicum diversitat arbor.>[100]

34] <(aromaticarum alvredus aromaticum nichil aliud est nisi dulce subtiliatum per eius naturam multam habet fragrantem materiam) et dicit quod causa odoris aromatici est siccum terreum subtile commixtum subtili aquoso et secundum eius dominium magis in una parte arboris quam in alia est una pars magis aromatica quam alia.>[101]

fol. 173v:

35] (Quod autem comestibile) Alvredus nota quod planta quandoque nascitur proprie quandoque per accidens. proprie quando plante calide nature nascitur in loco calido temperata in loco temperato. et frigida in frigido. Et hoc ex natura terre producentis materiam plante. Scilicet humorem et vaporem sibi similem in natura. per accidens nascitur planta calida in terra frigida quia ex frigiditate constringuntur pori eius superficiei et includitur aer quo calefacto aere exteriori movetur vehementer et vehementer suscipit calorem cum non possit exalare et humorem et vaporem attrahit quo vapore augmentato et[102] calefacto tandem prorumpit in plantam calidam. sibi enim simile producit. econtrario in loco calido nascitur planta frigida quia ex caliditate aperti sunt pori et vapor calidus et subtilis evaporat. qui autem frigidus est et grossus terre et aque vicinus adunatur et procedit in plantam. Unde frequentius in calida regione provenit planta frigida, quam in regione frigida et econtrario. Similiter in loco temperato secundum diversas aeris consistentias per accidens producitur planta quandoque calida quandoque frigida. cum vero planta aliqua in quocumque loco fuerit generata tantum simile attrahit ad suum nutrimentum. dissimile autem ut abhorribile repellit et hoc naturali electione appetitu et desiderio.[103] [top left]

36] Alvredus nichil est comestibile nisi ex caliditate et humiditate sit perfecte digestum et hoc ex materia subtili et digestibili et nisi sit digestum calore extrinseco violento.[104] comestibile.

Lenibus altis. Alvredus. Quia in planis locis equaliter habundat humiditas et hoc si assit loci dulcedo et aeris temperies. Similiter et in altis quia ibi est aeris temperies et humiditas dulcis propter spongiositatem vaporem dulcem attrahentem et ideo frequenter in montibus maior est fertilitas et melior. In valle enim difficile movetur aer. Unde ex conculcatione cito ibi putrescit aer et vapor grossus. Unde prava est ibi digestio hinc etiam est ibi humor salsus.[105] [upper margin]

37] plantam unctuosam Alvredus. ad hoc enim ut durabilis sit planta oportet quod bene digestum et unctuosum habeat humorem. Unde ille plante que habent

[99]Not A; R: fol. 197v. This gloss is more a report of Alfred's opinion than a direct quotation.

[100]Not D, A, L, or H. R: fol. 199r.

[101]The text within the parentheses is only in L, fol. 214r. The remainder is R fol. 198r. Not A.

[102]The edition inserts *multum.*

[103]This major quotation from Alfred occupies part of the top and left-hand margins of fol. 173v. It is marked with a grotesque animal.

[104]This first part is also in R fol. 201v, the second at fol. 202r.

[105]The *est* after *prava* is not in the edition, but the text (apart from punctuation) is very close. D (fol. 325v) marks the gloss with a large gibbet. R: fol. 202r.

humorem aquosum liquidum in digestum superveniente frigiditate cito arefiunt. hac causa caulis ultra triennium non durat tamen si ei inseratur incita[106] ex natura incite multa in stipite fiet decoctio et ita convertetur in materiam incite et ita durabit diu.[107] [left margin]

38] (Et planta quando dominabitur) Alvredus. ex temperie servatur plante crementum. ex nimia vero humiditate opilantur pori per quos nutrimentum debet ascendere quod tam in planta quam in animali in specie fumi et vaporis ascendit ut[108] ipse predixit in tertio capitulo secundi libri et ita nutrimentum cogitur descendere et non nutritur planta. Simile contingit ubi nimia habundat siccitas. ex siccitate enim constringuntur pori ne nutrimentum possit ascendere.[109] [lower margin]

39] (semine terminato) Alvredus. idest in sua specie perfecto et maturo et absque putrefactione conservato.[110] [right margin]

40] (loco convenienti) Alvredus. idest territorio et hec duo ut dicit necessaria sunt ad plante generationem.[111] [right margin]

41] (aqua moderata) Alvredus. humore temperato et plante convenienti.[112] [right margin]

42] <aere consimili alvredus. idest temperato quia si nimis sit calidus evaporabit calor naturalis poris apertis. si aer sit nimis frigidus suffocabit plantam. et hoc duo sunt necessaria ad plante nutrimentum.>[113]

43] (longitudine diei)[114] Alvredus. quanto aliquis locus est remotior a sole tanto est ibi dies longior in estate. Unde existentibus sub septentrione *idest polo septentrionali* diem habent continue per medium annum et per reliquum noctem. ibi ergo raro nascitur vel crescit planta vel animal. in estate enim non potest propter continuationem caloris. In hyeme non potest propter continuationem frigoris. [right margin]

44] <comprehendit humore scilicet non bene digerendo in una hora anni et nimis consumendo in alia hora secundum alvredum.>[115]

fol. 174r:

45] eodem modo Alvredus olee vel olive viscosam habent humiditatem unde difficiliter attrahunt. Unde uno anno vacant attractioni, alio fructus productioni, et ideo ut plurimum olee uno anno sunt steriles, et alio fertiles. eo tamen anno quo sunt fertiles folia producunt et flores ex materia liquidiori et digestioni obedientiori. sed non fructus, quia non parum digerunt.[116] [lower margin]

[106]Long (n. 23 above): *insita.*

[107]Also in R fol. 202r.

[108]H, D, A, and Long's edition (n. 23 above) insert *ipse.*

[109]This text in R (fol. 202r), H, A, and D agrees closely with that in Long's edition of Alfred's commentary.

[110]R: fol. 202r.

[111]The *ut dicit* is an insertion. R: fol. 202r.

[112]Long: *conservatiuo.* This is a gloss in H and a gloss in D. R: fol. 202r.

[113]Not A; R: fol. 202r.

[114]The lemma in the edition is loco a sole remota two lines earlier in the text of A.

[115]Not A; R: fol. 202r.

[116]A (fol. 174r) and R, not H or D. The text of the edition of Alfred's commentary is very close to this quotation.

46] <propter diversitatem Alvredus. quedam grossos et unctuosos habent humores. et etiam viscosos. et ideo non possunt subtiliari. et ideo non habent flores, ut ficus. quedam autem liquidos habent humores, et ideo carent floribus ut palma.>[117]

47] <in medio Unde Alvredus humor siccus unctuosus et viscosus in radice cum decoquitur prima digestione. cum vero decoquitur prima digestione in medulla transit in lac.>[118]

fol. 174v:

48] (eruntque ex illo spine) Alvredus. spine numquam fit in planta nisi cuius humor est viscosus quem cum propellit aer ut spiritus nutrimentum in corpore animalis nec possit ascendere propter opilationem ex viscositate lateraliter prorumpit[119] in conum et acutum. Sic omnis ignis et aer in forma piramidalis ascendit. [left margin]

49] (Viriditas) Alvredus. hec est ratio viriditatis extrinsecus in arboribus sicut et in omnibus terre nascentibus quia calor aeris plurimum habundans extrinsecus nutrimentum arboris scilicet humorem vel terreum vaporem ut plurimum trahit ad exteriora in quo humore cum sit multum aquositatis et debilis agens caliditas est color viridis et quod materia sit plurimum terrea, patet quia desiccata humiditate remanet cortex nigra. In foliis autem quibusdam maior habundat aquositas cum aliquantula terreitate. Unde et in eis non est adeo intensa viriditas quod patet cum arescunt fiunt citrina. Interius autem melior celebratur digestio propter temperatam humiditatem non superhabundantem. et ideo arbor alba est interius, vel secundum naturam nutrimenti. Ut dicetur inferius.[120] [lower margin]

50] (Figuram autem plante) Alvredus. Quedam planta magis tendit sursum quam deorsum et hoc quia eius materia aerea est magis quam aquea vel terrea. quia utique aeream habet materiam et directos poros et amplos, prosera sic fit[121] ut fractinus[122] et abies et ideo abies lenis est et mollis propter eius aeritatem. alia autem magis crescit deorsum quam sursum in quibus aquea habundat materia que opilans poros ne aer possit ascendere eum ponderositate sua conprimit deorsum. alia autem equaliter crescit sursum et deorsum in qua scilicet iste cause conveniunt equaliter.[123] [upper margin]

51] est autem prima digestio. Alvredus. in planta tantum sunt due digestiones prima sub[124] planta cum attrahit nutrimentum, secunda in medulla et hoc ideo quia planta grosse est substantie et parum distat ab elementis et suo nutrimento sed in corpore animalis multa est membrorum diversitas et remotio[125] a suo nutrimento et ideo in animali necessarie sunt plures mutationes et ideo ibi triplex est digestio. [upper margin]

[117]Not A; R: fol. 204r.

[118]Not A; R: fol. 204r.

[119]Long: *erumpit.*

[120]The edition has *colorata* after *nutrimenti.*

[121]Long's edition has *procera* and does not have *sic fit.*

[122]Long: *fraxinus.*

[123]The critical text ends with an additional *ut esculus.*

[124]Long: *in.*

[125]Long: *remota.*

52] (figure vero) Alvredus. figura plante provenit secundum quantitatem seminis et eius perfectionem, si non contradicat territorium. Si enim semen sit inperfectum et planta erit inperfecta ex eo nascens. Sed flos et fructus respondent nutrimento ex quo fiunt. et nota quod in materia animalis scilicet in spermate est digestio absque omni alio nutrimento adhibito et vegetatio et partium quarumdam generatio que ex solo spermate generantur. Unde secundum quosdam sicut in ovo ex vitello generatur fetus et albumen cedit in[126] nutrimentum *huius tamen contrarium vult aristoteles in decimoseptimo de animalibus. Vult enim ibidem quod ex albo ovorum est principium generationis et nutrimentum ex citrino.* Sic ex parte quadam seminis generatur fetus et reliqua pars eius est nutrimentum sed ex semine plante nulla fit generatio nec est in eo actualis vegetatio nisi prius attraxerit nutrimentum. Sed attracto nutrimento et aliquantulum digesto statim prorumpit in plantam.[127] [lower margin]

fol. 175r:

53] (Quelibet vero arbor) Alvredus. planta semper crescit in longitudinem[128] donec in ea vel ex nimia humiditate vel frigiditate vel duritie vel constrictione impediatur humiditatis ascensus et discursus quo impedimento[129] statim planta desinit esse. arescit enim. crescit autem continue quia directi sunt meatus humoris in planta, et omnes partes consimiles. Unde humor a superiori pore[130] exiens extendit planta in longum.[131] quia si alicubi erumpit humiditas, illic fit discursus. In corpore animalis non est tanta longitudo et ideo non vehemens est humoris discursus. nec etiam tam liber exitus in terminis animalis sicut et arboris. non enim habent humores liberum ascensum super capud. Sed ibi reprimuntur et obvolvuntur. membra autem nova non possunt generari in animali propter diversitatem materie, quia os vel nervus non potest generari nisi ex prima materia animalis. [upper margin]

54] (Quod autem folia) Alvredus. arbores que viscosos habent humores et difficiles digestibiles retinent sua folia que habent humores liquidos non retinent. [upper margin]

55] (Sed cum habuerint) Alvredus. planta que habet vehementem virtutem attrahentem semel fructificat quia semel perfecte attraxit. que debilem habet attractivam vicissim attrahit et similiter digerit sic et fructificat. [lower margin]

56] (Planta vero) Alvredus. Quatuor sunt genera plante arbor frutex herba et holus. In herbis autem et holeribus tanta habundat humiditas quod materia non potest coagulari nec solidari. Unde post aliquantum[132] tempus in herbis superveniente frigidi-

[126]For *cedit in* the edition has *est eius*; Long 160.

[127]The words in italics are not in the critical edition, but could possibly be an insertion, especially since Alfred does not usually give references that include book numbers, and that *De animalibus* was apparently first translated by Michael Scot shortly before 1220, after Alfred's time. In the case of gloss 15 we have to conclude either that only the first sentence is from Alfred, which would be very unusual in this style of presentation, or that Alfred did indeed have access to *De animalibus*, perhaps in Arabic.

[128]Long: *longum.*

[129]Long: *impedito.*

[130]Long: *poro.*

[131]The gloss here omits *Hac eadem ratione generantur novi rami continue in planta.*

[132]Long: *maturatum.*

tate repercutitur humor et arefiunt et ideo olera non durant ultra tertium annum.[133] [top right corner of margins]

57] (Venalitas)[134] Alvredus. Cum arbor crescit in calidissima regione eius nutrimentum in colore est intensum et in substantia spissum quod cum natura voluit digerere propter eius parvitatem circa eum intendetur actio caloris et ita provenit venetus color in arbore et eius lignum erit interius nigrum ut ebanus et sic secundum maiorem et minorem calorem fiunt omnia ligna inter alba et nigra. [right margin]

58] (Quod autem in planta) Alfredus. planta que habebit terream materiam erit in colore ut nigrum. que aqueam, erit album eius lignum. que habet materiam inter utramque temperatam erit lignum eius glaucum. [right margin]

fol. 175v:

59] Quod autem quedam Alvredus. quedam arbores grossos et viscosos habent humores et ideo non possunt subtiliari. et ideo non habent flores ut ficus. quedam adeo liquidos habent humores quod non possund [*sic*] digeri. et ideo carent floribus ut palma.[135] [top left margin]

60] (Planta vero que grossos) Alvredus. planta vero que grossum habet corticem et durum multum crescit in longum qua calor exterior parum attrahit de nutrimento in latitudinem quare interior vigens circa interiora multum potest humorem circa longitudinem extendere. [left margin]

61] (Sed planta que lac) Alvredus in plantis que habent lac fortis est prima digestio in radice ita ut unctuosus fiat humor qui cum decoquitur[136] secundo in medulla transit in lac quo vapor inde generatus ad exteriora transmittet. Sed cum non poterit coagulari et digeri in estate impediente calore incluso in viscositate ipsius qui ipsum dissolvit et ita coagulatione resistit superveniente autem frigiditate coagulantur perfecte. Similiter si erumpat intensa caliditate existente in aere coagulabitur. Unde numquam gummi coagulatur nisi caliditate vel frigiditate intensa. [left margin]

62] (Gumme vero calide) Alvredus. Gumme numquam coagulantur nisi ex nimia caliditate vel ex nimia frigiditate. Unde gumme que in aere temperato stillant non coagulantur. Sed tamen auctor videtur velle quod gummi numquam coagulantur ex frigiditate nisi ex humore lacteo et viscoso ut in premisso capitulo ostenditur caliditate autem coagulatur humor liquidus duumodo sit calor vehemens. sed humor liquidus calore mediocri non potest coagulari. [lower margin]

63] (Arborum vero quedam) Alvredus. quedam arborum ut buxus in estate est viridis in yeme glauca quia habet humorem viscosum in se in radice multam habet humiditatem et liquidam et ideo non cadunt folia. Unde adveniente caliditate repercutitur humor et habundat siccitas et fit color glaucus. [upper right margin]

64] (Fructus vero erit amarus) Alvredus. fructus in principio est amarus quia habundat in eo frigiditas et sic qui[137] hic dicitur amarus sapor vulgaritur dicitur[138] acidus tamen in hoc est differentia quod[139] si sit ibi frigiditas et siccitas cum grossa

[133]Fol. 175r.

[134]See Lulofs and Poortman (n. 22 above) 557 for the forms of this word in the manuscripts.

[135]Also R fol. 204r with slightly different wording.

[136]Long: *dequoquatur.*

[137]Long: *quia.*

[138]The critical edition does not have *dicitur.*

[139]The critical edition does not have *quod* or the following *ibi.*

substantia erit ponticus. Si cum liquida substantia et subtili, acidus vel amarus deinde perfecta digestione succedit caliditas et humiditas sine quibus nulla fit digestio et ita fit dulcis. [lower right margin]

65] Arbores que nascuntur. Alvredus. arbores que nascuntur in aqua acetosa attrahunt humorem acetosum sibi similem qui est frigidus et siccus. illudque arbor sibi incorporat digerit et facit dulce. reliquum autem minus digestum emittit in fructus et folia et ideo fructus eius primo fit acidus convalescente autem calore et humore, per digestionem fit dulcis. sed quia ibi pauca est humiditas et multa caliditas cito consumitur humor et succedunt caliditas et siccitas et fit fructus amarus. [lower right margin]

fol. 176r:

66] (Arbores vero que fuerint) Alvredus. arbores que nascuntur in loco temperato ante ver fructum producunt quia cum aer sit temperatus continuique[140] aperti erunt pori aderitque humor liquidus et digestibilis quare[141] levi calore poterit digeri ad fructus productionem. [lower margin]

67] Omnibus quedam arboribus Alvredus in principio generationis fructus habundat frigus in materia eius in quo si dominetur humiditas, fructus erit acidus vel amarus si siccitas, fructus erit ponticus.[142] [lower margin]

68] Mirabolanorum Alvredus. nota quod arbor mirabolanorum poros habet mediocres et habet virtutem digestivam equalem virtuti attractive. Unde humorem attractum statim digerit. Unde fructus in sui productione est dulci[*sic*]. communiter autem habundante calore extrinseco constringuntur pori sive pori[143] sive fructus sive arboris. et ita obstruitur via humoris in quo etiam includitur calor naturalis. Unde in fructum subit frigiditas et siccitas. Unde fit sapor ponticus. postea augmentata constrictione augmentatur frigiditas et siccitas in fructu. Unde et fit[144] intensior ponticitas. ad ultimum vero convalescente calore naturali ex opilatione pororum tandem vehementer prorumpit, poros aperit, et calore exteriori adiutus vehementer agit in fructum eum decoquendo et calorem et siccitatem inducendo. Unde fit fructus mirabolanorum amarus.[145] [top right corner of margins]

The Glosses: Comments

1-5] Clearly the teacher of the student annotator of A found Alfred's introduction the best way of locating the subject matter within Aristotle's physical doctrine. In place of this gloss in R, in contrast, is a passage from Boethius on the purpose of philosophy as a whole.[146] To teach the doctrines of ancient Greek philosophy in a thirteenth-century

[140]Long: *continue.*

[141]Long: *qui.*

[142]The final *fructus erit* is not in the critical edition.

[143]*Sive pori* has been inserted in error.

[144]The edition does not have *fit.*

[145]The edition does not have the final *fructus mirabolanorum.*

[146]Boetius philosophia non est possidendi gratia, sed quatenus ammoveatur ignorantia. Item animus affectuose diviciis intendens a perpetuorum contemplatione quorum cognicio est sapientia penitus evacuatur.

Christian society meant that a basic set of principles had to be asserted. Although *De plantis* is not by Aristotle, it uses peripatetic doctrines; and the university teacher's business was to accommodate the specialist area covered by the text both with the other aspects of Aristotle's physical philosophy and, above all, with Christian truth. The soul was central to both. The Judeo-Christian sources took the soul as the agent of immortality, and when the church needed philosophy to defend and spread its beliefs it adopted, firstly from Plato, some Greek doctrines of soul that gave it physical characteristics important in the life of living things. The use of Aristotle's physical philosophy in the thirteenth century was the final stage in the church's adoption of parts of Greek philosophy.

These five glosses act as an introduction to the question of the essential nature of plants. Having by the use of Alfred's commentary located plants in their place in the philosophy of the physical world, the teacher goes on to address the central question of the extent to which plants can be said to have souls.[147] He locates plants in this respect somewhere between animals and minerals, and discusses what their powers are. In using Alfred's commentary he reflects the period when Aristotle was suddenly coming to be preferred to Plato as the philosopher of nature. Some similarities of doctrine between the two philosophers helped such a change to take place, and Alfred is showing that cross-reference to the other newly-found physical works of Aristotle was a greater resource than could be found in Plato.

6-10] Two important physical powers of the soul were to provide the body with sensation and to allow it to nourish itself with food. The special problem with plant life was that plants clearly nourished themselves from the earth but had no sensation. For in animals it was only by means of sensation—that of hunger—that the faculty of nourishment was exercised. Moreover, hunger was a faculty of a special part of the animal body, the upper orifice of the stomach, that had no counterpart in the plant. Nor could plants have the desire for the Good which was such a feature of Aristotle's account of animals. Probably our teacher here found Alfred's commentary of use because it was at an appropriate, introductory level of explanation. Alfred's commentary was an introduction to issues being faced for the first time; this was useful for the later university teacher because he was introducing his pupils for the first time to the same issues. The elaborate commentaries of the great masters had a different audience.

11] Alfred was one of the first to face the implications of Aristotelian physical doctrine for fundamental Christian beliefs. On the one hand, in Aristotelian physical doctrine the powers of the soul were physical actions of the body and had their own organs (at least in animals), beliefs unacceptable to the Christian; on the other, for the Christian the soul was a separable entity and had certain faculties when separated from the body, beliefs incompatible with Aristotelian doctrine. Alfred is here expanding a hint in the text on this point, and clearly the teacher also found it useful.

12-16] In comparison to that of man, the soul of plants was so lacking in faculties that the question arose as to what "life" might mean in the case of plants. Life without sense is the image of death, says Alfred, and in man sense is the basis of the higher faculties of the soul, such as the reception and interpretation of sensible and intellectual species. The soul of man and that of plants are at either end of a range of complexity,

[147]According to Burnett (n. 18 above) 51, Alfred's view of the soul was deeply indebted to Avicenna.

and the problem of comparing them (and of what "life" might mean) is made easier by reference to Aristotle's work on animals and his description of intermediate forms. These are the hard-shelled animals that do not move (and do not therefore have male and female forms) but which have the senses of touch and taste. From some other source Alfred adds another intermediate form, snakes that are fixed to the earth but which can move their parts with voluntary motion.

17-21] The teacher continued to find Alfred's commentary useful on the important question of the soul, its faculties, especially sense, and how the faculty particularly of attraction (so important in nutrition) could exist without sense. Sense after all was a defining feature of animals. Alfred's commentary was useful in establishing the relative perfection of animals and plants, largely on the basis of the much bigger Aristotelian work on animals.

Alfred's commentary in the critical edition[148] moves directly from gloss 22, fol. 166v and Lulofs and Poortman p. 521 (28), to fol. 173v, Lulofs and Poortman p. 550. It omits, that is, a very large part of the text of *De plantis*, twenty-nine of the forty-six pages of the modern edition. But it is clear that Alfred was not silent on this part of the text. Our group of manuscripts contains quotations and opinions from Alfred's commentary on the central part of the text. After the first twenty-three, which as we have seen were found useful by the teacher, glosses derived from Alfred become fewer. There are twelve in all from the apparently missing part of Alfred's commentary, the last of them in chapter 15 of book 1. Our teacher did not have, or did not find useful, any comments by Alfred on the first six chapters of book 2, and the manuscripts contain no glosses from this section of the text. However, glosses 36 to 70 below use the *whole* of Alfred's commentary on the remaining part of the text. They reproduce the text more accurately than the early glosses (which tend to condense slightly what Alfred had said).

It is clear then that Alfred's original commentary on *De plantis* was larger than we thought, covering at least another thirteen chapters of the first book. At least fragments of the commentary on these chapters were available in the university where A was annotated. Perhaps this availability represented teaching at a time closer to the time when Alfred had written the commentary, which was probably early in the thirteenth century. Our textbooks of natural philosophy represent teaching later in that century, after the formulation of statutes that specify the Aristotelian works to be read; none of the *corpus vetustius* manuscript textbooks belong to a date later than the end of the thirteenth century. Perhaps by then the original commentary had been partly lost. The manuscripts examined by Long are of a different kind: not annotated teaching texts, but commentary written out continuously. Most of the manuscripts, and the one that was most reliable (from Durham), that Long examined date from the fourteenth century. Possibly the commentary as presented by Long was assembled from some such source as teaching materials, like the natural-philosophy textbook, after the full original commentary had been lost sight of. The twelve "missing" glosses are spread so thinly in the *glossa anglicana* that they would easily overlooked in such a process of assembly.

23-25] In the "missing" part of the commentary, Alfred continues with the topic of the senses as faculties of the soul and how this relates to the differences between animals and plants. His sources include the Aristotelian *parva naturalia,* where the spe-

[148]Long (n. 23 above) 155.

cial doctrines of the senses are worked out. Again the explanation is that the more elaborate soul of animals has more faculties, each of which requires special organs and materials to achieve its purpose, here the motion of vapors in sleeping and waking. The absence of such faculties from plants means the absence of the materials needed for the operations: plants do not wake or sleep.

26-28] The soul, which Aristotle called the principle of animal life, was the Form of the animal. When Aristotle used the term "nature" in connection with it he meant the "nature of the animal," not an external agent. The Form of the adult animal was the full expression of its nature, and what interested Aristotle was the means employed by the nature-of-the-animal to fully express itself. Thus the *generation* of animals was a prime explicand in the animal books. Alfred not unnaturally also took it to be a central question in the text on plants. Alfred is concerned with the material ingredients and conditions of the process of generating the fruit or, in other words, the material and efficient causes of fruit. The problem with plants (it was also a Theophrastean problem) was that fruits (and leaves) seemed to be a natural part of a plant, but fell off the tree in the autumn. No "part" of an animal did this, which led Alfred to define a part as belonging to the essence of plants and animals.

29-33] The comparison between animals and plants continued to be an illuminating one for Alfred and was clearly useful to the teacher whose pupils also knew Aristotle's *De animalibus* and whose curriculum by statute included some other Aristotelian works on animal life. *Explanation* of plants in teaching meant in part indicating the parallels with the better-known case of animals. The students were told what it was in plants that resembled the legs, feet, and hands of animals. Alfred's explanations are structural in a Theophrastean way rather than concerned with Aristotelian final causality; and this was found useful by our teacher.

34] As mentioned above, after this gloss the whole of the remainder of Alfred's commentary is covered collectively by the manuscripts. The text and distribution of the commentary among the manuscripts is given here, with the slight differences from the critical edition that occur. It will be seen that Alfred's commentary is concerned with the physical and material basis of Aristotle's philosophy of nature. There is much on vapors and humors characterized in various physical ways, on heat and cold, on the attraction of similars, decoction, putrefaction, the elementary qualities and the places and seasons associated with them, and so on. With this apparatus Alfred explains how spines are formed on some plants, and why all of them are green; how they grow to be different shapes and why they grow in different places. He goes back to Aristotle and his animals to compare eggs and seeds and to give material reasons for the greater diversity of the parts of animals. The omission of formal and final causality is again obvious, and it is clear that Alfred and the teacher who used his commentary accepted a largely materialist account of plants. It was of course knowledge that was not held for its own sake, but as the *glossa* said in opening, for the removal of ignorance or as part of the divine gift of philosophy.

Since this final part of Alfred's commentary is of the same order of size as the common *glossa*, we can compare the use of the two by the teachers of the students who annotated the manuscripts.

35] This gloss is placed in A at the top of column 1 on fol. 173v. Particularly in A, these special quotations are distinguished not only by their position but, as noted above, by little drawings, generally grotesque mixtures of men and animals. Such things were often used by English scribes[149] and are not merely decorative (and certainly not students' untrained doodles). This gloss is indicated by a dog/dragon figure.[150] The text is here very close to that established by Long. The manner of referring to Alfred is the same as in the quotations from the "lost" part of the commentary and strengthens the inference that the teacher had a fuller commentary than is available in the manuscripts studied by Long.

43] Unusually in R (fol. 202), the gloss is marked with a drawing, no doubt because it is a quotation. In H the gloss is displaced to the top right of the folio, for the same reason.

45] The gloss is located at the top of the folio in R, fol. 203r, and at the bottom of the margin in A.

48] The gloss is marked by a drawing of a man in a pointed hat, possibly a miter (fol. 174v col. 1).

49] The gloss has a special position, in the lower margin, reaching across the two columns of fol. 174v. It is marked with a drawing of a figure stepping out of the text into the left margin. The foot of the figure reaches down to another quotation from Alfred, immediately below.

50] The gloss is in the upper margin above column 2, fol. 174v, as the first of a pair of quotations from Alfred. It is marked with the same dog-headed serpent grotesque that marks the gloss to Quod autem comestibile on fol. 173v.

51] The gloss is the other one of the pair at the top of column 2, fol. 174v.

52] This is one of the pair of glosses marked by a drawing of a figure stepping out of the text, in the bottom margin of fol. 174v.

53] The gloss is located at the top of fol. 175r in the privileged upper margin, stretching across the two columns. It is marked by a drawing of a man wearing a crown (possibly a visual pun on "king" Alfred) who is pointing with either hand at this and a second quotation from Alfred located immediately below (gloss 56).

55] This gloss is located in the lower margin below column 1, fol. 175r.

59] The gloss is in the top margin of fol. 175v, marked with a drawing of a tonsured head.

62] The gloss is at the foot of column 1, fol. 175v.

63] At *caliditate* in the penultimate line the gloss omits *provocatur humor ad exteriora, qui tactus calore fit viridis. Adveniente frigiditate...* Almost certainly the glossator's eye has jumped from *adveniente caliditate* to *adveniente frigiditate* in the text he was copying. This suggests that he was copying from an exemplar of Alfred's commentary. This is suggested too by the fact that the agreement between these glosses and the text

[149]Similar grotesque animals can be seen on the Hereford *Mappa mundi,* dating from the end of the thirteenth century. The purpose there was to picture traditional grotesque "combination animals" like the centaur, and many of them must have come from an exemplar-book. See Roger French, "Putting Animals on the Map: The Natural History of the Hereford *Mappa Mundi,*" *Archives of Natural History* 21 (1994) 289–308. Exemplar or pattern books were sometimes compiled from what they had seen, by artists or scribes who wanted to maintain a library of images for professional use. Some such continued copying made it possible, for example, for artists to agree on what heraldic animals looked like. See also R. W. Scheller, *A Survey of Medieval Model Books* (Haarlem 1963).

[150]The visual image like the simple pointing hand or an elaborate multi-animal grotesque seems clearly designed to draw attention to something *not* within the apparatus of text and comment, where the "points" or divisions of the argument are marked by gibbets.

established by Long is closer than that between the various versions of the *glossa anglicana*. The latter vary in a way that suggests that they were fair copies of notes taken rapidly from a lecture. (For example, sometimes another verb of equivalent meaning is used). This gloss is placed, distant from its lemma, top-but-one in the inner margin of fol. 175v.

64] This gloss, like the previous one, is located at a distance from its lemma, and is one of a pair of quotations from Alfred's commentary in the margin below column 2 of fol. 175v. In Long's edition this and the previous gloss are a single comment, but here they are displaced to the top and the bottom of the column, with the *glossa* glosses located close to their lemmata in between.

65] This is the second gloss of the pair at the foot of column 2, fol. 175v.

67] This and the preceding gloss are a pair of quotations located below column 1, fol. 176r.

68] This last quotation from Alfred's commentary on *De plantis* is in the privileged position at the top right corner of fol. 176r, occupying both vertical ruled columns of the margin.

CONCLUSION

The arrival and use of Aristotle's physical doctrines in the West is rightly regarded as significant, especially within the discipline of the History of Science. Yet in a society where dispute about Christian fundamentals could lead to war, Aristotle's physical doctrines could be dangerous as well as useful. Alfred of Shareshill was the first Western commentator on the physical works and among the first translators. This paper argues that he adopted certain strategies in making the physical works acceptable in a Christian society and used them primarily in relation to doctrines of soul, a critical issue.

The evidence for this is drawn partly from a previously unsuspected common gloss shared by manuscripts in England annotated by English students in the second half of the thirteenth century. This reveals (i) further evidence of Alfred's strategy; (ii) glosses from his commentary which have been previously unknown and are absent from the critical edition; (iii) what the teacher found important in Alfred's original commentary; (iv) how the dangers of Aristotle physical doctrines were handled in the second half of the thirteenth century; and (v) some details of classroom practice, including new information on lectures and textbooks.[151] The evidence is drawn primarily from Oxford and covers the period in which the Aristotelian works were banned in Paris. It is argued that the cultivation of natural philosophy in Oxford was a resource when natural philosophy was reintroduced to Paris.

[151]In my article giving the whole *glossa* on *De plantis*, I make the case for the *corpus vetustius* being a teaching textbook (and not a stage in the reception of Aristotelianism): *Physis* (1997, forthcoming).

VIII

GENTILE DA FOLIGNO AND THE *VIA MEDICORUM*

INTRODUCTION

The great change in medieval Italian medicine, the addition of natural philosophy to vocational training, has been made clear to us by Siraisi in her study on Taddeo Alderotti.[1] The introduction of the Aristotelian *libri naturales* enabled Taddeo and his circle to present medicine as a university subject with a standing equal to that of law. The universal arts of Aristotelian argument could be applied to medicine and medicine as a science could be treated as a natural extension of Aristotelian natural philosophy.

Medical education in this period of change continued to be based on a small collection of tracts known as the *Articella*. The core of this collection was a group of at first five, and then seven Greek works in translations that were made from the Greek in the period before the wave of translations of medical texts from Arabic. The tracts in the Articella were largely introductory and prognostic; and the bulk of the actual teaching was made up of the now Aristotelianised commentaries of the masters.

Gentile da Foligno lived almost a generation after Taddeo and because it cannot be demonstrated that he was a pupil of Taddeo, Siraisi does not include a discussion of his work. It is argued below that Gentile helped to give Italian medicine a new character in the years after it was accepted in the universities in its Aristotelianised form. Broadly, I shall argue that Gentile's perception of what medicine was, based largely on the *Canon* of the Arabic author Avicenna, caused him to sketch out a *via medicorum*. This was a path for physicians to tread *qua* physicians. This implied a degree of medical autonomy that was theoretical, practical, professional and less Greek. (The commentaries of Gentile continued to be read for about two centuries, and I hope to argue in a future publication that the *via medicorum* was an important resource for anatomy and physiology.)

1. N. Siraisi, *Taddeo Alderotti and his Pupils*, Princeton University Press, 1981.

J.D. North and J.J. Roche (eds.), The Light of Nature. ISBN 90-247-3165-8.

GENTILE AND THE *CANON*

As observed above, the textbooks of Taddeo's time were largely Greek, introductory or prognostic and particular (not general). In addition there were specialised works like Galen's *De Interioribus (De Locis Affectis)*. Gentile appears to have been the first to complete a commentary on the *Canon*.[2] This was clearly different from that taught by other and earlier masters.

To begin with, the *Canon* was Arabic, not Greek. The shift in medicine towards Arabic sources involved not only the *Canon*, but the *Colliget* of Averroës, with which Gentile was familiar, and from which he drew parts of his conception about the nature of medicine. The *Colliget* was not translated until 1287 and its absence from the medicine of Taddeo's generation contributes towards the difference between that medicine and the medicine of Gentile. Avicenna and particularly Averroës can be seen as Aristotelian commentators, who had also a knowledge of the works of Galen that was greater than that of the physicians of Taddeo's and Gentile's time. Those physicians who were able to read Avicenna and Averroës were thus more aware of the differences between the doctrines of Aristotle and Galen.[3] Moreover, Galen's major reasoned account of anatomy and physiology, *De Usu Partium*, was known to Gentile, but apparently not to Taddeo's pupils[4] and on both topics there would have been seen a much greater degree of agreement between Avicenna and Galen than between either and Aristotle. In addition, Avicenna's own dependence on Galen meant that a study of the *Canon* was partly a revival of Galenism.

That the *Canon* was very much larger than any other text also contributed substantially to the difference between Gentile's medicine and that of earlier masters. He believed it contained everything that, when properly understood, was necessary for the education of the doctor. It was systematically laid out: this was valued by Gentile not only for its comprehensiveness, but because an ordered presentation was convenient for teaching and learning.

Order of presentation; reliance on Arabic sources and adoption of 'barbaric' terminology; reconciliation of the great ancient authors; subtlety of commentary: these are important elements in scholastic medicine. The picture we have of scholastic medicine is still coloured by the account of it given by the Hellenists of the 16th century, who ultimately won their propaganda battle with the scholastics. Thus the subtlety of argument, undoubtedly the result of the extensive use of Aristotelian logic by Taddeo and others, is still sometimes thought

2. Taddeo and Dino del Garbo were pioneers of such a study, but their commentaries were incomplete; Dino did not deal with books three and five. See Siraisi, *Taddeo*, p. 105.

3. See N. Siraisi, "The medical learning of Albertus Magnus" in James A. Weisheipl, *Albertus Magnus and the Sciences*, Toronto, 1980, pp. 379–404; 396, 400.

4. Siraisi, *Taddeo*, p. 101.

of as sterile and impractical. Order is seen as rigidity, technical terminology as inelegant, the elaborate structure of the analytical commentary as "stuttering". For a Hellenist like Leoniceno, Gentile was one of the more notable villains of scholastic medicine, the "old commentator" on that unreliable author, Avicenna.[5] Certainly Gentile contributed in a major way to scholastic medicine, however characterised, and his commentaries continued to be used until they were printed in the sixteen century.[6] But to understand this contribution we need not look at him through the eyes of a Hellenist.

THE *VIA MEDICORUM*

There are a number of ways then, in which Gentile helped to shape medicine in the period after its Aristotelianisation at the hands of Taddeo and his circle. What Gentile meant by the phrase *via medicorum* was, in short, book three of the *Canon*. In Gentile's view, book three contained all that was necessary for the education of the physician. It proceeded from anatomy through physiology to pathology and treatment; it covered all parts of the body; it was systematic in treatment and ordered in a manner convenient for teaching. It came to be the only book prescribed in the statutes for the *practica* course at Bologna (al-

5. N. Leoniceno, *Opuscula*, Basel, 1532: the "Errors of Pliny", pp. 29v, 43r. Leoniceno attacks the techniques of commentary. His parody ". . . primam ibi, secundam ibi, tertiam ibi . . ." refers to the elaborate structure of the *expositio* section of the commentary, in which the expositor looks forward in the text to identify salient points in the argument by means of quotations. On the structure of the commentary see R.K. French, "Berengario da Carpi and the use of commentary in anatomical teaching", in A. Wear, R. French and I. Lonie, *The Medical Renaissance of the Sixteenth Century*, Cambridge University Press, 1985. It is suggested by Ottosson that the first vigorous growth of the commentary in the late 13th and early 14th century came to an end with the black death and did not recover its vigour afterwards. Gentile died of the plague in 1348, and his commentators would thus appear to be some of the most elaborate of the middle ages. See P.-G. Ottosson, *Scholastic Medicine and Philosophy. A Study of Commentaries on Galen's Tegni (c. 1300–1450)*, Uppsala, 1982.

6. For example *Tertius Canonis Avicennae cum dilucidissimis expositoribus Gentile fulginate nec non Jac. de partibus Parisiense*, Venice, c. 1499 (in three volumes, including book 4); *Tertius Canonis Avicennae cum amplissima Gentilis fulg. expositione. Demum commentaria nuper addita videlicet Jacobi de Partibus super fen vi et xiii. Item Jo. Matthei de gradi super fen xxii quia Gentilis in eis deficit*, in two volumes, the first without date or place, the second being *Secunda Pars Gentilis super tertio Avic. cum supplementis Jacobis de partibus parisiensis ac Joannis Matthei de Gradi mediolensis ubi Gentilis vel breviter vel tacite pertransivit*, Venice, 1522. This *Secunda Pars* is continued in a third volume, covering books four and five: *Quartus Canonis Avicennae cum praeclara Gentilis fulginatis expositione* . . . . It will be seen that Gentile, called "the speculator" in the colophon of the first volume of the *Secunda Pars*, did not in fact complete his commentary on fen xxii. There is also an edition by Scotus' heirs, Venice, 1520: *Avicenne medicorum principis Canonum liber unum cum lucidissima Gentilis Fulg. expositione.*

though this undoubtedly endorses Gentile's view, we cannot tell if it is the result of it).

Gentile's proemium to book three helps us to understand why book three was so important to him. This proemium is bigger than that to the *Canon* as a whole and has an elaborate structure. It begins, as do most of Gentile's important expositions, with praise of God. This is not merely a formal gesture, a kind of grace before an intellectual meal, but a necessary part of placing Avicenna and the *Canon* in their context in the world. Gentile felt the logical primacy in first announcing God as the Creator of everything: not only of Avicenna and the *Canon*, but of the human body and of the understanding which a physician can bring to bear upon its illnesses and which a teacher and expositor needs in order to handle the texts of the authorities.

Similar reasoning was to be found in the Latin versions of the Arabic authors[7]: this may have added to their attraction for the 13th- and 14-century scholars, for whom Greek philosophy was, after all, pagan. Certainly the temporary condemnation of Aristotle in 1277 must have pointed to the Arabic alternative in medicine. In beginning with God as Creator, Gentile observes that the Aristotelians would not agree (because the peripatetic world was eternal, not created) and he draws support instead from the Arabs, Galen and Plato.

This placing of medicine in respect of theology was also seen later as a hallmark of scholastic medicine. To return to Leoniceno, he used "monkish" as a pejorative term for the scholastics, and in particular Turrisanus, the *Plusquam Commentator*, was "The Monk".[8] It seems likely that this aspect of scholastic medicine reflects the importance of the *studia* of the friars in places like Bologna. Here there was at least as much logic and philosophy as in the *studium* of the town; and within the broad framework of interpreting Aristotle in a way acceptable to Christian theology, it was the Dominicans who adopted a proselytising manner of teaching.[9]

So a medieval physician like Gentile, looking back on the history of his subject, found that it differed in many respects from philosophy. It was not so much a question of philosopher-physician disputes as of marking off a medical area out of bounds to the philosophers. Gentile's words make it clear that in creating the world God acted upon principles of Aristotelian causality, so a knowledge of natural philosophy was still necessary for the physician, and the physician following the *via* was not simply opting out of philosophy.

7. For example in Averroës' commentary on the *Cantica* of Avicenna (an important source for Gentile) and in Rhazes' *Almansor*. The first of these was printed in the second half of the *Secunda Pars* of Gentile's exposition of the *Canon* (see note 6) and the second, for example, in Basel, 1544: *Abvbetri Rhazae Maomethi . . . opera exquisitiora . . .* , also reprinted (Culture and Civilisation) Brussels, 1973.

8. Leoniceno, *Opuscula*, p. 158v.

9. I am grateful to Mr. C. O'Boyle for useful discussions on this point. See also Siraisi, "Albertus", pp. 386, 387.

In the proemium to book three, Gentile sets up his theological position as a proposition to be demonstrated from the authors. The entire proemium consists of the proof of two such propositions, and the second of these, and the unique one, is the *via medicorum*. It takes the form "It is not proper for the skilled physician to leave this path", and in analysing it in the manner of an expositor Gentile builds up the picture of what a skilled physician is and what is the path he must not leave. The proposition itself is taken from Haly Abbas, who intended the "path" to apply to his own book. Gentile thought, however, that it was more appropriate for book three of the *Canon*, as an improvement on the work of Haly. Although Gentile uses the sentence as a text, rather as a fragment of the scriptures would be used in the *ars praedicandi* or in one of Gentile's graduation speeches,[10] he nevertheless takes the idea – that a good text could be a *via* – from Haly's use of it. He was familiar with Haly's book, and we can usefully take Haly's opinions into account when examining what the *via medicorum* meant to Gentile. As a path leading to the state of being a skilled physician, says Gentile, the *via medicorum* systematically lays down the methods, aims and instruments of medicine. What follows in this paper is largely an examination of these aspects of the *via medicorum*: what Gentile meant by the skilled physician, the use of *ordo* in systematic exposition, the nature of medical knowledge, the means of achieving it and the practical fulfilment of the aims of medicine.

THE PHYSICIAN AS HISTORIAN

In seeking to define the term "skilled physician" of his proposition *peritum nullo modo deceat medicum hanc transgredi viam*[11] Gentile brings forward the opinions of a number of authors as to what constitutes the "best doctor". And in choosing the third book of the *Canon* as the *via*, he rejects other possible books. Likewise, in writing the medical texts available to Gentile, the authors often enough opened with an account of the shortcomings of earlier works. All this necessarily involved the selection of medical heroes and texts both in terms of the excellence of their art and historically. In other words, the medical man saw himself in an intellectual, practical and professional tradition, the nature of which was determined by its founding fathers and luminaries. Who these were depended, of course, on the selection of the individual medical man, but as we shall see there was by and large a consensus based round the old Greek authors.

10. See C.C. Schlam, "Graduation speeches of Gentile da Foligno", *Mediaeval Studies*, 1978, 40, 96–119.

11. Gentile, proemium to the commentary on the third book of the *Canon*; see note 6. Haly Abbas, *Liber totius medicinae necessaria continens . . .*, 1523, p. 7r.

In the view of those who discussed it, the *via medicorum* was a result of an historical process of development. Gentile took the phrase from a discussion by Haly Abbas that was largely historical, and his use of it for the third book of the *Canon* indicates that he believed that the development had proceeded beyond Haly Abbas' book. Haly is very clear about the earlier part of this development: the founding father of medicine was Hippocrates, who was the first to commit the art to writing. In treating most parts of the subject, Hippocrates was necessarily terse in expression – as in the *Aphorisms* – and so Hippocratic medicine requires explanation. Galen, the eminent, wise and honest, wrote fully; indeed, he was so prolix in enquiry and demonstration that his arguments against his opponents are examples of the "path of the sophists", says Haly.[12] Moreover, he adds, no single work of Galen's is directed to the whole of medicine.

It seems to be broadly true that the Arabs wanted from Greek medicine only what was needed for a better understanding and practice of medicine, preferably presented in a form convenient for teaching.[13] Haly thus gave qualified approval to Oribasius and Paul of Aegina, although he found that both gave too little attention to the Naturals, that is, the point at which medicine linked up to natural philosophy. The same criticism, combined with that of lack of order in presentation, is levelled at the "moderns": Aaron, Messius, Serapion the younger and, principally, Rhazes.

But Haly maintains that despite the shortcomings of earlier authors there was nevertheless an agreed body of knowledge on the nature of disease, its cause, signs and treatment. The principal disagreements between the authors had been questions of emphasis, not of kind, and it was therefore possible to present the basic premises of medicine concisely by omitting trivial disputes. Haly claims that his own book is built on such premises, strengthened by the techniques of logic and natural philosophy.

The agreed body of knowledge that Haly has in mind could of course be added to, and Haly argues that the cures and diets of earlier physicians that have been proved with time will form part of his discussion. So although Haly lays stress on logic and natural philosophy in the structure and sequence of exposition of medicine, yet proof of the efficiency of diets and drugs is empirical, and is to be gained over several generations, and while of great professional interest to the doctor, has no great interest for the philosopher. This will be discussed in more detail below, and here it is enough to argue that the historical consideration of medicine contributed something to the *via medicorum*.

12. Haly Abbas, *Liber totius medicinae necessaria continens*, p. 5v.

13. *Ibid.*, p. 5v. For the kind of material omitted from a Galenic text by the Arabs, see R.K. French, "De Juvamentis Membrorum and the reception of Galenic physiological anatomy", *Isis*, 1979, 70, pp. 96–109.

The rather moral tone of Haly's original sentence (at least in its Latin form), which appears also in the form given to it by Gentile and later writers, is also a professional aspect of the *via medicorum*. Haly lays down that the wise and proper physician – that is, he who treads the path – should behave according to the ethical principles of Hippocrates. The tyro should honour his teachers as parents, and his fellow students as brothers; the teachers should lead on their pupils to excellence and knowledge, without regard to payment for the teaching itself or for entry (for suitable candidates) to the class. These are ethics for the governing of a profession; and perhaps they relate, like Haly's ideal medical text, to the teaching needs of the Arab physicians. With regard to his patients, the proper doctor does not supply abortifacient drugs, or the means for suicide. He does not reveal patient's secrets, is pious, clean in habit and dress and suspicious of a smooth tongue. In respect of his own *scientia* he must read whatever books he can obtain and visit hospitals, where he may learn from other physicians about other books, and about the knowledge of cures they may possess. This again is empirical or rather experiential knowledge – Haly uses the Aristotelian term "accidental" to indicate it is not the knowledge of causes proper to the natural philosopher – to be gained cumulatively and co-operatively.

EXPERIENTIAL KNOWLEDGE

The rather moral flavour of the *via medicorum* as expressed by Haly and used by Gentile relates not only to professional ethics but also to the means of acquiring knowledge through experience. It was generally admitted that only experience could teach the effects of certain medicines and diets upon individual patients; it was also accepted among many that only sensory experience could properly teach anatomy. Such knowledge, particularly that of the action of medicines, was dangerously close, in the new profession of medicine, to being empirical; and inasfar as it related to medicine as an art and a manual craft (particularly in anatomy) it could not support medicine's dignity as a *scientia*, part of natural philosophy. This is not the place for a discussion of medical 'method" and the relations between physicians and philosophers, and we need only note that what I have called the moral tone of the *via medicorum* related to the professional code of the medical man, urging him to learn by experience, even though there was no philosophical basis for the knowledge so gained.

In his tract on doses and proportions Gentile explains that theoretical books are governed by the intellect, but the practical as it were by faith alone, by adhering to experience.[14] The use of "faith" reflects exactly the way the *via*

14. In Mesuë, *Opera . . . cum Mundini, Honesti, Manardi et Sylvii, in tres priores libros observationibus. . . ,* 2 vols., Venice, 1581–2. Vol. 2 of this contains Gentile's *De Proportionibus Medi-*

medicorum came to be used, particularly by anatomists: commitment to a higher truth that was not open to reason. Satisfactory practice of medicine will never, he adds, be gained by intellect alone, because the canons of practice are *experimentales*, not *scientales*.

Gentile can justify his view by reference to Haly Abbas and to Galen. If we look at how Haly treats the topic of experiential knowledge in connection with the *via medicorum*, we find that he too refers back to Galen. But what is a passing remark in Galen (he is dismissing Archigenes' reasoning as not leading to practical results[15]) becomes a major topic in Haly. For all his emphasis on logic in the presentation of medicine, he makes clear that logic alone will not make clear the nature of disease: it does not lead to causes, signs or treatment. Gentile, too, often presented as the arch-scholastic and known as "Doctor subtillissimus" and "Speculator"[16] (theoretician), urges sensory experience, and presented his tract on dosage as a means of enabling the practioner to walk the *via practica* until such time as he had gained his own practical experience.

It should be emphasised here that the *via medicorum* is not simply an aspect of the philosopher-physician question. The area in which the professional "faith" of the physician operated was beyond the grasp and purposes of the philosopher. Gentile gives an example in his commentary on Egidius' tract on the pulse.[17] Here he remarks that the philosophical definition of "pulse" is "a motion of the heart and arteries". But this is a definition *per causam*, for philosophers looking for causes, and is of little use to the diagnosing physician holding the patient's wrist. What is needed is a *definitio physicalis* that gives the essence of the pulse medically speaking – a (perceptible) motion composed of the motion of the heart and the motion of the arteries.

For Gentile, then, observation and experience are among the "methods" and "instruments" the doctor should employ as he proceeds along the *via medicorum*.[18] Here he also derives support from Averroës' discussion of theory and practice in the *Colliget*.[19] Averroës has the elaborate discussion we might expect of an Aristotelian commentator turning to medicine, which is firmly located within the *scientia–ars* relationship: there is no act of medical "faith". Practical medicine is the *ars experimentalis* of anatomy and the study of the actions of medicines. The *ars experimentalis* is difficult and lengthy (and in Aver-

---

cinarum Solventium et de Modo Investigandi Complexiones earum et ad Sciendam convenientem Dosim cujuslibet medicinae . . . , p. 232v.

15. Haly's reference seems to be to book one of *De Locis Affectis*. See Galen, *On the Affected Parts*, trans. R.E. Siegel, Basel (Karger), 1976, p. 21.

16. See the colophon mentioned in note 6, and Ottosson, *Scholastic Medicine*, p. 26.

17. Aegidius Corbelensis, *Carmina de Urinarum Judiciis et de Pulsibus cum Expositione et Commento magistri Gentilis de Fulgineo*, Basel, 1529. Unpaginated; sigs. O4 and P.

18. Proemium to the commentary on book three of the *Canon*.

19. Averroës, *Colliget libri vii*, Venice (Junta), 1553, p. 5r (book 1).

roës' time particularly, since anatomy was no longer practised, he says). It was indeed the *ars experimentalis* that Hippocrates meant when he said that life is short and the art is long. It is then the duty of theoretical medicine, adds Averroës, to give us the causes of what has been discovered through the *ars experimentalis*. Careful use of the *ars experimentalis* will give the physician principles to work by, but since he is handling largely "accidents" of matter (in the Aristotelian sense, as used also by Haly Abbas), he will not arrive at true causal principles. He can only arrive at a direct cognition or *demonstratio* of things, and in return for the causal principles supplied to this art by the theory of medicine, it supplies to theory knowledge of the material circumstances (particularly anatomy) in which theory has the *loca* of its subject. Lastly, theoretical medicine is distinguished from natural philosophy by Averroës by its aims, that is, the removal of disease, not merely understanding it. In short, Averroës made available to Gentile a sophisticated discussion about the relationships of science and art which Gentile (but not Averroës) uses to extend the notion of a *via medicorum*.

A rather different emphasis is put on the matter by Averroës in his commentary on the *Cantica* of Avicenna,[20] on which Gentile also draws. Here Averroës, in the course of disagreeing with Avicenna's and with Galen's definition of medicine, dwells more on the uniqueness of the science and art of medicine. Again, medicine is distinct from natural philosophy in that its purpose is more than simply to understand, and for its practical side, both reason and experience are necessary. What is special to the art of medicine is the physician's *scientia* or reasoning on the means, the "instruments", by which he will produce health. The manual operations by which this aim is achieved have the same standing as anatomy, for neither, Averroës insists, can be learned from words, for the images supplied by words are insufficient. Experience is the only teacher.

Medical "faith" in experiential knowledge is put in a slightly different way by Gentile in the phrase "medical *speculatio* does not transcend sense".[21] Here Gentile is commenting on the *Tegni* and his discussion about sense and reason comes close to what the historians have called the question of "method". It will suffice here to say that Gentile distinguishes between demonstration *propter quid* – from cause to effect – and demonstration *quia*, or from effect to cause. In the latter, knowledge of the effect is prior in the senses, and it is close to simple sensory observation, or observation of particulars.[22] If the effect is the action

20. See notes 6 and 7; the discussion is on pp. 101r–v.

21. Gentile may have come across this phrase in Taddeo's commentary on the *Isagoge* (*Thaddei Florentini Expositiones in arduum aphorismorum Ipocratis volumen. In divinum pronosticorum Ipocratis librum. In praeclarum regiminis acutorum Ipocratis opus. In subtilissimum Joannitii Isagogarum libellum*, Venice, 1527, p. 351r), but Taddeo is using it in a discussion about function. The phrase was later picked up from Gentile and used to great effect in an anatomical context by Berengario da Carpi. See note 5.

22. (Turrisanus) *Plusquam Commentum in Parvam Galeni Artem . . . Gentilis, qui primum*

of medicines on the body, like rhubarb purging bile[23] then demonstration *quia* is akin to the *via experimentalis*, the experiential way of gaining knowledge. Likewise Turrisanus' use of *quia* is close to direct observation, and seems characteristically medical.[24] In a similar way Taddeo and Turrisanus had a characteristically medical way of explaining medicines' effects that could not be derived rationally, but which were observed empirically. These two authors speak of "specific forms" whose working is essentially occult, that is unknown, but with observable effects.[25]

An important vehicle for the discussion of rational and empirical procedures was the first aphorism of Hippocrates. Hippocrates was of course identified by all medical men as the founding father of their profession, and he contributed greatly to the physicians' self-image and their perception of the medical tradition. Equally their perception of what was best in medicine led them to reinterpret Hippocrates to show that he was indeed, but perhaps in some hitherto unsuspected way, the true founder of medicine. The *Aphorisms* was arguably the most important Hippocratic book, particularly in an educational context, and the explanation of an aphorism was a standard part of medical graduation,[26] for which the student would be prepared in class by some such *expositio* as Taddeo's. In expounding "Life is short, the Art long, opportunity fleeting, experiment treacherous, judgment difficult", Taddeo says that "judgment"[27] can be rational or empirical,[28] and for "difficult" he presents the case of an ill man who takes a number of remedies, some of which benefit him while others are harmful: neither reason nor experience can easily demonstrate which is which. Demaitre suggests[29] that particular, experiential knowledge was rather more characteristic of the southern universities than of Paris, where general and rational knowledge had a greater emphasis. If so, then the first aphorism provided a model for a properly medical and professional empiricism. It is not known to me if Gentile interpreted the first aphorism in this way, but as we have seen, he was aware of Averroës' derivation of an *ars experimentalis* from it.

---

ejusdem Artis librum partim explicando partim dubitando declaravit . . . , Venice (Junta), 1557, p. 222r.

23. *Plusquam Commentum* (note 22), p. 222v.

24. Siraisi, *Taddeo*, p. 132.

25. Siraisi, *Taddeo*, p. 295.

26. Malagola, C., *Statuti delle Università e dei Collegi dello Studio Bolognese*, Bologna, 1888, pp. 438 *et seq*.

27. Hippocrates, *Aphorisms*, Loeb Hippocrates, London, vol. 4, 1967.

28. Taddeo's commentary on the *Aphorisms* (note 21), p. 2r.

29. L. Demaitre, "Theory and practice in medical education at the university of Montpellier in the thirteenth and fourteenth centuries", *J. Hist. Med.*, 1975, 30, pp. 103–123; 118, 119.

ANATOMY

The practice of dissecting the human body for teaching purposes in the universities began at some time during the lifespan of Taddeo and Gentile. It followed on the formal organisation of medicine as a university discipline and the reception of the *libri naturales* of Aristotle and the medical works of the Arabs. It is not the purpose of this paper to investigate whether it was Mondino, as his pupil Guy de Chauliac seems to imply,[30] who first devised a systematic course of instruction, or whether the dissections were derived from legal *post mortem* examinations.[31] The question is to what extent was anatomy part of the *via medicorum*?

Gentile said that anatomy was the fundamental subject in medicine and should be taught first, as the alphabet is taught first to those learning to read. Nevertheless, Gentile does *not* comment on the anatomy of book one[32] on the grounds that he is following established practice, which he calls the "common error".

In some statutes the anatomy of the *Canon* is expressly excluded.[33] It is possible that some form of anatomical demonstration on animal bodies, preserved human parts or even pictures[34] had been common since the Salernitan demonstrations, but as practical affairs were not material for commentary, the usual mode of teaching. We know from a rather later period that when dissections were performed, they were governed by strict rules of frequency and attendance. Very likely the anatomical demonstrations themselves antedated the regulations by many years; possibly then the exclusion of Avicenna's anatomy from the routine course of lectures simply reflects the convention that anatomies took place separately. Gentile's remarks would then be a criticism of when it was taught (i.e. not first). Gentile compensates for his lack of commentary on the systematic exposition of anatomy in book one of the *Canon* in his commentary on the particular anatomy of book three. Here, indeed, the anatomy does come first in the treatment of each part of the body. We may even speculate that the difference between Gentile's commentary on book one and that on book three reflects an earlier and a later period of medicine, in which anatomy played a different role. If Gentile wrote his commentaries in a sequential order, then perhaps he was teaching book one when there was a recognised gap in the Galenic anatomical literature,[35] and before the systematic teaching of Mondino

30. Siraisi, *Taddeo*, p. 112.
31. See also Siraisi, "Albert", p. 395.
32. See the edition of 1520 (note 6): fen. 1, doctrine 5, summa 1–v.
33. Malagola, *Statuti*, p. 275.
34. Siraisi, *Taddeo*, p. 112.
35. This was recognised by Bartolomeo da Varignana in drawing up a list of texts for an ideal course in theoretical medicine. Siraisi, *Taddeo*, p. 104.

had begun. By the time he began his exposition on book three, he was familiar with Galen's *De Usu Partium*, for he uses it as the first authority to establish the first of the two propositions which compose the proemium: the order, harmony and function of the parts of the body were evidence to Galen of the wisdom of the Creator. Gentile can hardly have been untouched by Galen's insistence on anatomy as fundamental to an understanding of the body.

This is borne out by Gentile's bibliographical essay on Galen's works.[36] Gentile often employed a "causality accessus"[37] in his introductions; that is, he liked to analyse the text under discussion into material, formal, efficient and final cause. He can do this too with Galen's works, and he arranges them so that as basic and first come Galen's treatment of the elements, mixtures, complexions and humours, followed by the anatomical works, primarily *De Usu Partium* and the lost *Anatomia Vivorum* and *Anatomia Mortuorum*. These all together relate, for Gentile, to material causality and the human body as the material subject of medicine. The synthetic building up from macrocosmic elements through the Naturals to the organic parts was a common rational presentation of anatomy. In second place among Galen's books, argues Gentile, are those that relate to formal causality. These are the physiological books like the *Natural Faculties*, the *Opinions of Plato and Hippocrates*, the books on the pulse and voice, motions of muscles and related works. In short, function comes after and depends on structure, at least in terms of the desirable sequence of reading Galen. Efficient causality is represented in Galen's works, continues Gentil, by *De Causis Procatarcticis*. Lastly, he says that Galen had no need to write on final causality (because such knowledge is contained in the knowledge of the effects of medicines, etc.), but that he wrote several books on the purpose of medicine, that is, those on the preservation of health, regimen and the prevention of illness. Taken together, this is a clear sequence of knowledge from structure, the "alphabet of medicine", to health as the goal of medicine.

ORDER

An important part of the third book of the *Canon*, as Gentile's *via medicorum*, was the arrangement of the material within the text. The question of *ordo* was an important one in medieval medicine, and one that is seen as characteristically scholastic. Gentile praises book three for its "beautiful order" that

36. It is printed in the Venice, 1483, edition of the *Articella*.

37. On the use of the accessus in medicine, see R.K. French, "A note on the anatomical accessus of the middle ages", *Medical History*, 1979, 23, pp. 461–468.

38. Gentile, the proemium to the commentary on book three; the beginning of the commentary on book one has much the same remarks.

"gives power to the memory" and makes similar remarks in introducing book one. The text for both is Aristotle's opinion in *De Memoria et Reminiscentia* that a natural or well-constructed series is easier to recall than one badly arranged. Such a series, says Aristotle, is "like the successive demonstrations in geometry".[39] Aristotle here distinguishes a necessary connection between the parts of the series and a customary connection; the major point he is making is that given one part of such a series, the following parts follow it in recollection, but that the mind is powerless without such a starting point. We can see why this Aristotelian text was so appropriate in Gentile's treatment of the *Canon*, and, moreover, in his own *expositiones* of the *Canon*. The text of the *Canon* was structured logically (and the *expositio* in exposing this structure could reduce its sentences to propositions), just as the "successive demonstrations in geometry" were logically linked. The *Canon* was not only structured logically in a series, but book three repeated the same mode of exposition for each part of the body in turn, so that the reader knew what kind of information he would find in which place, although the particulars of that information were new to him. To have such a sequence (of exposition) in his mind made the task of remembering the particulars easier, and it seems to be to this that Gentile applies the text of Aristotle, for geometry proceeds not only in a logically necessary series, but there is a common, and therefore repeated mode of exposition in different problems.

The importance of *ordo* lay in the institutional teaching of the Arabs and the Western universities. The Hippocratic and Galenic works had not been the product of schools and had not been designed for teaching, at least not the new kind. The medieval doctor looking back on the past of his subject and the author pointing out the shortcomings of earlier books saw Galen as prolix, specialised, digressionary and occasionally vituperative, and Hippocrates as terse and often obscure. What both needed in the new teaching context was order: a systematic approach that was comprehensive but not too large and employing a standard technique of exposition that would help the student through the text. The difficulty of bringing the students to an understanding and memory of the medical texts of the authorities is often expressed by Gentile, for example in the introduction to his exposition on the *Tegni*.[40] The purposes of *ordo* are clearly set out by Gentile in the opening of his exposition on the *Canon* as a whole[41]: Galen's medicine, although complete, is spread out over many particular books, and Galen was thus often obliged to repeat himself (the *ordo* of the *Canon* makes repetition unnecessary); where Galen attempted a general book, like the *Tegni*, there are omissions (the *Canon* is complete); the introductory

39. 452a.
40. Taddeo has similar remarks at the beginning of his commentary on the *Prognostics* (note 21).
41. See note 6: the edition of Venice, 1529.

books of Joannitius and Rhazes are brief to the point of obscurity (the *Canon* is detailed and lucid); and where lucidity and comprehensiveness demand a very large book, then *ordo* makes the task of the memory easier.

As we have seen, it was among the purposes of the *expositio*, the first stage of the commentary,[42] to expose the order of the text by analysing its logical structure: clearly a consistent and repeated *ordo* made the task of the expositor easier, and eased the load on his students' memories. The memory was also involved in recalling the intention of the author in his method of approach, so that the mind would be led from the general principles of organisation down as far as possible to the details of what was said. In Gentile's "causality accessus" method of analysing a text he sought the efficient, material, formal and final causes. The efficient cause was the author, the material cause was the human body, or medicines, in short the material topic of the book, and the final cause was health, or the prevention of disease. The formal cause of the text was its structure, its mode of exposition, the thing exposed by the expositor. Normally it was double, the *forma tractandi* and the *forma tractatus*. The *forma tractatus* was the division of the *Canon* into books, fens, tracts, *summae*, chapters and so on, while the *forma tractandi* was the mode in which Avicenna wrote. Broadly speaking, says Gentile, this was the resolutive mode, where resolutive can be taken to include definitive, divisive, narrative, exemplary and even compositive. These are not "methods", but modes of exposition, and Gentile uses the term "resolutive" because book three of the *Canon* is divided, like the body, into a number of organs *a capite ad calcem*, together with their diseases. *Ordo* then includes the repeated pattern of anatomy-physiology-pathology-treatment for each division of the body. It is perhaps this mode of exposition that Averroës complains of, attributing it to an excessive use of the divisive method of the schools, practised principally by the vainglorious men of Andalucian Spain.[43]

42. See French, "Berengario" (note 5).

43. Averroës, *Colliget*, proemium.

IX

The Medical Ethics of Gabriele de Zerbi

Introduction: How Ethical were Medical Ethics?

In this and a subsequent chapter in this book, 'ethics' will be used in a particular sense. The current interest in medical ethics is an interest in ethical problems. It might seem unproblematic that medical ethics have a history, and that these problems can be studied in the past. We might, for example, take the problem of abortion, and look at it historically. But then we would find that there have been times and places in which abortion provided no ethical problems. Such a history would be the history of a practice, not of an ethical problem. In other words, modern medical ethics derives from the particular nature of modern medicine and the society in which it exists. So a history of medical ethics is a history of medicine and of society and of the problems that looked ethical to them, but not necessarily to us. Looked at in this way it soon becomes clear that ethics have a function, for the group that practises them, other than the internal, explicit injunctions that are normally seen as 'ethical' in some abstract way. Most of the Hippocratic ethical works can be read as defences of the medicine of one group when threatened by another. Asclepiads and groups making use of presocratic philosophy and the methods of the sophists can be identified in texts like *Ancient Medicine, Oath, Law,* and *Decorum,*[1] books that lay down rules for the proper practice of real medicine; that is, the medicine of the group to which the author belongs. Ethics comprise a system of rules that not only characterizes the group, but which in directing the behaviour of the group contributes to its success. Whatever the source of the rules and however they came to be written down (if they were) it is unlikely that that they originated with this explicit intention of benefiting the group. Rather, if the cumulative effect of such rules, whatever their nature and origins, was good for the group, it survived. Other groups, perhaps in direct competition, may have had ethics that did not have this effect.

Looked at in this way we can see that it is the group, not the individual member, that is the beneficiary of its ethics. The members may have to make sacrifices to remain in the group. They enter and leave it, but the group persists. In this account, too, we can see why ethical rules are largely moral rules: they are obeyed not because of a rational awareness of any penalties, which would be the case if the rules were rationally derived for the interests of the group, rather they are obeyed because of the deeper-than-rational moral loading that a successful group can put on its members.

The Hippocratic ethical works provided a resource for those who later came to think about medical ethics. They did so primarily because they were concerned with the internal regulation of a group of medical men and the reputation of the group of the whole. Thus the Arab Haly Abbas found it useful to assert, as did the Oath, that the beginner should honour his teachers as parents and treat his fellow students as brothers; should select whom to teach and do so without payment; should not supply abortifacients or the means of suicide; should respect his patients' secrets; should dress cleanly and should be suspicious of a smooth tongue. To these plainly Hippocratic injunctions he adds one that seems to derive from the Arabic doctor's environment of practice, namely to improve his learning by visiting hospitals and talking to the doctors there. Haly's views in turn acted as a resource for Gentile da Foligno, the man who did a great deal (before his death in the plague of 1348) to bring Arabic medicine into the West while the New Galenism (described by Garcia-Ballester) was being absorbed and developed from other sources. Gentile developed a 'way of the physicians' – *via medicorum* – that was 'ethical' partly because it was technically ideal, like the New Galenism, and partly because it drew upon the Hippocratic ethical works, no doubt by way of Haly Abbas.[2]

Learning, Ethics and Reputation

When they rewrote the statutes of the student *universitas* at Padua in 1468, one of their philosophy teachers was Gabriele de Zerbi. He had been there about a year. Many of the statutes are concerned with the political structure of the *universitas* and in particular who was allowed to vote. (Zerbi was named among those on whom the obligation to vote was not to be enforced.) As for the statutes that governed the teaching and practice of medicine, they pay particular attention, in very strong language, to two special points, the regular performance of human dissections and to the control of unlicensed practice.[3] We shall return to these statutes in finding reasons to explain how Zerbi's ethics came to have the shape they did. (We shall also see how Zerbi's well-known book on anatomy is closely linked to his ethics and the statutes.)

Seven years later Zerbi moved to Bologna[4] where he taught logic, philosophy and medicine for eight years. The subsequent ten years that he spent in Rome brings us to 1494, when he moved back to Padua as the *ordinarius* in medicine. In the following year he published his little book on advice to medical men, the *De Cautelis Medicorum,* 'advice to medical men'.[5] This calendar of events likewise contributes to our understanding of 'ethics' at Zerbi's particular place in time, as we shall see.

The *De Cautelis Medicorum* is a textbook of ethics in the sense that it consists partly of advice, devices and strategies that the doctor can employ to enhance his reputation. The advantage that follows from this is not only the benefit of the individual but also that of doctors as a group and of a certain kind. The 'ethical' doctor leaves behind a reputation that will encourage the patient and his family to call a doctor a second time, rather than one of the different kinds of unlicensed practitioners.

The image of the doctor that Zerbi wanted his colleagues to maintain was – to deal with one aspect first – that of the serious and reliable doctor. To gain and retain the confidence of the patient, the good doctor should not take part in festivities; should not sing or dance, or play a musical instrument; and he should not hunt or use weapons.[6] In other words, Zerbi thought that a frivolous doctor would not be trusted by the patient. And neither would a loose-living doctor, who consorted with evil men. The patient's confidence in his doctor would also be diminished, said Zerbi, if the patients knew that the doctor took part in public affairs and consequently did not devote himself entirely to medicine: the authority of the doctor would be diminished and his medicine useless.

It was important for Zerbi that the doctor came from the right social class. It was in the nature of the vulgar, he argued, that they could not command respect, and as doctors they could have no authority and were not associated with learning. The doctor should therefore emphasize the signs of his class. His house, said Zerbi,[7] should be large and obvious, so that everyone knows where it is (and can reach it rapidly in emergency). His clothes and behaviour should be distinctly non-plebian[8] (decent, but avoiding the over-dressing of the doctor who sought success by merely pleasing his patient). He should not go shopping for food and household necessities, for he would be noticed by the vulgar, which would cheapen him. The Good Doctor does not cultivate land (by which Zerbi no doubt means that the doctor should not be associated with the rustic class and should not spend time on non-medical activities).

The doctor's position in the middle of the social scale meant that special parts of Zerbi's ethics are devoted to behaviour at his upper and lower class boundaries. This is most directly stated in his account of how to deal with plebians. This is not difficult, he says, because every plebian is ignorant and vulgar. But there are pitfalls even for the refined and distant physician, for in their ignorance the common people break up what the doctor says into contraries.[9] What Zerbi leaves unsaid here is that a coarse but penetrating wit might well have punctured the pomposity of the university-trained physician. He is indeed more explicit when dealing with the situation where other medical attendants bring unlearned assistants into a case on which Zerbi's Good Doctor is already at work. Such men, says Zerbi, 'are not solemn', and if – as often happens, he adds – they have a way with words and are men of shrewd native judgement, then they deride the solemn and learned opinions of the Good Doctor.[10]

Outside the sickroom the ethical doctor was not in such medically and embarrassingly close contact with plebians, and could afford to be distantly polite. Never be familiar with plebians, advises Zerbi, for it is sure to breed contempt. The reputation of the physician would suffer as a result; that is to say, he would prove less attractive to the class with the power to pay his fees. Do not even talk to plebians if you can avoid it, advises Zerbi, and if you are obliged to, never dispute with them but agree where possible and talk of things common to all men.

On the other hand, the physician, as middle class, had to cultivate an ethic that smoothed the boundaries between him and the higher classes. The Good Doctor, advises Zerbi, is not pompous, and can address all classes in the same way, exchanging courtly greetings with knights.[11]

The reputation of the doctor depended on success. It was, therefore, ethically important not to take on hopeless cases. Zerbi says quite precisely[12] that cases involving children, pregnant women and diseases of the eyes are likely to damage the reputation of the doctor and should not be taken on. No doubt high infant mortality and the technical difficulty of eye diseases accounted for Zerbi's gloomy assessment of these two kinds of case. The problem of pregnant women was that powerful remedies might result in miscarriage, when the doctor would be in danger of being accused of procuring an abortion. To avoid this in cases where it became necessary to treat a pregnant woman, Zerbi advises the use of phlebotomy only in the presence of a colleague; and the use of weak medicines, the preparation of which is to be entrusted to the family. Zerbi is here able to use the Hippocratic Oath and its prohibitions against abortifacients and poisons. Like the Hippocratic doctor, the Zerbist did not cut for the stone: not only was it Hippocratically unethical but also unlikely to be successful, Zerbi says. (Zerbi had his followers, at least in anatomy. Berengario da Carpi disparagingly called them *Zerbistae.*)[13]

Ethics and Money

The ethical problems of the doctor's fees were complicated. The patient was buying health and wanted to strike a good bargain. But medicine was a highly technical business – and the doctor took care it should remain so – and the patient was never entirely sure of what procedures of the doctor were appropriate to the final result, health. He knew very well that what he paid the doctor depended on how long the cure took, and how many times the doctor called, and he must often have suspected that the doctor came too often and extended the cure for the sake of a bigger fee. To maintain the doctor's reputation, it is, therefore, ethically important, Zerbi says, to cure as quickly as possible, for a lengthy treatment generates a bad name, particularly among the vulgar. Become the authority of the sickroom, advises Zerbi: everyone will obey quickly in order to save money.[14] The image of the quick and efficient doctor was enhanced by his use of expensive and thus apparently effective remedies. 'Expensive medicines cure quickly' is one of Zerbi's aphorisms; if they are given free, he says, they do not help very much.

The ultimate claim the doctor made to counter the patient's fears that he was paying too much was that the doctor's aim was not money but health. Zerbi adds (not from the church but from the Arabic author Haly Abbas) that the physician knows that he will be rewarded by God. It was, nevertheless, uncommonly useful that the doctor should also be rewarded by the patient. So much so that Zerbi describes as divine the kind of patient who, seriously ill, prays and pays at the same time. In contrast they are diabolical who, restored to health, refuse to pay and avoid the doctor afterwards. To

Zerbi's despair, it was commonly held that cure of a disease was due to the astrological influence of Mars: an odious belief, says Zerbi, and unremunerative (because the patient could use it as an excuse to refuse payment to the doctor).

Zerbi's advice is, therefore, to take your fee at an early stage, unless your patient is magnificent, curial, a relation or a pauper. It is proper to accept what is offered, however small (Zerbi no doubt means from a pauper): be *mercenarius* about your *mercedes*. But do not turn away a patient from whom you think you may not get a fee. Take the case, for pity's sake, because it is a Christian thing to do, and because 'it generates a laudable reputation' says Zerbi. Such a reputation would be destroyed, he adds, by any obvious pursuit, particularly at law, of a patient reluctant to pay. Yet all too often the doctors of the late fifteenth century did just this, and Zerbi bewails the fact that the result is that 'it makes our art look ignoble'.[15] Do not sue your patient, but seek the intercession of a third party, such as a friend or relative of the patient, or an apothecary.

But it is best, says Zerbi, to secure payment by means of your technical knowledge of medicine. Remember that when the patient is in pain and the disease is strong, he will readily offer promises to the doctor (and the doctor in return should pledge his best help). But when the weakness has passed, the patient retains little memory of the devotion shown by the doctor. So act opportunely in securing your fee in acute cases; and in recurrent fevers you will be given renewed opportunities with the return of the critical days. Receive your fee, Zerbi concludes, with all the modesty you wish, and as if the soul, while noticing, appears not to notice; or as if while your soul in its liberality declines the fee, the hand in its dexterity is extended to receive it. In short, do not appear to be greedy.

Ethics and People

Treating ethics as a code of behaviour that characterizes and informs the actions of the group, we should expect to see ethical problems at the places where the group meets others. This is particularly so if the other groups are engaged in competitive activities. Surgeons and physicians shared a common university training in Italy and were not professional rivals in the way that they were in Northern Europe. It is for this reason that Zerbi's ethics contain no advice on how the physician should deal with surgeons. But he does have things to say on apothecaries, students, different kinds of patients and the assistants and bystanders in medical cases.

The doctor's ethical behaviour to apothecaries is mainly a question of choosing a good one, a 'faithful' person, in Zerbi's words.[16] The greatest danger to the doctor is in the power and quantity of the medicines he orders, particularly the opiates and purges. The strength of these medicine is such, says Zerbi, that mishandling them can cause death. The doctor should be personally present when these are being made up. He should not write down in a single prescription the whole of what a patient will need. Indeed, says Zerbi, it is a good *cautela* to write nothing down, in case anything goes wrong and angry friends and relatives of the patient go to the apothecary's shop to find out what the medicine was. A written prescription in such a case would be a ticket to disaster in terms of reputation, says Zerbi.

A section of Zerbi's advice[17] is devoted to the appropriate behaviour of the medical man when another doctor is also in attendance on the case. If the medical man finds himself with a case that might arguably end fatally, it is wise to call in one or more colleagues. Perhaps they can add to the first doctor's knowledge of remedies, and certainly a fatal outcome will bring less blame to a small group of consulting doctors than to an individual. Society does not withdraw its reward, says Zerbi in his aphoristic style, but singularity more often brings infamy.

Part of the function of this ethical manoeuvre is thus to avoid a bad reputation. The same is true of Zerbi's advice about choosing a colleague who is to act in these circumstances. First make sure that everything is prepared, so that the incoming doctor and the practitioner calling him should not suddenly appear to need something. The new colleague should be senior, sympathetic to the patient and, in first place, 'faithful'. It is important that the colleague thus chosen, says Zerbi, should be learned in the *scientia* of medicine, which will make full and private discussion of the case possible. In this case the best course of action, says Zerbi, is to issue a single, joint *consilium*. We can see from the context of Zerbi's advice that the advantage of this was, again, that responsibility was shared and criticism deflected. The danger in issuing two *consilia,* particularly if differing in advice, and especially if written, was that the learning of the practitioners, their very claim to monopolistic practice, would be called into question. We have already seen the dangers to the learned doctor's reputation when the bedside is surrounded by impudent but clever quacks.

In the converse case, that is when the doctor whom Zerbi is addressing is called to another doctor's case, then the function of

Zerbi's ethics is the same. Here, too, the imperative is to close professional ranks and maintain a common reputation of learning and behaviour. Ask the first doctor if he has seen the patient yet, advises Zerbi. If he has, then praise some of his remedies and propose collaboration. If the first doctor's pupil is at the bedside, continues Zerbi, treat him with respect and do not denigrate him. Take him to one side and converse with him in a low voice and with a grave face: this will give the appearance of thinking deeply about the case. If the doctor coming into this situation finds that a mistake has been made then Zerbi advises that the correction should be made in private and never publicly. If you are obliged to disagree with your colleague, says Zerbi directly, tell only the friends of the patient and do not argue in front of others.

But there was an exception to Zerbi's expectation that given tact and a few rules of etiquette two learned doctors would act to preserve their common reputation. There is a danger, he says, of rich and proud doctors coming late to a case and while paying scant attention to the patient, imposing their own will and opinions. These were the practitioners, says Zerbi, whose practice it was to surround themselves with sycophantic empirics and plebians, who would shout down the learned and modest doctor. Who was Zerbi referring to? What group of practitioners were distinct enough from the university-trained, learned and rational group that Zerbi represented, to have a different system of internal rules, or ethics? Zerbi further describes such a practitioner as 'some professor of medicine to whom, by law and by merit, collaboration cannot be denied'.[18] So such a person professed medicine (Zerbi does not necessarily mean he taught it) and was clearly an able physician – to merit Zerbi's grudging admission, such a doctor must have met Zerbi's criteria of being learned and rational. Clearly, too, he had a legal standing at least equal to that of Zerbi's group. For Zerbi to mention the fact – and the resentment is clear – this was clearly some status, or even legal protection over and above that which Zerbi and his kind claimed as learned teachers and practitioners.

Zerbi's term for such one-sided collaboration is *collegium.* The activity itself is expressed by a verb, and Zerbi says those who *collegiant* publicly are damnable. What Zerbi is condemning is the tendency of the 'collegiating' physicians to aggrandize themselves at the expense of their own kind, and in front of third parties. This, says Zerbi, 'causes murmurs among the vulgar' and generates disrespect for doctors as a whole.

Zerbi's ethics here reflect a professional rivalry between politically different groupings of similarly educated physicians. Let us try to reconstruct his situation. Zerbi identified with the student *universitas* of Padua and its medical teachers. But the professional body in Padua was the College of Philosophers and Physicians, which gave degrees and licensed practice. It was not necessary to belong to the College in order to practise or even to teach. If Zerbi was not a member of the College, or, if a member, was not part of the powerful inner ring of older *numerarii,* he may well have resented the powers of granting degrees and of licensing practice – and for which they doubtless gave themselves airs – that the College had.

There is also another possibility. Padua was in the Veneto, under the control of rich and powerful Venice. Venice, too, had had a College of Physicians, from the early fourteenth century, which was concerned with the regulation of the professional practice of medicine. This, then, was an institution of a kind different to the Paduan *studium,* and was not at first concerned with education or the granting of degrees (there being no *studium* in Venice). But it claimed the right to give degrees at some time in the middle of the fifteenth century, and nearer Zerbi's time, at the visit of the emperor Frederick III in 1469 the Venetian College of Physicians was given the right to give eight degrees annually in arts and medicine. The ambition of the Venetian College was to extend its power and become a *studium,* examining students and granting degrees.

The *studium* of Padua clearly felt threatened. Almost certainly their statutes of 1468 (with which this chapter began) were designed to reinforce its privileges in the face of the ambitions of the Venetian College. By 1470 some Paduan students were indeed going to Venice for their degrees. (In the same way the professional College of Milan attracted students who had been educated in Pavia.) The student *universitas* in fact claimed the autonomy to co-operate with a professional College other than the Paduan for the granting of degrees to its students. There was intense rivalry between the Colleges of Padua and Venice on this account, and considerable strain between the Paduan College and the *studium.*[19] By 1489 the Paduan College was losing income and prestige to that of Venice. In other words Zerbi's 'collegiants' would have been especially 'damnable' if they came from the College of the politically dominant Venice, were the agents of the decline of the Paduan College and the seducers of the students of the *studium,* and were politically powerful within the profession in terms of practice and degrees. Zerbi's *ethical* dissatisfaction with their behaviour reflects perfectly the fact that the College was to an extent a *rival* grouping with its own set of values and behaviour. Indeed, the College in Venice had an explicit ethical code, with detailed advice on cases of which Zerbi complained, where two doctors were called.

In considering the doctor's behaviour to his patients, Zerbi seems to rely primarily on the Hippocratic sources. The 'ethical' doctor obeys the *Oath* when entering a house and avoids all injury to those therein.[20] Just as the Hippocratic ethical works seem to be sets of 'our' rules in opposition to those of 'them', so Zerbi has here a great deal of rhetoric against the flattering doctors, whose aim is to please by personal attention and agreeable treatments, and who succeed (says Zerbi) mainly with women and the vulgar, generating 'a hollow reputation'.[21] Perhaps Zerbi is drawing on Hippocratic sources with which he can, because of their authority, identify. It is not clear that he and his group were in fact facing a threat from such practitioners from outside the group. The same is true when he speaks of those doctors whose aims are simply evil. That is, there was much in the post-classical literature that was set out in the strongest terms against opponents who were necessarily 'evil', or in our terms 'unethical', and Zerbi can add to his rhetoric (for 'our' group) by quoting these sources. They are (in addition to the Old Testament) Averroes, Damascenus and Pietro d'Abano.

Women patients were a special sub-group. Not only were there the technical and ethical problems of women-related diseases (see above) but also the problems of the male doctor attending the female patient. Again, the source of Zerbi's ethics is the *Oath*. Do not even begin to think about libidinous approaches, says Zerbi.

Ethics and Learning

So far we have looked at Zerbi's advice to the doctor in situations into which the doctor's practice leads him, but which are not in themselves concerned with the technical content of that medicine. But the doctor's ethics did concern themselves with the technical content of medicine, in two ways. First, the doctor naturally believed that the kind of medicine he practised was the best. It would clearly be unethical to depart from the best medicine; and other kinds of medicine were also unethical. Second, Zerbi's kind of medicine was rationalist (in following Galen's natural-philosophical explanations) and learned. These two characteristics of medicine had been used in the high middle ages to justify the study of medicine in the *studia* as a true *scientia,* and Zerbi devotes much of his ethics to a defence of learning and to the training of the rational, learned doctor.

So Zerbi is defending *his* kind of medicine, taught in the university and battling to preserve its claims to monopoly in practice. Zerbi is at pains to demonstrate not only that this is the best kind of medicine, but that it is the only possible kind. It was consistent with, and linked to, other aspects of Zerbi's world, to his religion, his view of the social order and to his knowledge of other disciplines. To practise the best medicine, ethical medicine, meant to share these views.

To Zerbi, learned medicine was progressive. This was partly from necessity, for the physical decay of mankind, since the ancients, had allowed the appearance of new diseases unknown to the ancients (Zerbi was writing a few months after the first appearance of the *morbus gallicus*)[22] Old remedies were no longer always appropriate. Moreover, medical knowledge had been added to by a string of authors since Hippocrates and Galen had written, and Zerbi makes generous use of the Arabic authors and some of the commentators. Zerbi felt himself to be in a tradition of learned medicine, a tradition that had to be defended. He makes his defence by binding together all those aspects of his view of the world that would be shared by people of his group and class, who if not medical men, may well have been in a position to fight for the privileges which the learned doctor claimed. This binding-together is most evident in Zerbi's ethics, which show that the Good Doctor is ethical precisely because he behaves in accordance with a view of the world that a learned physician might be expected to have.

Let us look in more detail at the world-view of Zerbi's Good Doctor. He knows that it is of the utmost importance that the young should be introduced to good doctrine at an early age.[23] (Zerbi's elaborate analogy of a seed growing in good soil is founded on the Hippocratic *De Lege.*) The aim of education is to enable those who have completed it to lead a good life. This is a comprehensive goal, and includes medicine where the educated man wishes to become a doctor. The best way of living, says Zerbi, is by reason perfected by art. The sentiment is Aristotle's, and Zerbi has borrowed it from the *Metaphysics.* Good education, university education, was of course almost entirely Aristotelian. The reason that art perfected was the Aristotelian dialectic with which the arts course began. The student passed on to Aristotelian moral philosophy in the *Ethics* and *Politics.* Aristotelian natural philosophy, which normally came later in the arts course, contained the natural principles on which the theory of medicine rested.[24] Good medicine was an extension of natural philosophy, and good practice of medicine was informed partly by moral philosophy. For example, the doctor's ethical reluctance to discuss details of his patients' cases is overcome only by Aristotle's observation in the *Ethics* that discussion with someone capable of theoretical understanding should be completely frank.[25] Zerbi insists that the doctor's erudition begins with the grammar, rhetoric and dialectic of the schools and universities, with the four quadrivial arts of arithmetic, music, geometry and astrology, and above all, with natural philosophy. (Even his discussion of the medical *cautela* is informed by the four Aristotelian causes.)[26]

So the Good Doctor is *learned* in Aristotelian, and then medical knowledge, and he is *rational* in dealing in an Aristotelian way with the particulars of sense observation in his practice in relation to the universals that are in the mind. Do not, says Zerbi, give your attention only to universals, and despise particulars, for to do so is not the art of medicine.[27] Indeed, sensory observation will reveal to you things that cannot be put into words and cannot be written about in theoretical treatises.[28] The Good Doctor is he who has been well exercised as a young man in practice, having sought out hospitals and other places where there are many patients, diseases and skilful doctors. On the other hand, says Zerbi, do not give your attention wholly to particulars and despise universals, for that is empiricism.[29] In this way Aristotle furnishes the Good Doctor with both a theory of knowledge (what is first in the senses is not first in nature; there is nothing in the mind that was not first in the senses) and with a criterion for medical licensing (empirics have no knowledge of universals). Zerbi says, expressly from Aristotle's logical works, that nothing can be known without its first principles. But, he adds, while the foundation of medicine lies in its first principles, first principles are on their own useless unless brought down to particulars. (It is in acquiring new particulars that medicine was for Zerbi, as we have seen, progressive.)

The later part of this education of the Good Doctor, says Zerbi, takes place in 'celebrated universities'.[30] Zerbi has a great deal of rhetoric on the behaviour of students. He makes an elaborate simile illustrating that as the father is the cause in procreation, so the teaching master is the cause of the student learning a *scientia*. Zerbi's rhetoric, in its prefatorial and aphoristic style, enlarges upon how the students must learn from, respect and obey their teachers, paying due reverence to their authority and skill. Now, this is a natural thing to write for a man who has been a university teacher for most of his adult life; it is also something that would naturally appeal to those with power to help implement Zerbi's view of the doctor's duties and privileges. But it is more than this. In these words Zerbi is binding together other aspects of his view of the world. We can examine these by focusing on the central notion of trust, or faith. Ultimately the Good Doctor is the one who behaves 'faithfully' – he is *fidelis*. It is faith that the student shows to his teachers in accepting what they say, obeying them and revering them. It is this same faith that the modern, late fifteenth-century doctor gives to the old authors. Despite the change in the human body and the progress of knowledge, faith is to be given to the fathers of medicine – Hippocrates followed by Galen. When Zerbi was writing it was only a few years since Leoniceno had launched his attack on Pliny.[31] The result was a bitter dispute in which the defenders of Pliny argued that although he may have been wrong in places, it was improper to make such a violent and public attack on so great a name. Colenuccio,[32] the lawyer, pointed out that in a court a misdemeanor could be excused if the defendant was a great ornament to society. Leoniceno, in his opponents' eyes, lacked that faith and reverence that should be accorded to one of the fathers of the Latin tradition of learning, the *res latina*. Precisely the same thing was to happen when Vesalius attacked Galen when, after the bitter troubles of the early Reformation, Vesalius' opponents lent a distinct *odium theologicum* to their accusations that Vesalius 'lacked faith'.[33] Much of Zerbi's ethical advice centres on the 'faithful' doctor, who *erit non aliter quam fidelis*.[34] The doctor is the faithful companion of the body of his patient, suffers with him and rejoices in his health. To neglect him, to act improperly in his home, to do anything prohibited by common morality or special medical ethics, would be to break faith with the patient.

Another element that Zerbi is binding into his notion of 'faith' is the Hippocratic ethics of the *Oath* and *Law*. The *Oath* represents an initiation procedure. The entrant swears to obey it. He is enjoined to keep the secrets of the group he is joining. He swears to honour his teachers and to pass on freely the secret knowledge to their sons. Other Hippocratic ethical works suggest that this secret knowledge is believed to have had a divine origin: it characterizes the group that has it and is responsible for their success. Its origin and utility meant that it had to be protected from outsiders, the profane. Holy things are given only to holy men. The doctor who used the *Oath* in his own ethical system saw himself as being within a tradition of special knowledge that had to be protected and where the fathers of the discipline were the first teachers, to whom were due reverence and faith. It was in Zerbi's time that the medieval medical textbook, the *Articella,* came to include not only the *Oath,* but also the other Hippocratic ethical text that Zerbi used, the *Law.*[35] Both clearly – and *Law* expressly – relate to a time when there was no system of medical licensing, but because both deal with the initiation of doctors and the faith within the medical tradition, and because of the authority of the name of Hippocrates, Zerbi can use them to strengthen his arguments for learned medicine to be the way he wants it to be inside and outside the universities.

Another thread that runs through Zerbi's view of the world that goes to make up his ethics is religion. This too deals with 'faith' and the word never entirely loses its Christian meaning. We should not expect that it would, for in the fifteenth-century university there could be no division of kind between 'medicine', 'religion' or other similar categories. During the previous two centuries medical commentators (like Gentile) could rationally begin their expositions with an invocation of divine help on the grounds that God was the ultimate cause of everything, including the commentator and his text.[36] God (they said) followed Aristotelian causality in creating all things: we can see arts-course Aristotelianism as providing a deeper understanding of religious doctrine. Contemporary discussions of what constitutes knowledge often emphasize the singleness of 'philosophy' as all knowledge of the works of man and God. Its purpose was perfection of the soul of man in anticipation of temporal and eternal happiness.[37] This is consistent with and an extension of Aristotle's belief that the end of moral philosophy is happiness.

Zerbi, like his medieval predecessors, places invocation of divine help in first place when giving his opening account of how to achieve the good life (reason perfected by art).[38] The second instrument for this end is erudition: the physician must immerse himself in study, day and night (that is, ethical medicine is *learned* medicine). The third and last is to preserve one's reputation by observing the medical canons. These are broad ethical rules that are parallelled, says Zerbi, by the evangelic law. Again, the first of these is the invocation of divine help, the help of the legislator who created all things. The parallel is the text of Matthew: ask, and it shall be given; seek and you will find. Second is dedication to the task: the narrow gate that leads to righteousness. Third, avoid false doctrine. Here the text is the biblical injunction to avoid false prophets, that is, 'heretical doctrine'.[39] The parallel is a fine one: heresy and the teachings of false prophets are, of course, *other* people's systems of thought and belief and so, in the sense we are using the word here, deeply *unethical.* Medical heresy for Zerbi was empiricism, that is, unlearned and so unlicensed practice.[40] Here[41] Zerbi is tying tightly together 'correct', ethical, medical and religious belief by making a common enemy in medical and religious heresy.

Having discussed the natural attributes and acquired skills of the Good Doctor, Zerbi's second chapter is concerned with the most important *cautela* of practice, the doctor's behaviour to God. Again, medical and religious belief are not to be distinguished: the doctor, says Zerbi, is like a priest, and is divine in using the medicines that God has created on earth; and he is divine also in being he to whom divine things are revealed, in being, that is, a Hippocratic. Part of the ethical training of Zerbi's Good Doctor is to be made fit to receive such revelation. The revelation is the special knowledge of the doctor (Zerbi quotes the Hippocratic *De Lege* through the commentator Nicholas) but the training is late fifteenth-century Christianity.

The doctor was like a priest also in his practice. Urge the patient to confess, says Zerbi, arguing that a secret sin may be at the root of the patient's illness[42] (and so may be evil demons, the *alabin*). Zerbi says the Good Doctor invokes divine help in compounding his remedies and in writing *consilia*; before beginning treatment he says 'May God liberate you'; he remembers that it is God who cures, not the physician; in using antidotes he always completes his treatment by saying 'If God so wishes'; in making prognostications he is careful not to appear to usurp God's foreknowledge.

Prognosis

While taking care not to usurp God's foreknowledge, the rational physician nevertheless had good professional reasons for relying a good deal on prognosis. Prognosis was display. It was a display of technical knowledge and techniques that impressed the patient. It was a display that showed that the doctor knew about the kind of disease that the patient had, at the point where the patient's interest was at its greatest, that is, about what was going to happen. For Zerbi it was an essentially Galenic technique, for it was a display that demonstrated that the physician knew all about the patient's disease from its symptoms down to the fundamental facts of nature. Prognosis, that is, was part of the rational doctor's Good Story, by which his reason and learning impressed the patient. Rational medicine competed in the market-place partly on the basis of prognosis. It was an *ethical* practice in the sense we are using the term in this chapter: that it was controlled by an explicit set of rules (about when to do it and when not: see below); rules that characterized a group and contributed to its success.

Zerbi's ideal rational, learned and prognosticating physician made a careful entry to the sickroom. He did not hasten round to the patient's house, run up the stairs and make an unexpected entrance, hot and sweaty, but waited until both he and the patient were prepared for the encounter. Meanwhile he kept his eyes open for any signs of earlier treatment that might give him a hint about what the patient or a previous doctor thought the disease might be. The inspiration for Zerbi was Galen's account, in *De Locis Affectis,* of how he had immeasurably impressed the patient with his skill in prognostication on the basis of chance observations of things left in the sickrooom. Zerbi then advises the prognosticating doctor to take the patient's pulse, noting down the hundred and more differences he will feel. Contemporary medicine was well supplied with distinctions within the kinds of pulse and amply furnished with technical terminology. The doctor was making a display of his mastery of these technical matters, and Zerbi's advice is to spend a great deal of time doing it.[43] Then, says Zerbi, touch the patient's chest and abdomen, examine his tongue and teeth and if you like, smell his breath. Then with everyone present and the patient listening, describe the great medical usefulness of taking the pulse and say 'I will now examine the urine, for it is principally by these two things, the pulse and the urine, that the type of fever is understood, together with the origin of their cause, the *ratio* of life and the *professio* of death.' In other words, this is the patter of the rational physician selling his medicine by claims of rationality and a learned tradition: the audience is arranged, the name of Galen is invoked, the display of pulse-taking is rationalized by reference to causality, and finally it is claimed that this learning and reason lead to the solemn business of prognostication.

The benefits of making a correct prognosis were considerable. Zerbi calls them honour and glory. But the dangers were also great, and the doctor had to handle things carefully. Never discuss the significance of your findings about the pulse and urine in front of the patient, advises Zerbi. Leave the sickroom and let a little time pass. Consider everything you have been able to learn about the patient, from his symptoms, from his friends, by looking about the house, from any earlier medical attendant. Be very cautious about making a prognostication, says Zerbi, especially of death, for the patient's state of mind may make such a prophecy self-fulfilling. Indeed it is best not to make absolute predictions, he adds, and the wise medical man, like the astrologer, makes his prognostications conditional, saying something like 'Certainly it seems to me if things remain as they are and nothing supervenes ...'[44] The model for Zerbi is Galen's highly conditional judgement that a patient will escape the disease if he has a good doctor, is himself obedient, has diligent servants well prepared with all external necessities and if nothing unexpected happens.[45] If the doctor is uncertain about the outcome or if the disease is changing the doctor could take Zerbi's advice and answer questions obliquely: change the subject, reply indirectly or let drop a significant but uncommitted word or two. Zerbi concludes that on the whole it is best to make a rather gloomy forecast when uncertain. If the outcome is good, the doctor gathers up the glory.[46] If it is bad, the doctor avoids blame, either because he saw the danger early, or because the blame can be attributed to the failure of one of four conditions suggested by Galen – the failure of the patient to obey, the servants to be diligent, the external necessities to be correct, or the arrival of the unexpected.

Anatomy and Ethics

Six years after Zerbi produced his tract *De Cautelis Medicorum,* there appeared his textbook of anatomy.[47] Both publications are in many senses very novel. It is claimed that there were earlier works on ethics, but they are not so explicit or even so big as Zerbi's small tract. As for the anatomy, the contrast with what had gone before is more striking. The statutory text was Mondino's brief *Anathomia,* but this did not generate published commentary until Berengrio da Carpi in 1521. Most other anatomical work was limited to commentaries on the Canon by expositors like Matthaeus de Gradibus, Jacobus de Partibus and Gentile da Foligno.[48] Zerbi's *Liber Anathomie* is quite different. Nearly half of a million words long, designed for use in conjunction with public dissections, drawn from a wide range of sources, it is clearly intended to make some major statement about the nature of university anatomy.

What can Zerbi's anatomy tell us about his view of the world, which we have explored in locating and explaining his ethics? Let us return to Padua. The statutes of 1468 and their revised version of the early sixteenth century use unusually strong language on insisting on the suppression of unlicensed practice, and on the regular performance of the public anatomies. Some urgency was clearly felt about both matters, and mention is made of previous laxity. When Zerbi returned to Padua in 1494 after periods in Bologna and Rome, he was an *ordinarius* teacher, the teacher who gave the principal lectures. He was directly concerned with the teaching, the practice and the defence of university medicine. As we have seen, what made university medicine different from any other sort was primarily that it was learned. It claimed its authority from a tradition of learning that seemed to stretch back to Hippocrates and Galen. It was on a basis of this learning that the university doctor claimed also that his medicine was more effective than others and that this in turn gave him the right to claim a monopoly of practice. Galen, as a Rationalist, had constructed a medicine on the foundation of structure, from which a discussion about function, malfunction and treatment could link the patients' symptoms to the fundamentals of the natural-philosophical world picture.[49] Anatomy was the touchstone of learned and rational medicine. The spectacle of public dissections was much more than a way of teaching the Paduan physicans and surgeons about the inside of the human body. It was a statement about the kind of medicine that was taught and practised and about the identity of the people who taught and practised it. Nothing could be a more arresting spectacle than, in tightly controlled circumstances, placing a dead human body on a table and cutting it into small pieces, beginning with a sweeping incision along the length of the abdomen.

The place of anatomy within rational and learned medicine is reflected in Zerbi's book on the human body. It opens with a declaration of the nature and purposes of anatomy. These are largely philosophical. Anatomy of the human shows to the highest degree the skill and providence of nature, says Zerbi; knowledge of its parts is knowledge of a high order and is of benefit to the soul. Zerbi does not need to say that Nature is the mode by which the Creator worked and works in the world any more than he needed to say that academic study of Nature was a major component of the arts course and the main way in which rationalist medicine reached back to the fundamentals of the world picture. His readers would have been well aware of this consonance between Christianity and Greek philosophy.

In this way Zerbi saw that anatomy was fundamental to the kind of medicine (and of course it included surgery, for which anatomy was necessary) which he was trying to defend. It may be that the perceived threat was simply fom unlicensed practice. But he may also have been convinced of the importance of the *teaching* of proper medicine – his medicine – within the *studium,* where it would inform the practice of future doctors. The teaching of medicine was not part of the functions of the Colleges and perhaps Zerbi was trying to defend his kind of medicine against that of the

Collegiants. His defence was essentially practical. The anatomy text was practical, designed to accompany a dissection. The dissection itself was practical: not only would such an image, a characteristic of rational medicine, be much more memorable than mere arguments; but also Zerbi was taking effective action through his book and its associated dissections, to follow the urgings of the new statutes. His ethics too were practical – he says so in a formal discussion about their place in medicine.[50] And one of the ethical rules themselves is that the intending doctor should not waste his life in the theory of medicine. We can recall that another section of the new Paduan statutes reveal anxiety about the level of unlicensed practice, or in other words, the learned and rational physician was facing competition from other doctors. Zerbi's *De Cautelis Medicorum* can be seen as consistent with, even if not inspired by this corporate nervousness about external groups with their own systems of ethics. It explains to the university doctor above all how to promote and defend his own kind of medicine. It would make perfectly plain to anyone who had the power to promote Zerbi's ideal on what grounds rational, learned and university medicine claimed superiority. To summarize, anatomy, and public dissections of the human body, were very powerful displays of the fact that the medicine they represented was learned and based on a rationalist view that the structure, function and malfunction of the body was intelligible. Its practitioners also thought that this kind of medicine was also ethically the best, if only because it was clearly unethical to allow the practice of a different, and therefore worse, kind of medicine. For Zerbi and the men who gave emphasis to these parts of the statutes, learning and rationality were to be defended and promoted as much by anatomy as by ethics.

Conclusion: Ethics Old and New

We have seen that Zerbi's ethics were written down in all probability in response to a threat he saw to his kind of medicine in the 1490s. If these were historically 'local' causes, can we speak of an earlier history of ethics, perhaps even a genre or tradition? We probably cannot, certainly if we limit ourselves to written materials in which we might find explicit discussions of the physicians' professional behaviour. Even though Zerbi makes a virtue of naming his sources, his book is a compilation of fragments by other people on other topics.

One example must suffice. For Zerbi the Good Doctor was the *medicus canonicus.* It is this 'canonical physician' whose serious-mindedness was, as we have seen, sometimes punctured by the coarse wit of the vulgar. It was he, also, who suffered from the high-handedness of the 'collegiates', and in this case, Zerbi argues, there is a *modus canonicus,* a proper method of procedure to be followed by the canonical physician. The canons of medicine that he follows in the same way as he follows the evangelic law (see above) would thus seem to no less than ethical rules. But the *modus canonicus* is derived from the first book of Avicenna's *Canon.* At the point in the text indicated by Zerbi (fen 1, doctrine 1, chapter 1: de *subjectis medicine.*)[51] Avicenna discusses not ethics, or behaviour, or reputation, but how medicine can only be effective if based on the first principles of (an Aristotelian) natural philosophy, and that upon the 'first philosophy' or metaphysics. In emphasizing what the physician must know – and anatomy is very important – Avicenna tells us more about the history of what in this chapter we have called rational medicine, but is not writing about ethics. The 'ethical' use to which Zerbi puts his source is thus derived from its technical superiority, and is not inherited from an ethical component of Avicenna's medicine.

In the period after Zerbi and before that to which the later chapters of this book are devoted, we can look for a history of medical ethics primarily in the sense that it was naturally considered ethical to practise the proper kind of medicine – one's own – and unethical to do otherwise, or to allow other – unethical – groups to succeed. In the sixteenth century, especially, there were more groups, readily identifiable, to be considered than in the earlier period. Following Leoniceno's attacks on Avicenna, there were many who would not have considered Avicenna's medicine to be *canonicus.* These were the 'skilled Hellenists' as Zerbi and Berengario da Carpi[52] called them, who objected to all things medieval, to commentators and even to the Latin language. Perhaps even as early as Zerbi's book on anatomy, one of these Hellenists, Alessandro Benedetti, had written an entirely Hellenist anatomy (it was rather slim).[53] Undoubtedly the sponsors of the revived Greek medicine of the Hellenists and humanists rejected much of medieval medicine, and so their views of what it was 'ethical' to practise must have changed in part.

But in part, too, there were continuities that reflect the other aspects of the physician's life, the power of his religion, his defence of the learned tradition and his need to protect the reputation of physicians as a whole. These things are reflected in the structure of a set of medical ethics of an author a generation later than Zerbi,

Clementi Clementini, writing in 1535. His *Lucubrationes* are similar enough to Zerbi's *Cautela* for us to guess that by the sixteenth century there was in fact a recognized topic of 'medical ethics' in medical education. The inclusion of the Hippocratic ethical works in the essentially medieval *Articella* presupposes some form of commentary on them during teaching. And even though the new classicism of the Hellenists had led to the end of the publishing history of the *Articella* (almost at the same time that Clementini's book appeared) they would have had little reason to exclude from their teaching a discussion of Hippocratic ethics.

Almost everything that Clementini wrote can be related to Zerbi's work. There is space here to draw only a skeletal parallel. Clementini begins with the sacred nature of medicine. It is partly that the curative powers of medicines are God-given (the physician merely administers them); partly that the doctor should, at his first contact with the patient, use some of the formality of the priest to reconcile the patient with God, the author of disease as well as of medicines and health; and partly that the physician piously emulates Christ the Healer. Indeed, the physician should be to his patient as another God, benign, merciful, charitably treating the poor for no reward and even the well-to-do for Grace rather than fees. Be confident, urges Clementini, that such charitable treatments will be rewarded by God, who will provide the charitable doctor's necessities (and punish the uncharitable's sins) and, in fact, will act to the doctors as the doctor acts to his patients. But the professional demands of reputation and financial respectability are not to be ignored and Clementini slides easily and without irony into the practical results of charitable practice. *Constant* charitable practice will through experience produce a better doctor, and so a charitable spirit often leads to a better reputation and richer financial rewards; one grateful patient may well meet in his fee the lapses of others. As with Zerbi the basis of the doctor's relationship with the patient is 'faith' which the doctor keeps with his patient, involving charity, love and just treatment. Moreover, says Clementini, again without irony or conflict of ideals, such medicine cures more quickly; from duties and liberality the doctor gathers up praise and thanks.

Like Zerbi too Clementini places emphasis on the learning of the doctor. It is limited to advice to study hard and in particular to be certain of what the medical literature says about the variations in disease that occur in different places and at different times. However, in a striking contrast to Zerbi, Clementini argues that ultimately the Good Doctor is born, not made. It is by the influx of the stars that the best doctor is almost divine, with sound judgement and an ability to predict. To be sure, learning is a necessary part of the process, and Clementini says he has seen many a man born full of vice under a bad astrological sign and yet made good by a study of letters. Indeed, some such thing is hardly avoidable for, as he says, theoretical medicine is subject to Taurus and practical to Scorpio: both signs make medical men jealous and malevolent among themselves, and only a commitment to philosophical learning and to moral discipline can overcome these astrological disadvantages.

Although it was a commonplace of medical thought that the good doctor had certain natural attributes (such as a retentive memory and capable hands; Zerbi discusses such things) it was quite another thing to claim that a physician, as physician, was born rather than made. An extreme form of this view was held by Paracelsus: that medicine was God-given and traditional learning useless. No discussion of Reformist thinking is in order in this chapter, but again we are reminded that as the sixteenth century progressed a protestant way of thinking about the best, *ethical,* way of practising medicine was added to the other groups we have identified. Clementini hovers between the 'almost divine' nature of the attributes of such a physician and the very human similar ones that Zerbi had offered direct injunctions about acquiring. Such a physician does not become inebriated; does not mix with the ignorant or the rustic but, self-contained and solitary, avoids the contempt that is bred by familiarity; he uses knowledge of letters and especially of philosophy to avoid vices to so to stand out from the ignorant crowd and even to govern it; to such a man incurable cases do not happen, perhaps because of the near-divinity of his prescience.

But Clementini is as explicit as Zerbi and no doubt for the same reasons on what to do if the doctor does find himself with a hopeless case on his hands: do not tell the patient (it will only make him worse), but make clear the prognosis to the assistants. Having seen them now in Zerbi we can understand what is behind the rest of Clementini's related ethical injunctions. Do not, he charges his readers, make prognostications more than necessary, and certainly not before those who are merely curious. The outcome of diseases, like that of wars, is uncertain; and Clementini, like Galen and Zerbi, warns that the doctor cannot be certain of the obedience of the patient or the assistants. Clementini took the Hippocratic view that judgement is difficult and *experimentum* fallacious: although there is great fortune in prognosticating at times of great danger, and although he who can see what will happen on the basis of learning and experience, collects the greatest glory, it is best, concludes Clementini, to keep quiet rather than risk it. He, too, recognized the doctor's device (like all of these devices, expressed at more length by Zerbi) of representing a case as more serious than it actually was in order to avoid the blame of a death and to collect large fees and much glory if the outcome were favourable.[54]

So – finally – Zerbi's ethics seem to be one of the earliest expressions of a group's self-regulatory rules of the renaissance period. They incorporate, for obvious historical reasons, the rather more fragmentary internal rules of regulation of the various groups represented in the Hippocratic corpus. They give the historian more insight into the group-rules of physicians as a society than do the earlier 'pathway of physicians' of Gentile da Foligno or the equation between ethical and technical superiority made by the New Galenism, described by Luis Garcia-Ballester. After Zerbi the appearance of new groups of medical men suggests not only the below-the-surface formulation of new ethics for each of the groups, but also – as in the case of Clementini – the historical appearance (or continuity) of a self-conscious discussion about how medical men should behave.

Notes

1. Thus *Ancient Medicine* can be interpreted as a defence of experiential, dietetic and (its self-image) proper and originally divine medicine against fluent and personable opponents with a resembance to the sophists. The *Oath* can be seen as representing an admissions. procedure into a group very like that portrayed in *Ancient Medicine.*
2. See R. K. French, 'Gentile da Foligno and the via medicorum', in J. D. North and J. J. Roche, *The Light of Nature* (Dordrecht: Nijhoff, 1985) 21–34.
3. *Statuta Almae Universitatis D. Artistarum et Medicorum Patavini Gymnasii* (Venice, 1589). The reference to Zerbi is on f.61r. The statutes about unlicensed practice are at f.69r, where the civil authorities are urged to take new action. The new anatomy statutes are at 67v. It was directed that the new statutes should all be read out publicly in Italian to the sound of trumpets.
4. See J. R. Lind, *Studies in Pre-Vesalian Anatomy. Biography, Translations, Documents* (Philadelphia: The American Philosophical Society, 1975) 141–56.
5. Gabriel de Zerbi, *Opus perutile de Cautelis Medicorum, in Pillularium omnibus medicis Necessarium clarissimi doctoris magistri Panthaleonis* (Lyons: 1528). According to Lind (1975) 151, Zerbi's was the first systematic account of medical ethics, preceded only by more

fragmentary accounts by Arnald of Villanova, Alberto de' Zancari, Cristoforo Barzizza and Alessandro Benedetti.

6. f.lxiii r.
7. f.lxiii r.
8. f.lxxii v.
9. f.lxxii v.
10. f.lxx v.
11. f.lxxiii r; lxxii v.
12. f.lxviii v.
13. Jacopo Berengario da Carpi, *Commentaria cum amplissimis additionibus in Anatomia Mundini,* (Bologna: 1521), ff 307v, 310r.
14. f.lxviii v.
15. f.lxix v.
16. f.lxii v.
17. f.lxx v.
18. f.lxxi r.
19. See the useful account by R. Palmer, *The Studio of Venice and its graduates in the Sixteenth Century* (Padua: Lint, 1983).
20. f. lxi r.
21. ff.lxi r–v.
22. The widespread notion that mankind had degenerated was compatible with the respect shown for the classical authors by the humanists and hellenists. It was to be developed by the Parisian anatomists Sylvius and Riolan to explain how the modern body was different from that apparently described by Galen. See J. Sylvius, *In Hippocratis et Galeni Physiologiae partem Anatomicam Isagoge* (Venice: 1556), e.g. f.7v.
23. f.lvi r.
24. Natural philosophy in the universities began traditionally with the text and a commentary of the 'Eight books of the Physics', *Octo libri physicorum.* These general principles of natural change, were then explored through a range of Aristotle's *libri naturales* that dealt with subject matter of increasing complexity – generation and corruption, the heavens and earth, meteorology and finally the workings of the soul in animals.
25. f.lix r.
26. f.lv v.
27. f.lix v.
28. f.lvii v. There were two areas where it was generally agreed that theory was inadequate, and only empirical observation would suffice: the actions of certain drugs, and the complex shape of some parts of the body. See French, note 2 above, 21–34; also *idem,* 'Berengario da Carpi and the use of commentary in anatomical teaching' in A. Wear, R. French and I. Lonie, (eds) *The Medical Renaissance of the Sixteenth Century* (Cambridge: Cambridge University Press, 1985).
29. ff.lvii r; lix v.

30. f. lvii r.
31. N. Leoniceno, *De Plinii et plurium aliorum Medicorum in Medicina Erroribus* [Ferrara: nd.(*c.*late 1492)].
32. P. Collenuccio, *Pliniana Defensio* [Ferrara: nd.(*c.* early 1493)).
33. See Sylvius, *Isagoge*, note 5 above. See also B. Eustachio, *Opuscula Anatomica* (Venice: 1563). 165–73.
34. f.lxi v.
35 For example, *Articella nuperrime impressa cum quamplurimis tractatibus pristine impressione superadditis* (Lyons: 1525): *De Lege* is at f.x, the third work of the collection. The edition of Venice, 1523 contains *De Lege* towards the end.
36. See Gentile da Foligno, in beginning his commentary on Avicenna (note 48 below).
37. In this it was like the philosophy of many medieval accounts of 'the sciences'. Perhaps the best known and certainly one of the earliest is that of D. Gundissalinus (Gundisalvi), *De Divisione Philosophiae* (edited by C. Baeumker and G. von Hertling in *Beitrage der Philosophie des Mittelalters* (Munster: 1906) vol 4.
38. Prologue.
39. f.lv r.
40. f.lvii v.
41. f.lv r.
42. f. lxii v.
43. f. lxiii v.
44. f. lxv r.
45. f. lxv v.
46. f. lxvi r.
47. Gabriele de Zerbi, *Liber Anathomie Corporis Humani et singulorum Membrorum illius* (Venice: 1502).
48. *Tertius Canonis Avicenna cum dilucidissimis expositoribus Gentile fulginate nec non Jac. de partibis Parisiense,* 3 vols, (Venice: *c.*1499); *Tertius Canonis Avicennae cum amplissima Gentilis fulg. expositione. Demum commentaria nuper addita videlicet Jacobi de Partibus super fen vi et xiii. Item Jo. Matthei de gradi super fen xxii quia Gentilis in eis deficit,* in 2 vols, the first without date or place, the second being *Secunda pars Gentilis super tertio Avic. cum supplementis Jacobis de partibus parisiensis ac Joannis Matthei de Gradi mediolensis ubi Gentilis vel breviter vel tacite pertransivit,* (Venice: 1522).
49. See P. Brain, *Galen on Bloodletting* (Cambridge: Cambridge University Press, 1986).
50. f.lv v.
51. *Principis Avic. Libri Canonis necnon de Medicinis Cordialibus et Cantica* (Venice: 1527) 3.
52. Zerbi (*Anathomie* 7v) discusses the *Periti Elleni,* as does Berengario, *Commentaria,* 49r.
53. It seems likely that the first edition of Benedetti's anatomy was that

of Venice, 1502. Lind (1975) discusses the problem of identifying supposed ealier editions.

54. Clementius Clementinus, *Lucubrationes* (Basel: H. Petrus, 1535). All of these remarks on ethics are contained in Clementini's preface (unpaginated). Much of the text is concerned with the logical processes related to the gaining of medical knowledge. It may be part of a discussion involving scholars like Leoniceno on the opening words of Galen's *Tegni.*

X

Berengario da Carpi and the use of commentary in anatomical teaching

Introduction

The sixteenth century is widely held as a period of renaissance in medicine. Certainly there was a radical change in the style and content of teaching in the 1520s; and in anatomy this can be seen as the victory of the Hellenists over the men of the schools.

Some historical attention has been given to anatomy in the earlier sixteenth century, but much of it has been rather unbalanced. The principal reason for this is the historical eminence accorded to Vesalius, whose name is generally linked to humanism, renaissance, the beginnings of modern science and all the things that are good in common historical estimation.

In particular historians have attempted to group together the people who wrote anatomies before 1543 as 'preVesalians'. The implication is not merely that they were earlier than Vesalius, but that they were not so good as Vesalius. Thus Lind[1] speaks of the reasons (too much philosophy and not enough dissection) for their 'failure' (that is, their failure to be Vesalius). But the preVesalians were not striving towards a common goal, nor attempting to hit upon the proper method of proceeding. Some light can be thrown on what they were trying to achieve and what their conceptions of anatomy were by a closer look at Berengario da Carpi.

In fact a closer look at Berengario is long overdue. Historians have found it difficult,[2] because of its size, to tackle the *Commentary on Mondino*[3] of Berengario: this is the only major text omitted from Lind's collection of translations, yet it is almost a complete guide to the earlier anatomical literature,[4] is the first printed anatomy to be illustrated, and was the work identified by major figures like Fallopia[5] as that which initiated the revival of anatomy.

Many of Berengario's purposes in his teaching can be related to the commentary as a form. The commentary had been the vehicle of medical education for some two and a half centuries when Berengario produced his in 1521. The medieval commentary had a precise form, as is shown below, and differed in its structure both from its predecessors, like Galen's commentaries on Hippocratic works and those by the Alexandrian commentators on Galen, and from its successors, the humanist commentaries.[6] Broadly speaking, medieval medical education was based on a small group of short texts, the *Articella*, and increasingly upon the *Canon* of Avicenna. The substance of the teaching of different masters was commentary upon these texts.

The principal exception to this method of teaching was the anatomical demonstration. The essence of the dissection was that it was a *practical* affair. It was carefully controlled by regulations within the institutional arrangements of the university and formed a regular, if not frequent element of the curriculum. Probably dissections had been carried out since the Salernitan demonstrations[7] of the insides of pigs of the twelfth century. Human dissection seems to have begun in the late thirteenth century.

As a practical affair, dissection and the demonstration of the parts did not generate commentary. There was of course the necessary business of glossing anatomical terms as different authors became better known, and this extended to the establishing of sound texts and the correct attribution of works; but anatomical texts of the middle ages that had a direct bearing on dissection did not have the form of a commentary. Nor had there survived from antiquity any suitable text that might form the basis of a commentary. The only commentaries containing anatomical material were those upon book three of the *Canon*, which is much more than an anatomy text.

So Berengario was unique among his predecessors and contemporaries in producing a dissection-based anatomy in commentary form. Moreover, he was using the commentary – a device of the schools – at the time when the Hellenists were successfully making such great changes in medical education. A closer look at Berengario, then, should not only make available details of an unjustly ignored figure, but also illuminate the broader topic of the medical renaissance. We need to know details of Berengario that may help us understand his recorded actions; we should know what a commentary was, and why Berengario chose to use it; and we should try to understand how Berengario saw himself and his contemporaries.

Life

Berengario was born at Carpi in the early 1460s, for he was still a child, *satis puer*, in 1467. The records describe his father as a barber surgeon, but his practice indicates he had considerable skill in difficult cases and Berengario recalls two cases of badly fractured skulls[8] and a hysterectomy.[9] His father taught Berengario surgery as he grew up: while still a youth he helped to treat three serious wounds of the head, and later maintained that no one could learn to be a good surgeon unless he had spent his childhood at it. He seems not to have had a formal education in the early years and perhaps would never have been taught more than surgery had it not been for his friendship with the family of Lionello Pio, the *signore* of Carpi. Lionello's wife was Catherina, sister of Pico della Mirandola, and after Lionello's death, it was Pico's suggestion that his friend Aldo Manuzio should go to Carpi as tutor to the young Alberto and his brother.

The education of the future prince of Carpi then, was to be in the hands of a devoted Hellenist who had cut his intellectual teeth in a circle outside the universities. (The term 'Hellenist' has a particular significance in this chapter: see below.) The education of princes was of course a question much addressed by the Italian intelligentsia (and it was a question not only of teaching but of future reciprocal patronage). It was from such a network of personal contacts that the Hellenists waged their war against the academics. Aldo arrived in Carpi in about 1479, when Alberto was four and his brother two. Berengario in contrast, was about nineteen, and must have been a surgeon of some experience. By now he surely had mental habits that could not be entirely lost in the education he was to receive so (comparatively) late, and it seems likely that his later insistence on the importance of the senses of sight and touch in anatomy, his rejection of purely verbal demonstration of structure and his admiration for anatomists who were *artifices*, craftsmen, was owing to this.

We can gather something of Aldo's educational interests from his published 'letters' to Catherina Pio.[10] The favoured authors were Cicero, Horace and Quintilian, to be followed by the Greek studies so dear to him and to Pico. Alberto doubtless received great benefit from all this, but how rigorous Berengario's education was at the hands of Aldo is not clear. He says himself that his studies with Aldo were only of the 'rudiments of the gentler muses'. No doubt Berengario was later on pleased enough to be able to refer back to a period of instruction from a famous scholar, which, it has been suggested, he exaggerated, for critics like Haller have pointed out that Berengario's Latin style is not what we would expect from a pupil of Aldo. But as we shall see, Berengario's style was chosen for its purpose, and literary prose is restricted to his dedications.

We can assume that Berengario at least absorbed some Latin grammar from Aldo. This was characteristically humanist (for the particular use of the term, see below). The standard medieval authority was the two-thousand line versified *Doctrinale* of Alexander of Villedieu which, like the medieval lawyers' Code of Justinian, was treated as written reason and was committed wholly to memory. In contrast, Aldo *historicized* his subject by showing how language varies with time and by treating grammatical rules as codifications of practice, particularly that of the great classical texts. It was likewise a historical conception that 'everything that is worthy of praise' was first generated by the Greeks and subsequently passed into Latin.[11] The understanding of Greek became thus a matter of great importance, and it is easy to see that the Hellenists, with such a view, would come to see Latin as primarily the language of transmission, the language of the commentators.

We unfortunately do not know where Aldo placed medicine in his scheme of Hellenistic learning at this stage in his career. He was planning an edition of Galen at least as early as 1497 (the Greek *editio princeps* did not appear until after his death). However, Berengario says[12] that with Alberto and under Aldo's tutelage 'we had to dissect a pig', as if it were a considered part of Aldo's programme. Berengario was later asked to dissect a pig at the request of Ercole Gonzaga and in the presence of Pomponazzi and Bonamici,[13] but it is not clear that dissection and the knowledge it generated were parts of a humanistic or of a Hellenistic programme.

Whatever the details of Berengario's education at the hands of Aldo, by the mid 1480s (most likely) he was equipped to go to the university of Bologna, where he took the master's degree in arts and medicine in 1489. He was by now about twenty nine, unusually old for the degree, and again we may suppose he took from his surgical experience to the university and its systematic and largely theoretical medical courses, some firm ideas on the value of sense experience and manual operation. Probably too he had from Aldo an historical approach to his texts. His teachers probably included Manfredi (who taught astrology and was the *ordinarius* teacher of medicine) and Achillini (logic and philosophy). Manfredi's anatomy[14] is similar to Mondino's, is not cast in commentary form, and shows no evidence of Hellenistic tastes. Achillini shared anatomical experience with Berengario only later as a colleague, and Zerbi had left Bologna in 1483, almost certainly before Berengario arrived; but if Manfredi's was the only anatomical teaching Berengario received, it seems to have made very little impression on him for he never mentioned Manfredi's name in his published works.

By 1490 Berengario was back in his father's surgical practice. After 1494 when, it is said, the invading French army brought syphilis in its wake, Berengario began to use mercury in a – at least commercially – successful way in the treatment of the disease. It may well be that this treatment hastened both the beginning and ending of his teaching career: he must have been fairly notable as a successful surgeon to have been appointed in 1502 as the *ordinarius* to teach surgery at Bologna, and there is a persistent tradition (recorded by his biographer, Putti) that it was vivisection of syphilitic patients that led to his leaving the post in 1526.

He seems to have made surgical anatomy his prime interest and he based his teaching on the text of Mondino, his fourteenth-century predecessor at

Bologna. This, wrote Berengario, was the best text available, for it was short enough to be read in the necessarily short period of a dissection, and it covered all parts of the body. Above all, it was *practical* and *particular*. No other available text had all these characteristics: Galen's *Anatomical Procedures* was thought not to have survived and his *On the Use of the Parts* was not short nor particular, but general, teleological and lengthy. Galen's 'particular' books, like the *Anatomy of the Uterus* did not cover the whole body. The *Canon* of Avicenna was too unwieldy, said Berengario finally, and the commentators too diffuse and insufficiently practical. Berengario's first concern was to restore the text of Mondino to its pristine state, and then correct and amplify it for teaching purposes. These two stages are represented by his edition of Mondino in 1514 and the *Commentary* of 1521.

So in following Mondino and listing the shortcomings of the works of other authors, Berengario gives us some indication of what an anatomy text should be. Such a text should be practical in being closely linked to the manual operations of dissection, and should be particular in treating the parts of the body in turn, in terms of the particulars of sense perception rather than the universals of causality or general principles. Not every one had the same ideal, and we can usefully here look briefly at two anatomies published in 1502, the year of Berengario's appointment: as a new lecturer constructing a course, he probably read them. To historians who have read them they generally seem at either end of a scholastic–humanist spectrum.

These were the anatomies of Gabriele de Zerbi[15] and Alessandro Benedetti.[16] It is difficult to imagine two more different books. The difference is to be explained in the background of the authors and in their purposes in writing. Zerbi was a man of the schools: born in 1445, he had one intellectual foot in the manuscript age, and one of his tasks as a teacher was to bring together texts that were still expensive and hard to come by. He had taught medicine and logic at Bologna and had published his *Metaphysical Questions* before spending a period in Rome (when Berengario conceived an intense dislike for him). From 1494 he was teaching the theory of medicine in Padua. When he turned his attention to writing an anatomy, he was at least fifty five, and it is not surprising that the book is a thorough job by a professional teacher in a style of presentation that was not unique to anatomy. He declares that his purpose in publishing is to show that, properly understood, the principal authorities in anatomy do not disagree. The commentators are much quoted, and the whole work has the structure suggested by one of the earliest of them, John of Alexandria: each part of the body in turn is treated with the categorical–morphological *accessus* and the six observables.[17] Yet the book was intended to be a practical guide to dissection, as was Mondino's. The text is divided into alternate paragraphs of *textus*, 'to be read while the body is being dissected', and *additio*, to be considered at leisure between demonstrations. The book differs from Mondino's principally in the weight of authorities.

Benedetti's *Historia Corporis Humani, sive Anatomice* is very different. He too was a teacher (at Padua from 1490), but of practical medicine and anatomy. What makes his book so different from Zerbi's and Mondino's is his notion that anatomy is entirely a Greek affair. To have practised medicine for sixteen years in Greece, as he did, does not necessarily make a man a humanist, but it might well dispose him to become a Hellenist, with a knowledge of the language and a liking for the culture. As we look at figures like Benedetti and his circle of acquaintances we shall do better to call them Hellenists (rather than humanists) because this is how they saw themselves. Another Hellenist of this circle was Giorgio Valla, an important figure with a library of texts that was a magnet for other Hellenists like Leoniceno and Antiquarius. The members of the circle naturally supported each other's endeavours: Valla, discussing with Benedetti the latter's intention to write a history of the military campaigns of Charles VIII against Naples, urged him to model himself on the classical historians. Valla read the manuscript, and it was arranged that it should be printed by the humanist printer Aldo Manuzio. The arrangement not only gave Aldo the opportunity to print a work of which he approved, but it also gave him access *via* Valla and Benedetti to Venetian society.[18] In a similar way it was Antiquarius who urged Benedetti to publish his very Hellenistic anatomy.

Benedetti's dedication of the *Anatomice* makes his position very clear: he is to derive all his information from Greek sources, putting to one side the moderns who have tried to steal from the Greeks the honour of discovering medicine. Benedetti's terminology is studiously classical, and there is no mention of the commentators, their devices of exposition and their saving of the authors. His anatomy is certainly intended to be practical – he describes the construction and use of the anatomy theatre – but the message of the book is that anatomy is the *prisca anatomia* of the ancients which Benedetti is setting down in Latin for convenience of teaching. As a piece of Hellenistic propaganda, Benedetti realized the book would meet with the criticism of the great bulk of medical men brought up on Avicenna, and he loftily avoids the issue by declaring the book is intended not for them but only for the Emperor Maximilian, its dedicatee.

Turning back to Berengario, the scant evidence suggests that he was successful as a teacher. In an unidentified year between 1503 and 1512 he had ten or a dozen pupils, a number regarded by the university as satisfactory (his colleague, teaching surgery, had three, which was 'too few'). In the margin of these records, the university's 'reformers' noted that the teaching of surgery *non est multum honorabilis* but that it was popular with foreign students, those from across the Alps. (Other sources tell us that Bolognese medical education was popular among Poles and Germans. Berengario had at least one Spanish student, and perhaps the German Lange.) The same margin note says that student numbers would justify finding a temporary replacement for Berengario, but no one with his abilities could be found: *nemo practicus noscitur in hoc studio*. Perhaps these notes were written in 1512, for early the next year Leo X formally required the Bolognese authorities to release Berengario to go to Florence to treat one of Leo's relatives. Part of these arrangements was that Berengario was to have a replacement during his absence and that he was to be paid his normal salary. Before 1512 (when he died) Achillini could probably have replaced Berengario as a practical teacher, so almost certainly we are dealing with the year 1512–13.

What interests us especially about this episode is that surgical teaching was not highly regarded, not popular with the Italian students and perhaps only tolerated at the academic level of the *studium* because it brought foreign students into the town. Surgery clearly did not have the dignity of the other subjects of the arts and medical courses, and Berengario observed that physicians of his time disdained to be called surgeons. A professional teacher who had given courses on the natural philosophy common to the arts and medical courses could be naturally called up to teach medicine and anatomy, as an extension of the topics he was already teaching. In contrast, however, Berengario either could or would not teach other academic topics, and he must have felt himself in a somewhat isolated position in the *studium*: a confident and successful surgeon who was entrusted with the treatment of the pope's relations, a successful teacher, but not a member of the college of doctors and without the academic standing of his colleagues (at least in their eyes). This may well have combined with long-standing and firmly held convictions about the nature of anatomy formed in his early surgical experience to produce in him a suspicion of some of the sophistications and procedures of academic anatomy. Further evidence of this is perhaps found in his choice of Mondino as a teaching text. Although the traditional source of Italian anatomical teaching at least until the time of Curtius in the 1530s (a fact reflected in statutes), the text of Mondino was not an inevitable component of teaching, and neither Manfredi nor Achillini based their teaching on it. Zerbi disapproved of Mondino, and the Hellenists of course passed over him in a pained silence. But for Berengario (7v), Mondino was a craftsman like himself, for whom anatomy was to be conducted by hand: *secundum manualem operationem*, said Mondino. The edition of Mondino that Berengario brought out in 1514 and the *Commentary* itself seem to indicate a student-oriented[19] practicality that was neither purely academic nor Hellenist.

Whatever position Berengario chose to take up in relation to others who had an interest in medicine and anatomy, we must suppose that he saw the alternatives and rejected them for good reasons. To put him into a category of 'scholastic' or 'humanist' would be to impose a historical straight-jacket which would not explain anything. Although much of what Berengario wrote could be considered 'scholastic', we need not feel surprised, for example, that he shared the 'humanists' feel for classical culture. We know that in the year in which he published Mondino he bought an ancient stone torso, and two years later he bought a larger house in which to keep his collection of *objets d'art*. Five years after publishing the *Commentary on Mondino* he commissioned a pair of silver vases from Cellini in Rome, and when they were ready he shrewdly took away with them the drawings from which Cellini had worked. They therefore could not be copied and Berengario was able to pretend they were genuinely classical. In the circles in which he moved this was a compliment to his taste and, when the story got back to Cellini, his own stock in his circle of friends rose at once as the first man for a thousand years able to make such objects. There is no reason to suppose that such tastes came upon Berengario late in life, and no doubt he thought the same before the publication of the *Commentary*. He was approaching sixty when he began to write it, and he had long had the habit of accepting works of art in lieu of professional fees.

The Commentary on Mondino

The Venetian presses of Scotus and Junta continued through Berengario's lifetime to publish the commentaries on the *Articella* and *Canon* that formed the teaching material of the medical schools of Padua and Bologna. In publishing his own anatomical knowledge as a commentary Berengario was aiming at the same academic market. The form of the commentary encouraged a full and rigorous discussion of both morphology and procedure, and Berengario seems to have chosen the form as the one that first, did justice to the questions and which second, would most effectively convince the reader. His commentary was unusual in that its subject was an author comparatively recent and homely, in the non-academic typographical appearance of the book and in some of its purposes (all of which are discussed below). Nevertheless, the *Commentary on Mondino* has a structure that had been common to commentaries for two hundred years.

A medical commentary in Bologna would normally take such a form as follows. It would begin with a proemium praising God and the book under review. Berengario does so in the dedication and at the opening of the text. The first commentary would seek to place the subject matter of the book in its context in natural philosophy as a whole, perhaps through a device like the *accessus*. Here Berengario discusses the status of anatomy as a *scientia* and its relation to natural philosophy. The traditional commentary then began with an analysis of the book as a whole; for example the Bolognese commentators Taddeo Alderotti[20] and Gentile da Foligno[21] preferred to see the whole work in terms of a fourfold Aristotelian causality. In this place Berengario has some parallel general remarks on the necessity and use of anatomy, its 'final' cause. After the first, subsequent commentaries were invariably devoted to each section of the work, so that those standing at the head of a book, fen, doctrine or chapter would analyse the flow and stages of argument of the text, indicating to the reader the subdivisions of the text. The ultimate subdivisions of the text were perhaps only a sentence or two long, and each is identified within the preceding commentary by a quotation (within some typographical device serving the purpose of inverted commas) of its *incipit*.[22]

Thus the reader knew in advance which would be the fragments of text to be found embedded in the commentary and the whole exercise was designed to make clear the sequence of events in the text. Up to this point the exercise was an *expositio* designed to throw light on a difficult text (Taddeo says[23] picturesquely that the *expositio* is a light that brings out the colours of the text), and those whom we call commentators called themselves *expositors*.[24] Berengario and his predecessors as expositors characteristically subdivide the text in a hierarchically ordered way, so that the first level of division may reveal, say, six parts, the description of which by the expositor always begins at the second part, followed by the third and so on. The expositor then returns to the first part for a further level of subdivision, again with the second part receiving the first analysis. The purpose of this is that the expositor can preserve a continuity of analysis through the hierarchy, and so that by the time he has reached the end of his first *expositio* he has fully analysed the *beginning* of the text and can move on in subsequent expositions to the subsequent and already identified fragments of text.

Because Mondino's text was readily understood, Berengario allows it to stand in chapters without fragmenting it. He does however move through the stages of the *expositio* as outlined here, frequently concluding abruptly with the remark that Mondino's words are clear and should be read.

Having made his *expositio* in this form, the commentator would then bring forward a number of other aids to understanding the text, generally drawn from external sources. This would normally include an examination of the way in which the author used his terms. Just as the medieval disputation proceeded by the opponent (among other things) 'distinguishing' the terms of the proposition – that is, showing that the terms can have meanings inconsistent with the subsequent reasoning – so here the commentator explains in what specialized sense the author is using a term and how other authors may be using it in a different sense without necessarily contradicting each other. Where the *expositio* as described above has broken the text down into fragments of about a sentence in size, these can be treated as propositions and the whole text can thus be exposed to the rules of logic.

The commentator has now proceeded as far as he can in elucidating the text; the *expositio* is at an end. But the newly lucid text can now be seen, perhaps, to contrast with some other authority, and perhaps there are inconsistencies within it that cannot be resolved by the techniques of distinction. The next stage in the commentary form is thus the introduction of *quaestiones* or *dubia*. (The older commentators or their copyists or editors listed these *dubia* separately. Berengario does not do so, allowing the text of Mondino to be the guide to the contents of the commentary.) Here, then, Berengario brings forward the opinions of the authors for comparison and (generally) resolution. He, as a commentator, is reporting to the reader what the major issues in the field are. Sometimes, when the topic is a large one such as the formation of the foetus, the sheer bulk of Berengario's treatment is such that the commentary form is lost. He calls these *digressiones* (518r) – that on generation is about a hundred pages in length.

But more often the commentary form is retained and Berengario completes his review of the opinions of the authors before announcing any major discovery of his own, such as the structure of the vertebrate (490r) the existence of voluntary muscles within the nasal cavity (466r) the structure of the ventricles of the brain (444r) and the absence of the Galenic *rete mirabile* (459r). The novelty of these assertions necessarily meant that Berengario was in conflict with the authorities; it also meant that such bald and unsubstantiated assertions were unlikely to convince the reader. For these reasons Berengario generally introduced his assertion, or proposition, as something that would have to stand the examination of the learned and be seen separately by other skilled anatomists.

Berengario is not merely inviting his readers to 'see for themselves'. Rather, he is putting forward his anatomical discoveries as *propositions*, not because he is not convinced of their truth, but because the only way to convince others of that truth was through the stringent requirements of academic procedures. The formal structure of his commentary would have been perfectly clear to Berengario's readers, and they would have been perfectly familiar with the logical procedures of commentary, disputation, rhetoric and dialectic. Above all at the two points where Berengario could introduce his own interpretation of structure – in resolving a conflict of authority, and at the end of each comment – his readers would have felt the need of some form of *proof*.

But what kind of proof could be applied to morphological *structure*? The commentator was on traditional ground in dealing with the writings of the authorities, which could be treated as 'opinion', the premisses of the dialectical syllogism. Dialectic logic then has the business of demonstrating the falsity or truth of 'opinion' and the validity of related arguments. The process was akin to that of the disputation, with its technique of 'distinction'. Berengario is 'distinguishing' when he draws out of a single term, for example *siphac*, several meanings, not all of which fit the context and argument. Taken very strictly, *strictissime*, (50v) *siphac* means *peritoneon* (95v), but it means something else when taken merely *stricte* or *communiter*. Likewise *mirach* is used *large* and *stricte* to mean the whole abdominal wall, or simply the skin, fat and muscles (50v).

But all these are purely verbal techniques, and offer no 'proof' of structure. Certainly they could be very useful, particularly in association with detailed scholarship, to clarify the authors' texts, resolve their conflicts and so 'save' them. Berengario often calls his resolution of a conflict of authority a 'determination', the term used when at the end of a disputation the master decided in favour of one or the other disputing students; at other times he uses technical terms of rhetoric, and in both cases he seems to be invoking academic procedures to lend support to his conclusion. Now, his conclusions could be of three kinds: an assertion that an organ or part was this or that shape; an assertion that a part was *not* there, despite authority (like the Galenic *rete mirabile*) or an assertion that a part was there, but could not be seen. As we shall see below, Berengario expressly excluded the last kind of assertion as improper for anatomy. Among other things, this meant that he could not 'prove' the existence of a part from the existence of a function assigned to it.

In order to find some kind of 'proof' for the first two anatomical assertions, Berengario turned to the practical side of medicine. The commentators he had read had argued since the late thirteenth century that there were some areas of medicine where only sense-experience could lead to knowledge.[25] While it might be possible to treat the text of the *Aphorisms* in a completely syllogistic way, the only way to *know* the action of a medicine upon an individual was by experience. Berengario as a surgeon was above all a practical man, and as he many times announced his intention of writing a book on surgery, we might even see the commentary on Mondino as a 'theoretical' work, preliminary to the real business of medicine. But it would be quite wrong to think that Berengario's practical instincts led him out of scholastic anatomy and into a new methodology based on sense perception. He had chosen the commentary form and was addressing the academics in their terms, and any contributions he thought he was making were to their science. In seeking to substantiate his conclusions he used what we might call 'practical logic'.

This practical logic was *demonstration*. Derived from the simple physical *demonstratio* or *ostensio* (479v; 438; 351r) of the school anatomy, the term carries over some of the force of logical or even geometrical demonstration (450r). In general terms it meant for Berengario 'conclusion': in dealing with an insoluble problem in the field of generation, Berengario gives almost a complete bibliography of authorities and cries 'Oh! that I could demonstrate which of the foregoing opinions is true!' (139v). In this sense the word is close to *determinatio* of a disputation. Thus Berengario cannot 'determine' another conflict of authority on generation (227r) or another on the action of the heart (355r).

But the main force of the word *demonstratio* to Berengario is that it speaks directly to the senses. 'Proof' in anatomy is to expose the structure to the sight and touch, ideally to a number of observers, and at least in such a way that the reader can perform the dissection and employ his own senses (216r, 254r, 494r, 259v). Many eyes make proof; and when, in its proper place, Berengario introduces a new discovery, he puts it up as a proposition to be examined in the usual academic way and to be given a final *determinatio* or *demonstratio* by repetition (466r, 444r).

The image of the disputation provided by Berengario's commentary is strengthened by the place given to *sensus* in his method. Sense, he says, will always be his master, *magister* (that is, in providing a *determinatio*) and his guide, *dux* (that is, in investigation: 4r, 434v). More often sense is the ultimate arbiter, the *judex* (443r, 259v, 83v). Where sense has been unable to provide a final *determinatio* the question remains *sub judice* (239v, 227r). The legal analogy is present too in the very frequent use of *teste sensu* (and the occasional *necessarius est visus testificatio*: 75r). *Ad sensum* is used several hundred times.

In short, what is demonstrated to the senses is also proved to them (73v, 74v). In contrast, Zerbi uses *rationabiliter* as Berengario uses *ad sensum*, and 'proves' the warmth of the spleen syllogistically (Zerbi 22v). For Berengario the ultimate use of demonstration as proof was in the form of sensory experience that we call experiment. In the school anatomies hollow organs were often inflated to demonstrate their shape. The same technique could also prove that the organs had, or did not have, channels communicating to other organs. A major use of the proof by experiment for Berengario was the resolution of conflicts of authority. An example will make this clear: one such dispute concerned the sequence of appearance of organs during the development of the foetus, and was the result of the very different accounts of generation given by Galen and Aristotle. By Berengario's time it was also important to know at what period in its development the foetus received its soul and its animal virtues. Inspection of the early stages of the foetus could go some way to answering these problems by showing what organs had not yet developed: was the liver the first to develop, as Galen said, or was it, with Aristotle, the heart? Secondly, did the foetus, which received ready-made faculties and nourishment from the mother, need the organs responsible for these faculties while still *in utero*? For example, receiving pure concocted blood from the mother did the foetus need kidneys? Did it urinate?

Berengario realized that the only way to settle these old questions was through sense experience, the teacher or *magistra cui credendum est* (248r). But such experience was very difficult to obtain because it could only be gained from aborted foetuses 'which we see only on the rarest occasions, and with difficulty, because of the practice of our women, who refuse to show anything except secretly and with difficulty' (248r). At length and by means of furtive payments to midwives, Berengario gained the experience he desired about the early appearance of organs. Pursuing the question of development to the point where the foetus may be thought to urinate, and considering the possible role of the foetal membranes in collecting the urine, Berengario found himself in flat opposition to Galen. The only way to 'save' Galen was to assume that the relevant text was corrupt, but Berengario did not really believe that this was the case (253r, 254r). Berengario proves his case in the way outlined above:

> . . . what I have said agrees with true sense; I have seen it many times and shown it to many scholars. Today, that is, 17th May, 1520, I have shown in a single anatomy (of a woman who died in the eighth month of her pregnancy, unable to give birth) and before many trustworthy doctors and scholars, that everything I have said above is very true (254r).

Pursuing the matter still further, Berengario asserts that the foetus does eject waste material in the *later* months (257v) and in particular that it expels urine through the same route as the adult, and not through the umbilicus as Avicenna has it (259v). That this is true only of the later foetus Berengario demonstrated by forcing water from a syringe into the bladder of a foetal dog, whence it passed to the umbilicus. He found this always to be the case with the early canine foetus, but the bulk of his human foetal material was at a late stage of development, and the pathway could not be found. Again Berengario resorted to *experientia*, compressing the bladder of a nine-month foetus and finding no transfer of fluid to the umbilical region. Thinking that there might have been no urine in the bladder, Berengario injected a 'notable quality' of water from a syringe into the bladder through the penis and repeated the experiment, with the result that the water emerged only along the route by which it had entered. There still remained the possibility that the water had merely chosen the most obvious of alternative pathways, and so Berengario repeated the experiment, this time tying a ligature round the penis after the water was injected to prevent reflux. The same result was obtained. Finally Berengario injected the ureter within a kidney to demonstrate the normal flow of urine, and explored all possible pathways with a small silver probe (260v). He offers similar experimental proof of his analysis of kidney function (178v) and the connections of the gall bladder (153r).

Anatomia sensibilis

We have now looked at a number of reasons why Berengario might have chosen the commentary form, chief amongst them the need to adduce a proof to convince the academics – *scolastici, scolares* – to whom the book is addressed. As a commentary in form it goes far beyond the brief text on which it is based, and we can distinguish between the form and the content of Berengario's book. The content is his idea of what anatomy should be: the purpose of anatomy is, simply, the possession of anatomical knowledge, but the acquisition of knowledge, through the procedures of anatomy, is far from simple.

In discussing anatomical knowledge and its acquisition, Berengario draws upon the tradition of commentary that contained anatomical material, that upon book three of the *Canon*. Broadly speaking, the *Canon* came to be the biggest single authority in the two centuries before Berengario, and although, as in other fields, the logical and physical works of Aristotle provided the principal tools for academic business, in medicine the substance of the topic was provided by the non-Aristotelian *Canon*. Aristotelian natural science could in principle extend to medicine as well as to the rest of the natural world. Yet there were no Aristotelian works on medicine itself, and medical men took the substance of their discipline from elsewhere. This substance did not extend to other parts of the natural world, and the natural result was that the medical commentators of the *Canon* felt that medicine was a province with clearly marked boundaries, outside which it should not tread, but within which the writ of the philosophers did not necessarily run. In particular, book three of the *Canon*, providing a complete conspectus of medicine from anatomy to treatment, became the *via medicorum*, the path to be trodden by the medical man.

This is illustrated by one of the earlier commentators, whom Berengario quotes extensively, Gentile da Foligno.[26] The first part of his commentary on book three of the *Canon* is the common exercise on the wisdom and goodness of God. It is God the Creator who is presented to us, *artifex istius mundi*: God the practical craftsman. The advantages of this presentation to the medical man are clear, for the *medicus* can fit into his world picture the western theological tradition, the church fathers and, from within his own profession, the divine and creative Nature of Galen and the creating and protective Allah of the Arabs and Avicenna himself. Nowhere is the hand of God more evident than in the microcosm, which is the body of man and the special concern of the physician. God presented in this way is very different from the abstract ultimate Good of Aristotle, presiding over an eternal (not created) world. Gentile's views allow for God to have created the world through the mechanisms of Aristotelian causality and categories, and so an Aristotelian natural science is still possible in the world at large. But in the *via medicorum*, the professional preserve of the medical men, physical reasoning was not the most appropriate. Book three of the *Canon* was vocational and practical; it was the *only* text specified in the Bologna statutes of 1405 for the *practica* course.[27] Gentile's commentary develops the theme of the skilful doctor never stepping aside from the *via* and reaching medical virtuosity by treading the path from the practical business of anatomy to the equally practical application of remedies. Gentile's remarks refer to the educational training of the physician: the implication is that while the philosophers may have a satisfactory account of the *causes* of the parts of the body, or of the mode of action of medicines, the only way to acquire knowledge of the shape of a part or the actual action of a particular medicine is by experience.

These practical features of the *via medicorum* as outlined in Gentile's commentary clearly appealed to Berengario, and he picked them out of Gentile's largely non-practical context. He then greatly developed the doctrine within anatomy. He used the term *anatomia sensibilis* to indicate a method of teaching *and discovery* that yielded a body of knowledge enclosing in its boundaries only those structures perceptible in practice to the senses. By definition other *kinds* of questions, in themselves legitimate (like those concerned with the 'origin' of parts) were excluded. For example invisibly small parts are *imaginabiles* (for example 344r): not 'imaginary' but perceptible to the mental faculty that perceives *images*. This is the faculty of reason, which Berengario identifies with imagination because of its power of handling images. This power he says, distinguishes the *sensata*, brought in by way of the *sensus communis* from the external senses, from the *non sensata*, which are composed images partly drawn from the memory and seen, then, by the internal sense or 'eye of reason' (426v, 444r, 446r) which has no place in anatomy: *anatomia non notat insensibilia* (427v). Berengario energetically denies the existence of Galen's *rete mirabile*, which had played so important a part in these functions in traditional psychology: he claims to have opened hundreds of heads in search of it and claims Galen *imaginatum fuisse*, misled by reason, not wishful thinking (459v. Compare the misled Aristotle, 64v).

There were a number of other questions which now fell outside the boundaries of anatomy: perfectly proper questions, but not to be asked of the anatomist. If much-disputed questions as that of the origin of the nerves (brain or heart?) were pressed upon the *artifex sensibilis*, they had to be answered by him – indeed by all *medici* – 'at the brain' where they can be observed (346v). Nevertheless, the 'physical' (philosophical) reasons for supposing the heart to be sentient, says Berengario, are strong, and can even overcome the medical reasons. It remains the duty of anatomists to 'speak medically', and it is quite outside the bounds of anatomy to save both opinions and declare that sentience is *virtualiter* in the heart and *actualiter* in the brain, as the commentators had done. Almost as an act of faith Berengario declares himself to be a medical man and therefore incapable of leaving the *via medicorum*, which is a pathway across the 'whole ocean' of such disputes (68v): it is the job of the theorizing physicians and philosophers to deal with these questions (475r). The tone of Berengario's words closely recalls Gentile's 'Peritum medicum non decet transgredi hanc viam'.[28] A related question concerned the origin of the veins. Both Galen and Aristotle had argued for an 'origin' of the veins (in the liver and heart respectively) on the functional basis of a faculty flowing out from a central organ. Berengario is thinking in morphological terms (and not in functional or embryological ones) and he argues that there can be no 'origin' of the veins *nisi improprie et metaphoriae*, 'unless speaking metaphorically' (161v).

So at its simplest and most fundamental level *anatomia sensibilis* was the anatomy of what could be seen. But the acquisition of such knowledge was far from simple. No one dissector could by his own unaided efforts come to a knowledge of the whole body, and necessarily had to derive some information from elsewhere. The 'science of the nature and function of the parts' says Berengario (6r) grows co-operatively, by the addition of new knowledge to old, so that we are like boys on the shoulders of giants, able to see further than they. Berengario was aware that even Galen had said that others would come after him to add to the stock of knowledge (7r).

The necessity of deriving some information from sources other than the body, combined with his insistence of sense perception, led Berengario to examine very carefully the roles of observation and reason in anatomy: how can we *evaluate* information from other sources? On their own, even the senses can be deceived, and many anatomists mistake one part for another (7r). Simply to identify and put a name to the parts of the body, the anatomist must be a master of the literature and of the problem of historical terminology; he must also discuss the problem with other learned anatomists. Where sense and authority agree, all is well, but where it can be seen that sense cannot be made to agree with the authorities, they must be rejected. Berengario constantly refers to the practitioner of *anatomia sensibilis* as an *artifex* (for example 346v), the craftsman working with eye and hand. This craftsman can learn from others: the dispute over the alleged opening of the pubic bones at birth could be settled if anatomists would visit carpenters and see how doors and windows are made so that they will open (493r). The sutures of the cranial bones is best understood by examining the carpenters' dovetail joints (417r). The entire body has been put together by God, the *primus artifex* (367r) and so can be understood by lesser *artifices*. Because of its divine origin, nothing in the body, says Berengario, is made in vain (219v–210v). It also follows from this that the body has not changed substantially since its Creation and although aware of variation of the body (14r) (for example, the gluttony of modern man has reduced the size of the caecum (115r) to a mere appendage), Berengario had good reason to believe there was an unchanged normality of bodily structure common to ancients and moderns.[29]

The role of sense observation in *anatomia sensibilis*, said Berengario, was to be extended in a number of ways. A knowledge of comparative anatomy should be gained by the dissection of different animals and of both sexes in each case. The females should be dissected at different stages of pregnancy, and much attention was to be given to the structure of the foetus, in which many things were clearer than in the adult (46v, 53v). Animals should also be vivisected (6v). Dissections should be repeated, for one organ is necessarily destroyed in revealing another. Hollow organs can be inflated, and bones and fibrous parts dried for leisurely inspection (484v, 489r). Berengario while writing to refute the earlier commentators sat with a dried specimen of the vertebrae in front of him (484r). These are largely teaching devices; the research aspect of the use of the senses is discussed next.

Berengario often distinguishes public from private dissections. Public anatomies were the customary university dissections, attended sometimes by citizens (222v) and always by students, for whom Berengario says he is writing the *Commentaria* (192v, 287v, 305v). These were the inexperienced *scolares* who can be often led 'into the pit' by the blindness of teachers, and the school dissections they attended (*in gimnasiis publicis* 479v) were concerned with the traditional 'three venters' and their contents, and were necessarily brief affairs. Their function was to reinforce in the memory the words of the accompanying text with visual images, or to make clear the shape of organs that could not be adequately explained in words (the *clarificatio eorum qui in occulta sunt* of John of Alexandria[30]). Berengario adds that such 'common' anatomies cannot show a large number of things, firstly, the bones, muscles, nerves, blood vessels and fibrous parts, all of which need special techniques for their demonstration: boiling, maceration in running water, drying. The common anatomies were generally limited to a single body, and many organs were imperfectly demonstrated in being destroyed in order to reach another organ (119v); for example the top of the cranium was generally sawn off, making it difficult to see how the dura mater is attached to it (422v). The observing students were very often misled in such a complex dissection as that of the brain. When Berengario talks of private dissections, in contrast (424r), he implies that he was dissecting to decide a particular point, like the presence of water in the torcular of Herophilus, or the existence of the Galenic *rete mirabile*. Many bodies were to be secured in private dissections for the sake of a single organ (438r) and Berengario's vivisections of animals, undertaken to decide on such points as the presence of water in the pericardium (439r), must also have been private affairs.

In other words *anatomia sensibilis* was also a set of practical precepts for anatomical *research*, the generation of new knowledge about the body. In contradicting the major authors it provoked the students of the school anatomies into reading the texts of the authors and performing dissections and vivisections in order to discover the truth (398r). *In anatomia* stated Berengario, *locus ab auctoritate contra sensum non habet veritatem* (413r), and sense observation, gained in the cemetery and by boiling the skulls left over from ordinary anatomies, will free the student from the confusion induced by reading the authorities. If the new discoveries of *anatomia sensibilis* are provocative, so much the better in stimulating intellectual activity of the *scolares* (494r).

New medical knowledge was also to be gained in another area: some diseases were reckoned to be new, because modern man, it was often thought, either by degeneration or from the effects of an undisciplined regimen of life, was less hardy than the ancients. Doctors in northern Europe found for example that there was no classical description of scurvy or scrophula, and in the Italy of Berengario's time syphilis, believed to have been brought in by French troops in 1494, had no classical precedent. The dissecting surgeon or anatomist was therefore on his own, and was necessarily making pathological discoveries. In 1521, the year of the *Commentaria*, Berengario reissued Hutten's book on the guaiac treatment, and Benvenuto Cellini records that Berengario made a great deal of money while in Rome in 1526 by the mercury treatment. Berengario intended to discuss the disease in the book on surgery (308v). As a surgeon and as an anatomist he must have wondered about the internal pathological changes: here was an *aegritudo* without classical precedent, the last of the routine observables in a dissection (according to Guy), and a category best observed in vivisection (according to Mondino). Berengario was well aware of the changes in pathological appearance brought about by death (5r, 118v), and the consequent advantages of vivisection. Fallopia records the persistent rumour that after his stay in Rome, it was a charge of having practised vivisection on a syphilitic patient that cost Berengario his post in Bologna. A man with apparently homicidal tendencies in respect of his colleagues and political enemies (as noted by Putti)[31] may indeed have been too prompt in bringing to the dissection table a body in which life still lingered.

But what of 'reason' in *anatomia sensibilis*? When Berengario says at the outset in the *Commentary* that he will be guided by 'sense [observation], the authority of the divine Galen, and various reasonings' (4r) what did he have in mind? So far we have seen that he attempted to limit the part played by reason in anatomy; and to this we can add that he rejected the idea of the 'eye of reason'. This was a technique sometimes used to argue for the existence of invisibly small or subtle parts, like the veins or humours that nourish the transparent cornea, or the invisible superfluities of the spine (497v) on the grounds of the manifest nature of their *function*. This could easily be related to the Aristotelian principle that true knowledge of a part was not generated by the particulars of sense observation or morphology, but included the more general principles that lay behind the particulars, of which the most important was function. All university-trained physicians, we may suppose, were familiar enough with 'reason' of this sort, and the argument from function was much more widely used in anatomy than inductive and observational techniques that could equally have been derived from Aristotle. A model of a deductive argument from function had been provided by Galen, who had argued that nature did nothing in vain and that therefore the apparently blind pits on the surface of the cardiac septum are not useless. Their only conceivable function was to communicate with invisibly small pores from one ventricle to another: therefore this must be their function. We may recall that it was his attention to morphology and rejection of the argument from function that led Berengario to dismiss as inappropriate to anatomy any discussion of the 'origin' of the veins.

The answer to the question of Berengario's 'reasons' is probably to be found early in the text of the *Commentary* where he spends what at first sight seems a surprising amount of space on the 'similar' parts and their qualities. The similar parts were the homogeneous and fundamental parts of the body, described by Aristotle and constituting the first step of any synthetic treatment of anatomy. The qualities of the similar parts were similarly Aristotelian and fundamental. Yet some of the commentators and Berengario himself held that in the body no similar part as such was perceptible because each was inextricably bound up with others in the construction of the parts. It would seem that the similar parts constituted just such a part of theoretical anatomy that Berengario the *artifex*, the surgeon, would reject as improper to *anatomia sensibilis*. And how far were the theoretical qualities perceptible to the senses? In the pages where Berengario discusses the similar parts and qualities we do not see these as so much medieval mud sticking to the shoes of a traveller striving valiantly for the dry ground of the renaissance. Berengario goes deep into the question of the perceptibility of the qualities and similar parts because this was anatomy's principal link to theoretical medicine. All disease at root was a qualitative imbalance and so the complexion and temperament of the parts was of great importance. If anatomy was to be of help to physicians as well as to surgeons, it must deal with the qualities. Berengario concludes that the similar parts do in fact predominate in actual organs to the extent that their elementary qualities are perceptible to the touch (but that the commentators' seven degrees of comparison were absurd).

In seeking in this way to link anatomy with theoretical medicine, Berengario is not of course trying to make anatomy theoretical, but to demonstrate that it is the observational basis for the understanding of health and disease. And just as importantly it was necessary in an institutional and academic setting to show that anatomy was not just a manual art, but related to a *scientia*. Medical commentaries since the thirteenth century (at least) had argued in a similar way that medicine itself had the dignity of natural philosophy: these were at least partly professional arguments used in defence of young faculties of medicine. In short then, these 'reasons' of Berengario were part of *anatomia sensibilis* not in telling him more about the body but in making clear anatomy's external relations.

Part of *anatomia sensibilis*, in addition to establishing a relationship between the body, text, sensory experience, reason and authority, was the establishment of a sound text. A good anatomy text, of whatever age, was one that agreed with the body; and a text was bad either from the fault of its author (or his circumstances) or because it had suffered in transmission and translation. It followed that corrupt passages in otherwise good texts could be identified and *corrected* by the use of dissection. Practical anatomy was also an answer to the interminable disputes of the authorities and a guide to the correct attribution of texts to their authors. An example of Berengario using dissection to establish the correct reading of a text occurs in the case of the abdominal wall: Berengario has three authorities, the printed works of Haly Abbas, a manuscript version, and a version quoted by Nicholas, all of which differed and which Berengario decides between on the basis of dissection, providing a woodcut to illustrate the sensible anatomy of the part (85r). Berengario's first duty as a commentator, of course, was to restore the text of Mondino to its *pristinum sensum* (102v), for he says parts of the original are missing, other parts are expanded and the sequence of others has been changed (103r). Berengario's technique is to establish Mondino's mode of exposition as a whole, the *totus processus*, and to argue back to the opinion behind the suspect passage, avoiding a literal translation. Thus where Mondino appears to say there are ten contained organs in the abdomen, Berengario argues that it is a corruption introduced by the commentators who have been misled by Mondino treating thirteen organs under only ten textual headings.

Illustration. The *Commentary on Mondino* is one of the first illustrated printed anatomy texts. The modern mind so naturally seizes upon the idea that an anatomy text should be illustrated that it is difficult not to see Berengario as taking the first essential step. But for Berengario, of course, it was not in the least natural that an anatomy text should be illustrated, since no treatment of any length of the body before him had been illustrated, and in particular the structure of the commentary form did not admit of non-verbal elements.

Rather than taking a first step towards an ideal, Berengario's use of illustration was an answer to his own problem of presenting anatomy. *Anatomia sensibilis* was the anatomy of visible things, and visible things can be drawn, and engraved on to a wood block. The essence of his emphasis on sensory experience in teaching and discovery within *anatomia sensibilis* was that sense would reveal and commit to the memory shapes that could not be described adequately in words: illustration was a printed *anatomia sensibilis*. Thus the complex shape of the vertebral processes, or that of the ventricles of the brain (494r) defy full verbal description. We have seen that within the commentary form Berengario attempted to bring forward a mode of *demonstratio* that would convince his readers, and in the *Commentary on Mondino* in 'proving' that (for example) the uterus does not have seven cells, he provides not only a description of its actual shape but also a printed *praesentalis ostensio* – a woodcut – of the demonstration he would have made to his students in life.

Another reason for providing woodcuts was that the *Commentary on Mondino* described parts of the body that were not reached in the school dissections. Thus the bones were not normally boiled free from flesh in the public anatomies, and were not seen by the students: Berengario provides woodcuts of the articulated skeleton and detailed illustrations of the bones of the hands. As a surgeon he is aware of the greater medical usefulness of such a presentation, in comparison with the older anatomists' concern with the total number of bones (he is thinking of Achillini: 517v). Other woodcuts are designed to show where to let blood, and how to avoid cutting muscle when excising tumours, both better seen than described. (The limitations of the technique were the skill of the artist and more particularly of the block cutter, and the woodcuts in Berengario's *Commentaria* and *Isagoge* are somewhat crude, and he remarks that the print of the vertebrae does not represent the reality of structure.)[32] Other of his illustrations were intended also for the use of artists who, like the surgeons, would have been thought of by Berengario as *artifices*. Again we see Berengario, as a *practicus*, relating himself more closely to the medieval surgeons who had illustrated their works (Guy de Chauliac and Henri de Mondeville) than to his contemporaries, whether Hellenists or 'aggregators' (see below).

Berengario first used illustration in his book on cranial fractures to illustrate the trephine. He tells us he used the instrument on Lorenzo Medici and part of the message of the book is the need for a full armoury of instruments and a skilled hand. But Berengario's trephine was a *cranked* instrument very similar to a carpenter's brace, and quite distinct from that of the prime surgical authority of the time, Albucasis, which was straight rod rolled between the open hands. It is very much easier for a reader to grasp the idea of a crank and of the complex shape of its cutting tools, from an illustration than from a verbal description, and this is one of Berengario's reasons for including the woodcut. Characteristically, he is concerned with the variety of names and of the structures they represent: *terebrum, terebellum* and *trepanum* are all 'trephine' but all differ structurally. To avoid creating confusion in the surgical reader – *ne operatores ambulant in tenebris* (90v) – Berengario publishes, in the book on cranial fractures, a *catalogue* of names *with illustrations*.

Another reason for Berengario to use illustrations was that Albucasis himself had illustrated his text on surgery and instruments and so Berengario's own library provided a model (from his will we know that Berengario not only owned a copy of Albucasis but that he considered the book fundamental to medicine).

Scholasticism and humanism. So far in this chapter we have seen Berengario as an individual presenting his own view of anatomy in accordance with his aspirations and circumstances. Can we fit him into the usual picture of humanists and scholastics? What do these terms mean in the context of medicine and particularly anatomy? To attempt to answer the question we must first look briefly at the nature of medical scholasticism.

The Italian universities before the early thirteenth century enjoyed a prescholastic period during which they supplied largely vocational training in the skills of government, trade and the professions (the *ars dictaminis*, mathematics, law and medicine).[33] Scholastic techniques were introduced from the north (principally Paris) and by student demand. These techniques were probably most closely associated with the growth of the study of the *libri naturales* of Aristotle, which gave a natural–philosophical or 'physical' content of the vocational training.

The 'physical' subjects were closely associated with medicine and were generally taught by medical men. Aristotelian natural philosophy could be made to underpin the whole of medicine, but only after some problems had been solved. The first was that these works of Aristotle did not always agree with extant medical knowledge, partly derived from Galen. Second, the largest single authority in medical education quickly came to be the *Canon* of Avicenna and this too had to be reconciled with Aristotle and Galen. In particular (from our point of view) while the general principles of anatomy were tackled by Avicenna in book one, its topographical detail was dispersed through book three and the anatomical commentator had to re-assemble it (the topographical anatomical *summae* of book one were omitted from the medieval curriculum).

So medical scholasticism was at least in part a technique of dealing with texts. These were products of alien and sophisticated culture, and they naturally created problems in the medieval Latin west. To understand these texts, and to teach them, medieval scholars devised systematic methods of enquiry and presentation. The simplest was perhaps the topical question and answer of, for example, the Salernitan questions.[34] A more complex question-doubt-resolution routine is exemplified by Peter of Abano's *Conciliator*, also arranged on the basis of topic. An elaborate approach to individual texts was the *accessus ad auctores*, a set of formal questions asked of the text by the commentator in his introduction. Designed to explain the works of Aristotle and relate them to the rest of knowledge, the *accessus* came to be used in many areas of the school curriculum including, as has recently been shown, medicine. For our purpose it is important to note that a form of the *accessus* that is closely related to the Aristotelian categories was used by John of Alexandria in commenting on Galen's *De Sectis*. This gave rise to a *physical* 'accessus' – the observables in the body – when human dissection began in the middle ages (see note 17).

The overall purpose of the scholastics was to present knowledge in an ordered whole which could accommodate new knowledge and which was structured for ready teaching and learning. The world picture became largely Aristotelian, medicine and physics having a common substrate. The agreement between the related divisions of knowledge was ensured by drawing out the 'true' meaning of the texts. In such an ordered scheme ancient authors apparently differing in their opinions were 'saved', that is, shown to agree by revealing their 'true' opinions. Close logical analysis of the texts was one means of doing this. This scholasticism varied from subject to subject. The *accessus* ranged from the anatomical to the legal. In the study of the Bible, the question of saving the authors, so important in medicine, could not arise in the same way, and scholastic study was a question of drawing out essential meanings and moral parables by close application to the text. Legal scholasticism centred on the Code of Justinian, which was treated as 'written reason',[35] and again close study of the text was necessary in order to apply it as closely as possible to society. Given the importance of this one author and text, the lawyer did not have to save his authors as the physician did. The last of the traditional higher faculties was canon law, which developed as an assemblage and codification of papal decrees: in this case the given text was fragmentary and the scholar worked from internal evidence to build up a wider scheme. The role of the commentator, then, was different in all these branches of study. The medical commentator had not only his important texts (the *Aphorisms* of Hippocrates had been used in medical education from antiquity and approached in weight of authority the fundamental texts of the other major disciplines) but was obliged to reconcile his important authors. Moreover, the physician had to carry his precepts into practice, and the anatomist had the dissected body to place in his overall scheme.

Correspondingly, the humanism which replaced these forms of scholasticism differed as much as they. Perhaps the only feature we can identify with confidence as common to them all is a sense of historical distance the humanists felt between themselves and the ancients. The associated desire to recapture classical culture led to the use of classical models in rhetoric, and the pattern of arguments used by Cicero was opposed to the formality of the rules of the *ars dictaminis*. The legal humanists came to see the Code of Justinian as the product of an ancient imperial culture that was quite different from the cities of Italy and therefore inapplicable to their society. The scriptural humanists now saw that Paul's letters to the Romans had to be understood also in the circumstances of Roman political power. In the 1440s Lorenzo Valla showed that the church's 'Donation of Constantine' was a forgery: he did so on historical grounds, by pointing to anachronisms. A related weapon of the humanists was philology, or more precisely, historical terminology, the establishment of the meaning of a word at the time it was written. This concern with language was linked to the humanists' cultivation of a purely classical prose style, from arts-course rhetoric to technical exposition in the higher disciplines.

Armed with this historical awareness, the humanists began to see that the commentators, seeking to apply the Code of Justinian to contemporary society or seeking the real religious message of the words alone of the scriptures, were engaged upon an enterprise that looked increasingly foreign to the humanists' own aims. They attempted not only to show that the commentators had misconceived the nature of their sources, but that their techniques were mistaken. The humanists naturally objected to the fine logical distinctions made by the scholastics in penetrating the 'real' meaning of the text, and to their readiness to construct neologisms to explain these distinctions. These neologisms often included ugly indeclinable words from Arabic sources, and the humanists were tempted to step right over the Arabs and commentators back to the Greek and Roman sources.

These changes were spread over a long period of time, but some important ones occurred in the period when Berengario was reading and teaching. Thus the legal humanism of Valla and his followers crossed the Alps to France only in the first decade of the sixteenth century, in the hands of Budé. Valla's denunciation of the Donation of Constantine became known to a visiting German, Ulrich von Hutten, while he was in Bologna in 1512 or 1517.[36] When he returned home von Hutten published this *exposé* with 'explosive' results in reformist thinking.[37] von Hutten seems to have met Berengario in Bologna, and when he had gone, Berengario reissued Hutten's book on the guaiac treatment of syphilis, a disease that interested them both. We have seen that Berengario was acquainted with other important figures and their techniques in the intellectual battles of the day, and the fifteen years of his productive lifetime was a crucial period for the humanists' battle.

It seems that the extent to which medicine could be 'humanized' was limited. A 'humanist' physician would be aware of himself as being historically severed from the classical world and certainly to place his authors in a time scale suggested by this would be of value, but he could not historicize his texts in the same way as the legal humanists were doing. Taking the aphorisms of Hippocrates as an example again, however much they were seen to be the products of an alien society, they applied to physical and unchanged individual people, not to a changed set of relationships between people. The same applied *a fortiore* to anatomy: a good anatomical text carried the same message as the body itself. For the same reason it was not easy to dismiss the commentators, whether their subject was the anatomy of the *Canon* or the densely aphoristic Hippocratic writings. In other words these commentators were engaged in the *same kind* of activity (despite the uncouthness of their language) as the 'humanist' physician, because the ultimate object of enquiry was the truth about the physical human body. Moreover, the *Canon* seemed more complete than any Galenic work available[38] and study of it was indispensable. The 'humanist' physician might do what he could to avoid barbarity of language, but the Ciceronian style that suited rhetoric so admirably was not easily suitable for dissection guides and descriptive anatomy (Vesalius was to lose a number of readers for this reason). The humanists' tool of historical terminology was of great importance in a descriptive science like anatomy, but it had to be based upon Arabic as well as Greek terms; in using it the humanist physician found not only that he was engaged upon the same kind of enterprise as the scholastic commentator, but that the commentators had been doing it for about two centuries.

Hellenists. These general remarks may serve to locate Berengario and his contemporaries, but when we come to try to force them more tightly into this background, we find we cannot. We are obliged to suspend our historical categories. Berengario saw himself as an *academic*: he calls his colleagues and pupils *scholastici* and *scholares.*[39] But we cannot call him and them 'scholastics' because the term still has the pejorative sense attached to it by the later humanists, implying that such people were characterized by a want of practicality in an excess of dry and sterile argument. On the contrary, Berengario saw himself as extremely practical, devoted to the principle of the superiority of sense observation over reason, and at the same time heir both to a rigorous academic tradition that had established rules for the evaluation of knowledge, and to the best medieval surgeons.

Nor does Berengario use a term that we can translate as 'humanist'. Instead he contrasts the academics with the Hellenists, one of the principal spokesman of whom was, for Berengario, Leoniceno. It was argued above that Aldo Manuzio may have been responsible for some of Berengario's 'humanist' traits; and we should recall here that these Hellenists formed a circle of acquaintanceship with widespread influence. When Berengario pursued Demetrius Chalcondylas for the text of Galen's *Anatomical Procedures* he was mixing with members of this circle: Bonamici was a pupil of Musurus, who followed Aldo as Alberto Pio's tutor. Chalcondylas himself and his teacher, Theodore Gaza, were not merely Hellenists, but were *Greeks.* This serves to remind us why northern Italians of Berengario's generation saw Hellenists rather than humanists amongst them. In short, while for a long time elegant and classical pieces of the Latin authors had been used by some university teachers the Greek interests of the Hellenists have quite a different origin. Behind this was the Council of Florence of 1439 when a Byzantine delegation spent some eighteen months in Italy. Hard pressed by the Turks, the Byzantines sent the group in an attempt to unite the Greek and Italian churches, and so secure Italian military help in the East.[40] In thus negotiating with the Latin west the Byzantines were putting to one side a political antagonism that dated back from the Crusaders' capture of Constantinople: it was simply that the Turks were a more present danger. But many of the Byzantines were impressed enough with Florence to return later; and in turn the Florentines were not only equally impressed with the unfamiliar philosophies of their visitors, but also continued to be aware of the advantages of friendly relations with the Byzantine East. There were thus also political and economic reasons why the sons of north Italian nobles, who had been previously trained in the arts of seamanship and commerce, should be taught Greek.

So both before and after the advancing Turks captured Constantinople, Byzantine emigrés were a feature of life in northern Italy. Where they contributed to a growing Hellenism, their cultural interest lay primarily in the Greek language. To the Hellenists Latin was simply the language in which Greek ideas were to be expressed for convenience, without a great cultural inheritance of its own. It was also the language of the commentators. Thus fifteenth century Hellenism was very different from the humanism of the previous century.

Berengario's charge against the Hellenists, as far as their activities touched medicine, was that they had chosen the elegance of the study of antique letters and had abandoned the wide reading, thorough scholarship and rigorous standards of argument of the academics. We have seen that Benedetti anticipates some of such criticism in his little Greek anatomy, and it is certainly true that to regard anatomy as purely Greek reduced the necessary reading to Galen and fragments from Hippocrates and Soranus. In contrast Berengario argued that the good anatomist must above all be a master of the literature. His own commentary assesses the work of nearly a hundred authors; of these Galen was clearly the most important for Berengario, for his name appears in the commentary more than fifteen hundred times, three times on every folio. Avicenna, whom the Hellenists resented as stealing Greek glory, is quoted over a thousand times by Berengario (and Aristotle about six hundred times, Zerbi two hundred and the commentators and lesser Arabs each between one and two hundred times).

Berengario's attitude to the Hellenists is illustrated by his dispute with Leoniceno, one of the *periti Eleni* (skilled Hellenists) in the phrase of Berengario and Zerbi (49r and Zerbi, 7v). Berengario approved in principle of Leoniceno's attempt to establish a sound Greek terminology (40v, 42r, 480r, 486v, 495v) but argued that to ignore the Arabic authors would lead to error. Thus Leoniceno uses the term *epigastrion* for the entire abdominal wall, evading the vigorous academic debate about the identity of the Arabic *siphac* and *mirach* and the Galenic *panniculus carnosus*, all of which seemed to academic anatomists to be parts of the abdominal wall. Consequently *epigrastrion* was unsatisfactory to Berengario.

Again as a Hellenist striving to write in pure Latin, Leoniceno translated the *peritoneon* of Galen's *Commentary on the Aphorisms* as *membrana abdominis interior* because there was no single-word Latin equivalent to the Greek and because he did not wish to use the 'barbaric' Arabic term *siphac*. Berengario insisted not only that *siphac* was a perfectly proper anatomical term that precisely expressed the meaning of 'peritoneon' but that Leoniceno was unjustified in inserting additional words into the text, words moreover that introduced confusion by restricting the meaning to an *inner* membrane. The argument (104ff) had a very real surgical importance, for Galen's text asserts that if the omentum penetrates the abdominal wall, it necessarily putrefies, and Berengario as a practical surgeon understands this to mean if the omentum reaches the air: to penetrate merely an interior membrane (as occurs in the zirbal rupture) is not necessarily to putrefy. Arguing from observation and due consideration of the Arabs, Berengario feels himself to be in a stronger position than Leoniceno, who is concerned primarily with 'good letters' (*viri profecto omnium bonarum litterarum consumatissimi* (105v)). Leoniceno's reply[41] is textual, without reference to observation or Arabic authors. However elegant Leoniceno's 'good letters', it seemed to Berengario that they constituted mere unverified *authority* and that Leoniceno's method was therefore at fault. In particular he objected to Leoniceno attacking Mondino (the *artifex sensibilis*) *per auctoritates et non per sensum* (154v).

Berengario's position is that, given a knowledge of the literature, both in terms of its content and its *historical* sequence, we can understand how errors have arisen and give due weight to the important authors: there is no need to short-cut the Arabs, for we can sift their contribution to anatomy if we use the critical aspects of *anatomia sensibilis*. In particular although Galen's *On the Use of the Parts* had been known in Greek and a good Latin translation from the early fourteenth century, and was a natural focus for the attention of medical humanists with an interest in anatomy, yet more popular and easier to read was an abbreviated and corrupt form of the work that had reached the West through Arabic.[42] This must have seemed very different to the Hellenists of the renaissance, and Leoniceno denied that the two had the same origin (89v). But Berengario had read both works thoroughly and could see that the sequence of argument was the same, despite the battered state of the text of *De Juvamentis Membrorum*. That is, he considered that he had recovered the *via Galeni*, the essential Galenic doctrine (akin to the *totus processus* of Mondino: compare 34r) which was the criterion against which the shortcomings of the corrupt text (which he realized were acquired at the Greek–Arabic stage of transmission (89v)), could be judged.

In anatomy at least, the Hellenists did not have that historical approach to their texts which has been seen as such a feature of humanist scholarship. What inspired the Hellenists was the belief that they were recovering a true *prisca anatomia*; true, because Greek. In contrast Berengario did historicize his texts, realizing that their content must be understood in terms of the circumstances of their composition. Aristotle, said Berengario, lived in an age when anatomy was not highly developed and so was ignorant of a great deal; Galen too was often wrong in little things (for example in his description of the veins: 162r) as in big, notably in his description of the *rete mirabile*: 'I too' cried Berengario confidently 'have a keen eye and hand and suitable tools' (459r). Other authors in Berengario's view had suffered the accidents of history as their texts have been lost or corrupted (166r). Berengario had perhaps in mind Galen's *Anatomical Procedures*, for he had read in Galen's *On the Use of Parts* of Galen's first, short version of the text and his plans for a fuller version. Perhaps Berengario had not yet realized that the fuller version was represented partly in the Greek text with the medieval name of *De Anatomicis Aggressionibus* for he often bewails the loss of Galen's particular and practical anatomy (that is, in the style of Mondino) and he spent the years between 1521 and 1529 tracking down the Greek version and improving Chalcondylas' Latin version of it for publication.

Berengario continues by placing the Arabic authors in their historical context. The first of the *cardines* of medicine after Galen, he says, was Rhasis, followed by Haly Abbas and Avicenna (162v), and their different historical contexts including their different purposes in writing, for Rhasis was much more practical than Avicenna and Haly, who were less inclined to use observation than theory, and so repeated many errors (165r, 168v). Moreover, adds Berengario, although Avicenna depended heavily on Rhasis, it was Avicenna who became known first in the West, and the *Canon* was widely accepted without its derivative nature being understood. Its status ensured that subsequent anatomists simply 'made books from books' without recourse to observation.

An important part of the techniques of establishing sound texts was the study of historical terminology, seen throughout the *Commentary* and particularly in the anatomical 'catalogue' or glossary, which occupies some forty pages in the earlier part of the work. Berengario's statement that the purpose of listing anatomical terms accurately is to establish their meaning *as used historically by the authors* could hardly be bettered as a 'humanist' programme, but of course much of Berengario's philological enquiry is directed at the important Arabic authors. The reader, says Berengario, must make every effort, *ultimo conatu*, to discover which authors have used a term, and what it can mean in different contexts, in order to understand the 'mind of the author' who uses the term (15v, 29v). The essence of the technique is to grasp the idea in the author's mind, and not to be over-concerned with the literal appearance of words, over which some scholars waste their lives (61r). Having done so, terminology can be simplified in two ways: first, a good Latin word from an approved author will replace all synonyms, as *adeps* indicates 'fat' well enough to render all the synonyms unnecessary (54v, 55r), and second, barbarisms and corruptions will be avoided. But, says Berengario, it is in the end only by means of observation that we decide which is the better of two texts. Again Berengario points to the difference between *Du Usu Partium* and *De Juvamentis Membrorum* as an example (153v). In the larger work, Galen compares the insertion of the ureters into the bladder to that of the bile duct into the intestine (so that a flap acts as a valve) but the corrupt version makes the comparison with the insertion of the bile duct into the *gall bladder.*[43] Berengario accepts from observation that *De Usu Partium* is correct, and that the error of the corrupt version is one of translation, probably at the Greek–Arabic stage (89v). Moreover, since similar errors occur in *De Juvamentis Membrorum*, Haly Abbas and Avicenna, it must be assumed either that all three texts have suffered corruption in the same direction, or, more likely, that Haly and Avicenna depended upon *De Juvamentis Membrorum*, and did not have available either *De Usu Partium* or the opportunity of sensory observation. Since all the moderns, adds Berengario, 'walk with Avicenna', they are all in error. Many of the elements of *anatomia sensibilis* are involved in Berengario's examination of the question of the insertion of vessels into the gall bladder: Berengario wonders, *miror, ac longe miror*, how Nicholas, Zerbi and all the modern *cardines* of medicine have been deceived by *authority*, since to *observation* it is clear that the insertion is perpendicular, not diagonal; *reason* would suggest a diagonal entry (on the analogy of the ureters) because such an insertion provides a valve that prevents reflux, but this must be denied in the face of observation. There is no middle way to 'save the authors' except by saying their texts are corrupt; and the good anatomist will see by *dissection* that Berengario is correct, and can confirm his opinion by *experiment*: squeeze the gall bladder and the bile moves easily into the bile duct and intestine (there is no valve) (152–3).

Similar considerations persuaded Berengario that the text of Avicenna then common, that of Gerard of Cremona (91v) was corrupt in places, in particular where concerned with the structure of the abdominal wall. The result is that Mondino and all the modern authors are in error (49v), deceived by authority. However, the text available to some of the early commentators, particularly Nicholas, was superior, and Berengario concludes (92v) that it was possible to restore the text of the Gerardine translation by adopting Nicholas' report of certain passages *and by dissection*. More generally, the older commentators, says Berengario, had inferior texts, often from the Arabic. Thus Dino, Gentile, Ugo and Nicholas had only the old, ex-Arabic translation of Aristotle's '*De Animalibus*' (232v) which has *zirbus* and *mirach* interchanged in sense as the components of the abdominal wall, while the new translation (by Theordore Gaza (232v)) more correctly identified as *De Partibus Animalium*, had 'membrane' (103r–v) in a correct usage.

This *historical* evaluation of texts, translations and technical terms was, far from being a 'humanist' activity, the very substance of what the commentators had been doing since the translations had been made. The commentators had always been critical of the translations. Taddeo called Constantine the African a 'mad monk' incapable of good translation. Taddeo preferred the translations of Burgundio of Pisa, but was obliged to base his commentary on Constantine's text because it was so widely used in teaching. As better translations were made they were ofted added to the older, so that, for example, some of the printed commentaries include three translations, the latest being perhaps that of Leoniceno. As Berengario observes, Jacobus de Partibus was aware of the identity of *De Juvamentis Membrorum* and *De Usu Partium* and of the reasons for their different appearance (388v); Gentile recognized corruptions in the text of Avicenna (111) and considered whether or not *De Juvamentis Anhelitus* was correctly attributed to Galen (137v–138v). Peter of Abano questioned the Galenic attribution of *De Spermate* (220v); Jacobus de Partibus saw *siphac* as a good modern Arabic term, replacing the antique Arabic 'superscripts' (glosses) *berbentinem*, *alberiteron* which are clearly Arabic attempts to handle the Greek *peritoneon* (and which were *auditu horrenda* to Berengario). This improvement within Arabic terminology was seen by Berengario as a process parallel to the later coining of neologisms by the Latins to generate concise technical terms. We can see from Berengario's text that such terms could be Latinate in form or adoptions from the Arabic, and we have also seen what Berengario considered the advantages of a precise terminology of this form. The Hellenists, needless to say, considered both adopted Arabic and new Latin terms as barbaric, and translated from their Greek in circumlocutions when there was no Latin counterpart.

We can now see more clearly Berengario's view of the Hellenists. He was aware of a great amount of scholarship and a shrewd historical awareness of anatomical texts that had begun at least as soon as the early fourteenth century. The fruit of this scholarship was still to be reaped in Berengario's time, especially with his own critical techniques, which in their practical nature were not necessarily sympathetic to the Hellenists. This scholarship was academic, comprehensive and businesslike, but without the elegance of 'good letters'; but to avoid it, at least in anatomy, was a failure to grasp the nettle: without such scholarship it was all too easy to fall into elementary errors such as supposing that Galen did not make mistakes (and all that was needed for truth was a sound text) or being unable correctly to attribute works of Galen that had suffered in transmission (like Leoniceno and *De Juvamentis Membrorum*).

Aggregators and barbarians. Having looked at how Berengario saw himself in relation to the Hellenists, we must examine his opinion of other identifiable groups among his contemporaries. As suggested above, Berengario saw himself as an academic. Some of the outward signs of academic medical teaching were the heavy folios of double-column, black-letter printed commentaries and text of the *Articella* and *Canon*. This format identified them as academic; Zerbi was not 'unfortunate'[44] in his printers, but undoubtedly chose the format to suit his readership. The sheer bulk of these Venetian folios represents a considerable publishing investment, that could only be recouped by steady sales to a large educational market. The disappearance of these folios from the publishing programme of the houses of Scotus and others from the 1520s was the victory of the Hellenists.

But although an academic Berengario did not identify himself with the bulk of school anatomical authors. His admiration was reserved for the practical texts of Mondino and Guy de Chauliac, who, he said, like himself had practised *anatomia sensualis* (464r) while no-one else among the moderns did so. Guy, Berengario further explained, was the *maximus anatomes* whose work was read in the public anatomies of Montpellier as that of Mondino was read in those of Italy (171r). Like Mondino, Berengario addresses his text to the practical *operatores* (for example 78r).

Berengario particularly objected to those modern anatomists who undervalued sensory experience and dissection. Those who compiled their anatomies from books alone Berengario called *aggregatores*, a term that indicated most of the commentators and which was derived from the literary habit of collecting simple recipes. Zerbi in Berengario's eyes was the *magnus aggregator* (307v) who had in Bologna a following of 'Zerbists'. These often clashed with the 'Partists', the followers of the fifteenth-century commentator Jacobus de Partibus (310r); clearly Berengario felt as distant from them as from the Hellenists.

Lastly, since Berengario, the Hellenists, the aggregators and the commentators all had their different views on what anatomy was and what an anatomy text should be like, we may usefully enquire into what at first sight seems to be their common enemy, the 'barbarians'.

Zerbi, the academic aggregator, is clear enough on the point: Guy de Chauliac, the medieval surgeon, and his kind. Although Zerbi regarded him as a useful author (for he quotes him often enough) yet he observes that Guy is barbaric in his language, using medieval terms like *pincherium* (Zerbi 47v) to express the capacity of the bladder. Probably Zerbi was also aware that Guy used his native French. Zerbi himself did not cultivate a high style of prose, and was not above using neologisms (like *cerebri factiva*, 'brain-making' 38r) but he did his best to keep his language as Latinate as possible. Thus where Berengario invariably uses 'Haly' for the Arabic author, Zerbi uses the compound 'Haliabbas' which he can decline: it has the ablative form 'Haliabbate'. Even 'Averroys' is given the ablative 'Averroy' by Zerbi (30v, 33v) while 'Rasis' (for Rhasis) becomes 'Rasi' (32r). The normally indeclinable 'siphac' becomes 'siphacia' in the nominative plural (12v).

Zerbi's attitude to Guy was not shared by Berengario, who admired him as one of the few practical authorities. Like Mondino, Berengario consciously avoided an elevated prose style as unsuited for practical descriptions and where possible tried to 'walk like Celsus among the Latins' (393v). His own view of barbarisms differs from that of Zerbi and from that of the Hellenists. He defends his own usage in telling us that Arabic terms rendered into Latin characters (like siphac and mirach) although undeclinable are not in themselves barbaric, and that barbarisms are *corruptions* of a pure original introduced by the errors of copyists, translators and printers (45r, 46r). 'God preserve me' he pleaded 'from the translators' use of unknown names for known structures' (78v). Some of the *horrida nomina* that have found their way into Averroës' *Colliget* are so fearful in sound that Berengario cannot bring himself to use them (30r). As examples of corrupt terms we may take Berengario's list of variants produced by the Greek *peritoneon* passing through Arabic into Latin: *beriteron, berbetinem, berterin, alberiteron* and *albentirion*. The proper forms in the three languages says Berengario are *peritoneum, siphac* and *membrana*, and good scholarly anatomy reveals the identity of the *idea* behind the three different words by relating it to structure.

All such names derived from the Arabic, whether corrupt or not, were regarded by the Hellenists in their search for the pure Greek form as barbaric. Their barbarians were the academics and medieval surgeons. Berengario, who felt sympathy with both these groups, naturally felt that the barbarians were some other group. Yet when he was urged (he says)[45] by Bonamici, Pomponazzi and Ercole Gonzaga to publish his edition of Chalcondylas' translation of the *Anatomical Procedures* he seemed to share the Hellenists' views on barbarisms. In giving the book 'a true birth into Latin' he spoke with a characteristic Hellenistic rhetoric of the 'pure fountains of the Greeks' and of the 'very turbid streams' of the barbarians. This rhetoric was addressed to Ercole who, we may suppose, understood and approved of it. These barbarians were not Arabs, however. Berengario's barbarians are some of his contemporaries, those who draw their *remedies* (even though the context is the *Anatomical Procedures*) from the turbid streams. For the 'lack of skill' of these barbarians, Berengario uses *imperitia*, a word he elsewhere seems to relate to *empiricus*, 'an empiric'. In either case what is implied is a lack of thorough training, particularly anatomical; the training provides skill, and the anatomical knowledge provides the basis for a *rational* practice of surgery. This lies behind his attack, in the dedication of the *Commentary*, on the *cardines* of the medical faculty, ignorant of anatomy. Much more revealing is the text of his book on fractures of the cranium. He supposes that one of the most reliable surgical authors, because one of the oldest, was Celsus. He accepts the Arabs' historical judgement that by their day most of the old surgery had been lost, so that (by implication) both Arabs and the commentators were at a disadvantage. Nevertheless, *magnus* Guy de Chauliac (12v) was an ideal practitioner combining surgery, medicine and natural philosophy (30r). But since Guy's time, says Berengario, things have deteriorated, and physicians are not willing to undertake a long period of surgical training (ideally from childhood), and surgeons with good manipulative skills are rarely well-read. Learned physicians, he explains (29v) disdained to be called surgeons, but were very conscious of the money to be made in surgery; in this perplexity they pretended to be surgically knowledgeable, and covered their ignorance by pretending also to be too faint-hearted to operate: they attended patients, taking with them stout-hearted if ignorant *chirurguli* who performed the operation and shared the fee, 'the blind leading the blind', as Berengario observed.

These *chirurguli* in Berengario's eyes were empirical, ill trained and mostly Jewish. Most of the ancient authors had sought cause and effect (60v) (that is, they were rationalists) but the ancient sect of Empirics (who held that a knowledge of anatomy was neither useful nor decently gained) flourished principally among the Jews (58r), and although Berengario says some of them have not been negligible, yet none of them have become famous. Berengario has in mind his father's great friend Jacob the Jew, who treated Ercole, Duke of Ferrara; he also has in mind Master Abraam, to whom he resented playing second string in the case of Lorenzo Medici. Although he was not above obtaining the receipt for his own cranial ointment from Jacob by deception (Jacob imagined him to be of the ducal family), Berengario became most indignant over the claim of the empirical Jewish surgeons who believed that a depressed fragment of the cranium could be raised by the use of ointment alone. These ignorant empirical idiots (64r) are Berengario's barbarians, so different from the anatomically learned *scholastici* (103v).

XI

PLINY AND RENAISSANCE MEDICINE

The previous chapters of this book have discussed the greater or lesser fallibility of Pliny as a reporter of the natural world. The broadly critical tone of much Plinian scholarship of the last two or so centuries takes its origin from the renaissance and in particular in Leoniceno´s attack on Pliny in the last years of the fifteenth century. In an age characterised by attempts to recover, restore and above all admire the texts of classical civilisation, such an attack would seem to pose something of a problem. The historian of medicine might see in the episode similarities to Vesalius´ later attack on Galen, so often seen as the first successful attempt of the nascent science of anatomy to throw off the burden of ancient authority.(1) What then was the nature of Leoniceno´s attack: was it the first stirring of a medical renaissance?

The Natural History in the renaissance

As Eastwood has explained in his chapter on astronomy, parts of the **Natural History** were excerpted during the middle ages and used as texts devoted to a single topic. This is true also of medicine and related topics, for herbals were constructed from parts of the work, and the so-called **Medicina Plinii** is a collection of remedies for diseases listed from head to toe. (It was compiled perhaps as early as the fourth century; there is an edition of 1509 from Rome.)

The **Natural History** itself was one of the more popular texts of the renaissance, with 15 **incunabula** editions and at least 43 editions during the sixteenth century.(2) What interested the physicians of the time were Pliny´s accounts of various kinds of **materia medica**, particularly those described above in the chapters by Scarborough and Morton. Additionally, those interested in the structure of the human body found Pliny a useful source for good Latin terms for structures often also, and confusingly, known by their Arabic and Greek names. The problem of nomenclature was acute: in expounding the medical uses of herbs Greek medical texts generally gave only very brief physical descriptions of the plant, insufficient for the physician, particularly those of Northern countries distant from Greece, to identify it with plants growing in the field. Nor could he be sure which plant names in his own vernacular matched those in Greek, Latin and Arabic. William Turner found almost total ignorance about medicinal plants among the Cambridge physicians of the 1520s and could find illumination about the plants in Pliny (he owned the edition prefaced by Erasmus) only in Italy, Germany and Switzerland, with the new naturalists and philologists.(3) The **Natural History** was no doubt useful here, for Pliny was thought of as near enough a contemporary of, and familiar with the Greek sources, which he conveniently listed. His Latin terminology could be taken as authoritative translations of the Greek, and as an Italian he was no doubt familiar with the local and presumably near-Greek flora.

So when Leoniceno opened his attack on Pliny, he was not criticising a minor or obscure author. It must have been seen as a serious matter in the scholarly world. This chapter will sketch out the course of the dispute that arose from Leoniceno's attack and then discuss some of the reasons behind it and the attitudes taken by a number of different people in two areas of medicine: it is not intended to give a bibliographically complete account.

The argument(4) began with an exchange of letters between Leoniceno and Politian. Leoniceno had expressed some criticism of Avicenna and some medieval authors, and he had also accused Pliny of confusing the Greek herb **kisthos** with ivy, **cissos**. Politian replied in January 1491, concurring in the criticism of Avicenna, but chiding Leoniceno for attacking so notable an author as Pliny on such slight grounds. This prompted Leoniceno to publish in the following year a detailed criticism, **De Plinii et Aliorum in Medicina Erroribus**, concerned primarily with herbs and fruits in medical use.

This pamphlet brought two very swift replies. The first was the **Castigationes Plinianae**, begun by Hermolao Barbaro some time before, but now modified to meet some of Leoniceno´s critcisms.(5) The second was a much more direct response, the **Pliniana Defensio,** written expressly to refute Leoniceno by the lawyer Pandolfo Collenuccio.(6) While it was still in press he read Barbaro´s commentary, and the two authors added a joint appendix to the **Defensio.** Leoniceno sought to justify himself in a letter to Barbaro who, however, died before Leoniceno had finished it. It became a second ´book´ of the **De Erroribus** in the edition of 1509.(7) The third book of that edition is another letter, to Franciscus Tottus, in which Leoniceno rather half-heartedly returns to the attack on Pliny on the occasion of the discovery of a new manuscript. The 1509 edition is completed by two more letters of Leoniceno, the first of which had originally been published in 1498 and in which Leoniceno developed an earlier critique about the identity of the vipers used anciently in making theriac with the **marassi** of fifteenth-century Italy.

At first sight the dispute appears to have been a technical wrangle about the identification of the components of medicines. This had its important practical side, and indeed Leoniceno´s expressed reason for attacking Pliny was lest the great powers of medicinal substances be wrongly used and jeopardise life (the point was made again by the editor of the collected tracts of 1509). But inevitably the practical business of identifying plants became, in the ensuing dispute, a question of terminology within the literature; just as (Leoniceno maintained) Pliny had confused **kisthos** with **cissos** because of the similarity of the words (rather than of the plants).

But behind the technical detail of the dispute there lay Leoniceno´s perception of the **kind** of author Pliny was. Likewise Leoniceno´s opponents attacked him and defended Pliny not only on technical detail but for the motives behind and the nature of his attack on Pliny. This will be examined in more detail below, but we can note briefly here that as a Hellenist, Leoniceno saw Pliny´s work as sometimes clumsily derived from the superior Greek originals of Theophrastos and Dioscorides. It was in seeking pristine medicine that Leoniceno attacked Avicenna at the beginning of the dispute and the medievals Gentile da Foligno and Mondino dei Luzzi at other times. For Leoniceno they were all Latin interpreters. Similar reasons led him to attack Celsus, a figure in a position similar to that of Pliny in being an isolated Latin writer borrowing his material from a large number of older and more authoritative Greek sources. The belief in the superiority of the Greeks informed Leoniceno's attitude to medicine. For example, in reporting the disputations at Ferrara about **morbus gallicus** he went against the widely held belief that it was a new disease by insisting that whatever its causes were, they were natural (it was not divine punishment); and it was unthinkable that the same natural causes had not operated in ancient times as recently. It was equally unthinkable that the ancients had not perceived these and the resultant disease, and the reason we cannot read about the **morbus gallicus** in the ancients is simply that this is a vulgar name and the ancients called it something else, since forgotten. Once again, continues Leoniceno, Pliny is wrong, this time in asserting that new diseases had come to Italy in his own time: it was only, said Leoniceno, that there were not then enough skilled Greek doctors in Italy to recognise such things as being known to the great Greek authors; and the forgotten diseases were held to be new.(8)

Humanism

These are the bones of the controversy initiated by Leoniceno's attack on Pliny. To illuminate some of the reasons behind the actions of Leoniceno and his opponents and followers, I want to maintain a distinction that is not always made, particularly by historians of medicine. This is the distinction between Hellenists and humanists. In maintaining this I want to argue that the usual polarity between 'scholastic' and 'humanist' medicine is a false one, and that the relationship of medicine to such categories is often misunderstood.

The Italian **studia** in the early period of their existence taught vocational subjects including medicine and law. An essential part of these studies was the vocational use of rhetoric in a preparation for employment in affairs of government, politics and trade: the writing of letters and speeches, the **ars dictaminis,** taught by the **dictatores.** In general in the Italian middle ages no great use was found for the classical authors, and there were few classical models for these literary exercises. No commentary on a Latin poet or prose writer existed before the second half of the thirteenth century.(9)

In contrast in France there had been an interest in classical texts since the ninth century, and there was a considerable amount of classical study at Chartres and Orleans in the twelfth century. Italian humanism of the later thirteenth century was partly an importation from France. The new ´humanist´ teachers in the **studia** were the professional successors of the **dictatores:** they held chairs of grammar and rhetoric (later also of prose and poetry) but unlike their medieval antecedents they taught from examples of classical Latin prose.

The important point of this for us is that humanism was not only a style of teaching, but a style of teaching **certain subjects,** like the **ars dictaminis** it succeeded. Kristeller(10) points out that the term ´humanist´ arose, perhaps from student slang, to match the term ´canonist´ (for the teacher of Canon Law), ´jurist´, ´legist´ and ´artist´. The older term for the group of subjects taught by the humanist was **studia humanitatis,** embodying the idea of a liberal education, borrowed from Cicero and Gellius. By the first half of the fifteenth century the **studia humanitatis** included grammar, rhetoric, history, poetry and moral philosophy. The humanists used classical Latin models extensively in teaching (with a little Greek) and produced great quantities of commentary employing their historical and philological techniques of criticism. A number of subjects were excluded, then, from the **studia humanitatis:** medicine, law, natural philosophy, logic, metaphysics, astronomy and theology. Yet in the second half of the thirteenth century some of these subjects were also undergoing great changes. In particular (for our purposes) the reception of the natural-philosophical works of Aristotle opened up a large new field of study. In medicine the Latin translation of the **Canon** of Avicenna quickly came to occupy a major part of the teaching course. Both of these important sources lay outside the **studia humanitatis,** not only by reason of their subject matter, but because neither had been written in Latin and so could not provide models of Latin prose. The same is true of other, earlier translations from the Greek, which were concerned with technical subjects like medicine, astronomy and mathematics. An important text in this group is Galen´s **De Usu Partium,** translated by Niccolo of Reggio in 1317, but earlier available in Greek to such scholars as Peter of Abano (who claims to have read it).

The natural-philosophical works of Aristotle, the **libri naturales,** were taught in the **studia** principally by medical men. Indeed, the peripatetic world picture came to be the basis of the theory of medicine (partly through Galen's interpretation of Aristotle). Now, these processes, the assimilation and teaching of Aristotle's physical works, involved close examination of the text and the locating of each of them in its proper place in natural philosophy as a whole. All this was carried on by means of Aristotelian modes of argument and presentation: in a word, scholastically. Scholasticism had (like humanism) arrived in the Italian **studia** after their early vocational period (and perhaps also from France). To remember that in Italy scholasticism was no older than humanism and was principally distinguished from it by the subjects it taught will help the medical historian (in particular) to divest the term 'scholasticism' of some of the pejorative sense that still clings to it (as a result of the humanists' renaissance battle against it).

What relationship, then, did medicine have to humanism? It seems likely that in the century or so between the death of the great scholastic commentator Gentile da Foligno and the birth of Leoniceno (in 1428) medicine had absorbed much of what humanism was able to offer to it. In the Italian universities where arts and medicine were taught side by side it would be surprising if the humanists' interest in classical texts, and a philological and historical scholarship had not had some impact on medicine. Certainly by the last decades of the fifteenth century there is abundant evidence(11) that medicine shared the three great characteristics of humanism: it had its classical texts; philological scholarship strove to reconstruct the meaning of words as used by the authors in their own time; and a strong historical sense helped the medical men see the products of the past as formed by historical circumstances.

Indeed, the writings of medical men from Gentile to Berengario da Carpi (who as we shall see engaged in controversy with Leoniceno) betray little antagonism between humanists and physicians. Much clearer is the clash of interests and purposes of the natural philosophers and the medical men, for there were many natural questions to which they could not give similar replies. Since medical theory was based on Aristotelian physical principles the philosophers felt themselves qualified to pronounce on medical questions, at least in giving true causes; the medical men could not deny that medicine was part of philosophy, because Galen had largely Aristotelianised medicine; but nevertheless the medical men held that in at least two main areas of medicine - anatomy and the action of drugs - only sensory experience, not logical demonstration, could lead to true knowledge. The attempt of the medical men to establish a professional preserve against the philosophers - a **via medicorum** - is hinted at in Gentile(12) and clear in Berengario. These points - the subject-based nature of humanism, the partly humanised medicine of the later fifteenth century, the uneasy relationship of philosophy with both medicine and humanism (which did not come to grips with it until this time)(13) - set in greater contrast the last of the groups we have to discuss, the Hellenists.

Hellenism

The people whom history presents to us as taking part in purely intellectual disputes must often have been moved by more immediate and compelling motives. Such was the case with the Hellenists of the fifteenth century. Many of their actions can be explained on the basis of their political circumstances. For many of them were not merely Hellenistic in outlook, but were, in person, Byzantine Greeks. For our purposes the story begins shortly before the introduction of humanism and scholasticism into the Italian **studia**. In 1204 the fourth crusade sacked Constantinople and a ´Latin Empire´ was set up over Byzantium. The Italian cities, and particularly Venice, made great use of the new commercial markets that appeared, and Venice for a long time retained colonial possessions in the East. For the Byzantines the affair generated a long-lasting hatred of the Latins, whom they saw as culturally inferior ´barbarians .

Constantinople was regained (in 1261) by Michael VIII Palaeologus, and there followed a ´Palaeologan renaissance´ which emphasised the Greek culture of the Empire at the expense of its Roman origins, for ´Roman´ was the designation of the Western barbarians. But this was soon followed by increasing pressure from the Turks to the East. Byzantine emigrés even appeared in Italian cities. Finally the Byzantines were compelled to put to one side their hatred of the Latins in an attempt to save their state from extinction at the hands of the Turks. During the Council of Florence some 700 Greeks spent eighteen months in Italy in an attempt to unite the Christian churches of Rome and Byzantium and so secure Western military help for the defence of the East. This military aid failed to materialise and The City fell to the Turks in 1543.

But the Council of Florence had effects on the relationship of East and West that are of interest to us. First, the Italians were duly impressed by the culture and philosophy (particularly Platonism) of the Byzantines. Second, despite their lingering belief in the cultural inferiority of the West, many of the Byzantines were impressed with the vigour and wealth of the Italian cities. Some of them stayed in Italy after the Council and others returned, to be followed by more of their compatriots up to and after 1543. Venice´s Greek possessions survived the fall of Constantinople and so in addition to the intellectual attractions of the new philosophy from the East, there were sound practical reasons of colonial administration and commerce for the younger sons of the nobility to be taught Greek.

The history of the teaching of Greek in the West also reflects these political and commercial circumstances. Although the first Western chair of Greek was established in Florence in 1361 on the urging of Boccaccio, it is argued convincingly by Geanokoplos(14) that the real beginning of Greek studies dates back to Chrysoloras, who had been at the Council of Florence and who took the chair of Greek at Florence. One of the advantages of setting up chairs of Greek is said to have been the practical one of of recovering and practising Greek medicine;(15) but it is likely that the political and mercantile advantages were at least as clear. This is illustrated by the chair at Venice, held from 1504 to 1506 by Nicolaus Leonicus, who had studied with Chalcondyles, a pupil of Chrysoloras: this was not a university post but was attached to the Ducal Chancery School for the training of civil servants for the Venetian Greek possessions.

For their part, the teachers of Greek used their positions to express their nationalism and sense of cultural superiority. Before the fall of Constantinople these teachers spoke from their chairs of the necessity of saving their beleaguered countrymen; and afterwards, they called for help for emigres or even for the establishment of a new Greek state. Thus Bessarion, a veteran of the Council of Florence and now a cardinal, opened his house to other Greeks and called for the formation of a collection of Greek manuscripts for the preservation of Greek learning. Pletho (whose Platonism had been so interesting) had an ideal of a new Hellenic state; it was to have been a new Greece, not a new Byzantium (which had been criginally Roman). The cultural superiority felt by the Greeks is clear in Chalcondyles´ introductory address to the university of Padua in 1463. Despite some mock humility he makes it clear to his audience - one might say offensively clear - that he believed that everything of value in Latin culture had been given by the Greeks.(16)

These then, were the Hellenists, and it is helpful if we see them, at the time when Leoniceno was attacking Pliny, as a distinct group with certain things in common. They were certainly seen as a group by the medical men, for example by Berengario and Gabriel de Zerbi.(17) If we look at medical writing at the time we can distinguish **academic** medical men, who taught in the universities and who had absorbed much of both the scholasticism (they called themselves **scholastici**) and the Latin humanism of the universities, from the Hellenists, who were largely outside the universities, whose prime concern was being Greek, and who in a number of cases (like Chalcondyles)(18) began with only a rudimentary knowledge of Latin and its culture.

Before looking in more detail at the fate of Pliny at the hands of the medical men, we should note one more characteristic of Hellenism. In emphasising the Greek origin of all good things, the Hellenists were obliged to step back, over the Roman foundation of the Eastern Empire, to Athenian philosophy and science. Ancient Greek science was the **prisca scientia**, borrowed but not properly used by the Romans, and stolen by the Arabs. Like the Western humanists, the Hellenists´ business was to recover the culture of antiquity, but unlike their Western counterparts they saw Latin only as a language of transmission, and not a language in which the **prisca scientia** resided: it was the language of the commentators. But Greek philosophy antedated Christ and was pagan; in emphasising their Greekness, the Byzantine emigrés sometimes seemed more Hellenist than Christian. It has been suggested that Pletho´s ideal of a state of Hellenes involved the disestablishment of the church.(19)

In a similar way the classical sources for Western humanism were largely non-Christian. Hellenists and humanists agreed broadly on the range of topics proper to the liberal education they sought to establish on classical models, excluding medicine and the other topics listed above. In contrast the academic medical man saw himself in a tradition of scholarship that concerned itself with topics (like medicine itself), authors (like Avicenna and the commentators) and a period of history (the high middle ages) most of which were excluded in the search for a **prisca scientia.** The academic medical teacher of the partly humanised medicine of the time used the humanists´ tools of philological and historical criticism on the texts of the medieval Latin and Arabic writers; and as a technical writer, he even viewed the Hellenists with suspicion in choosing the elegance of antique letters as an easier option than the rigours of academic scholarship.(20)

It can also be argued that the academic medical man was more concerned with the Christian middle ages than were humanists and Hellenists. The arrival of the Aristotelian **libri naturales** and of Avicenna´s **Canon** produced generations of commentary which was still essential reading for medicine in the early sixteenth century. Of course, Aristotle´s natural science had to be modified, for example by dropping his claim that the world was eternal and by introducing a (rather Platonic) creator God, who better fitted Christian doctrine. God could then be represented as creating the world using principles of Aristotelian physics.(21) Avicenna´ Platonised Aristotelianism was also acceptable.(22)

In certain circumstances the Christian objection to Aristotle´s cosmology could be paramount. This happened at the reformationist university of Wittenberg in the early sixteenth century. In general, the arts course in European universities was almost entirely Aristotelian, beginning with the universal arts of argument and proceeding to their application in the sciences. Physics was the first science, the general study of the principles of physical change, and the student then proceeded through more complex sciences of actual physical motion, passing through meteorology to Aristotle´s **De Anima** or perhaps **De Animalibus.** The internal coherence of this scheme was great, and the early parts of the course were necessary stepping stones for the later; and after the final Aristotelian works the student was ready to proceed naturally to the still more complex study of medicine. Indeed, so rational and widely adopted was this scheme that it must surely have been a decision of some moment to abandon Aristotle in favour of Pliny for the early arts course at Wittenberg.

The reasons behind this decision were surely to do with Wittenberg´s role in reformist thinking. Passionate concern with the principles of religion may be assumed among those attempting to reform the church, and such concern would highlight the ways in which the usual Aristotelian teachings of the universities were not strictly Christian. We saw in the previous chapter that astronomy did not necessarily provide evidence for Nauert´s thesis about the protestant background to these changes at Wittenberg, but there is abundant evidence that the **Natural History** was used by Milich at Wittenberg because it could provide a basis for science that was more agreeable to the principles of religion than Aristotle´s physical works.(23) Milich´s argument is that the **Natural History** is about nature, and a knowledge of nature leads to a knowledge (**agnitio**) of God. With Pliny´s help, souls are led to true religion, which is defended by the stout walls of the **Natural History.** Milich can use both a text from St Paul (that divinity is so close in nature that we can almost touch it) and a Platonism (philosophers are ´just´ in being led by nature to God) to maintain an argument from design to Designer.

Milich´s purpose is to use book II of the **Natural History** to replace the physics of Aristotle in teaching his young students. This was a considerable undertaking, given that in the usual university course the whole of the later curriculum rested on the basis learned at this stage: what is there in Pliny comparable in scope and logical rigour to the basis and development of Aristotle´s physics? Answers had to be found, because it was quite clear to Milich that Aristotle´s physics was unsuited to describe the actions of divine will in creating and maintaining the world. The fundamental argument against Aristotle was that the world was not, in fact, eternal, as Aristotle maintained, but created: Milich spends much space on this, rehearsing the arguments in an academic way. Chief amongst them is that efficient causality cannot stretch back in an infinite chain, but must at length depend on a First Cause. Notice that in trying to sweep aside Aristotelian physics, Milich cannot however do without causality, efficient, formal, material and final: God is the efficient creator of the world and His purposes for it are its final cause; material and formal causes Milich finds in Plato. Further inadequacies of Aristotelian physics for Milich is the peripatetic denial of a Creative power, **nihil ex nihilo fit,** and the necessary relation between cause and effect: fire is obliged to burn. No, asserts Milich, a Creator can produce matter from nothing as He can equally suspend the operation of the elements and their qualities.

The basis of a **real** physics for Milich is God's creation of the world as a habitat for man. Final causality involves the providential design and usefulness of nature for man, by means of understanding which man comes to know God. The sequence of efficient causes from the First Cause to effect is Necessary Causality in Milich's theological physics, and he finds it necessary to defend his real physics against the pretended physics of the Epicureans, who would deny efficient and final causality. Milich's causes operate firstly on 'nature' in the general sense of the laws by which the world operates, and secondly on **particularis natura** of bodies, or their temperament, derived from their elements, qualities and faculties. For all his metaphysical re-orientation, Milich is back here to the standard components and powers of the natural world, by which the physician for example, would understand such Naturals as innate heat.

In short, Pliny's admiration for nature as the habitat of man was much more sympathetic to Milich than Aristotle's world of 'philosophical' causes. While there were religious reasons for this, this is not the place to enter into a discussion of whether the Wittenberg lectures on the **Natural History** was due to the Protestant view of things. But it should be noted that the people whom history normally calls the new natural historians of the sixteenth century (such as Gesner, Turner, Belon, Rondelet) all read the **Natural History** in the same way as Milich, and conceived it to be their duty to come to a knowledge of God through a study of His creation, the natural world. And in fact few of them were untouched by a protestant theology. Milich's concern for the education of his young students is not only that they should appreciate the religious utility of the **Natural History** but that they should do so in the usual academic way: his commentary is based on the common practice of scholars, the "scholastic disputation".(24)

Leoniceno and Pliny

It is against this background of Hellenists, humanists and academics that we can profitably ask why it should have been Leoniceno who attacked Pliny. The answer seems to lie in his personal interpretation of the Hellenists' message.

Nicolo Leniceno began his Greek studies at the age of fifteen with a relative, Ognibene Leoniceno. Through Ognibene, Nicolo was not far removed in a line of teachers and pupils from Chrysoloras, the Byzantine emigre and first great teacher of Greek in the West. We have no direct evidence of the transmission to Leoniceno of the passion with which the Byzantine emigres argued for the cultural superiority of their civilisation, but the circumstances are suggestive. Chrysoloras had been at the Council of Florence as one of the Byzantine delegation, and the urgent political needs of Constantinople must have quickened his sense of cultural identity and of history. The Byzantine delegation first met at Ferrara, Leoniceno´s town, when he was ten, in 1438, and it difficult to believe that the significance of the events was not explained to him. When he began his Greek studies five years later, it was still ten years before the Emperor and his subjects chose to die at the hands of the Turks in the City where their ancestors had lived for eleven centuries rather than abandon it.(25) (In that year too, the Byzantine Theodore Gaza began to teach at the reformed **studium** of Ferrara.) When Constantinople fell, Leoniceno was undoubtedly the master of the language, and it is not difficult to believe that the loss of a civilisation deepened in the minds of the Hellenists - including Leoniceno - an awareness of its merits and the importance of its records. Leoniceno took his doctorate in that year, 1453 (and performed the usual academic exercises alternately in Greek and Latin).

Apart from these hints as to Leoniceno´s Hellenism, we should note that he combined it with medicine (and mathematics and philosophy). It was not perhaps the most natural of combinations. Just as Western humanism did not in its origins and use naturally extend to the sciences or philosophy, so the Palaeologan Greek renaissance was not primarily an affair of the technical subjects. Of course, the authorities of the **prisca scientia** of the Greeks included Hippocrates and Galen, and so the Byzantines like Chalcondyles could still when faced with medicine maintain the superiority of their culture.

In general however, the humanists and Hellenists avoided the technical subjects of medicine and philosophy. The Hellenists often identified themselves as writing with eloquence´, by which they generally meant ´in Greek´. Those who knew Latin only, they said, ´stuttered´ in their expression, and nowhere more so than in expressing the matter of the technical subjects. The practitioners of these subjects sometimes retorted that the Hellenists were mere grammarians, unable to cope with the rigours and discipline of academic subjects like medicine and philosophy.(26) It seems to have been the case that many of the Hellenists (rather than humanists) were outside the universities and university based professions, so that ´academic´ can be opposed to ´Hellenist´ in this way too.(27)

Leoniceno, however, was not content that the Hellenists should make only eloquence and good letters their proper field of study and asserted that the time had come for the Hellenists to tackle the technical subjects of medicine and philosophy.(28) He taught his own students (such as Tottus) both medicine and the liberal arts,(29) and no doubt saw himself as a model philosopher and physician who like his great antecedents Plato and Galen conducted his business in Greek. He stigmatised his enemies as being without a knowledge of medicine or Greek and referred even to fellow Hellenists as ´mere grammarians if they did not have medical knowledge. Merula was a mere grammarian (30) in Leoniceno´s view because he worked on Latin rather than Greek texts (and was the teacher of Leoniceno´s enemy, the Patron of Pliny, whom we shall meet below). Even so Greek a person as Theodore Gaza, the translator of the Aristotelian zoological works, who had been appointed to the **studium** of Ferrara at about the time when Leoniceno bagan his study of Greek, was a **grammista.**(31)

In urging the Hellenists to extend their empire over more educational fields Leoniceno was giving a new direction to what was already a vigorous campaign for Hellenistic studies in education both within and outside the universities. The handful of people who did in fact combine Hellenism with medicine or philosophy felt themselves even more than the Hellenists as a whole to be fighting a crusade against an inferior but vastly more numerous enemy. Their self-image was never far in fact from the last defenders of Constantinople. Menochius wrote to Leoniceno in 1503, urging him to continue with his translations of Galen, fearing that if they were to come to an end "...just as the barbarians of Turkey destroyed a great part of Greece, so the medical barbarians of our age will confound confusion and will lacerate Galen with their inept translations".(32) Leoniceno spoke of medical and philosophical Hellenists as 'the few' who were 'proven in war'; Tricaelius presented Leoniceno to the reader in military terms as the victor over rustic barbarity(33): in the Hellenists' rhetoric the barbarian Turks were readily equated with the barbarians who had overrun the Roman Empire and imposed a medieval gloom over Italy's literary studies, and with the Arabs, who had stolen from the Greeks the claim to have discovered medicine.(34) Leoniceno and his circle addressed each other in their letters and dedications as those alone who had the ability and, above all, duty to combine eloquence with medicine and philosophy and so free Italy (or the republic of letters, or medicine or philosophy) from the barbarians (or the rustics or the monks).

There are many ways, then, in which Pliny fell short of Leoniceno's ideal. He did not write in Greek; indeed he was not Greek. Certainly he read Greek, but that only meant that the bulk of the **Natural History** was taken from Greek sources. And these sources, in the topics in which Leoniceno chose to attack Pliny, were the older and more authoritative Dioscorides and Theophrastos.(35) Leoniceno maintained that unlike Theophrastos, Pliny had no adequate scientific method, and that unlike Dioscorides Pliny dealt with words rather than things. Nor did Pliny have any special knowledge of philosophy and medicine, essential components of Leoniceno's ideal scholarship. At best, Leoniceno said, Pliny was a grammarian or orator(36) and later claimed that most people read Pliny for his vocabulary and style rather than for the technical content.(37) And it was in fact only the Latin eloquence of Pliny, whom Leoniceno calls with Hellenistic condescension Pliny the Latin Man,(38) that saved him from coming into the same category as the barbarians. Pliny, said Leoniceno, was 'in the same game , **in eandem aleam**, as the barbarians.(39)

In reading Pliny, Leoniceno as a Hellenist physician could hardly have found sympathetic Pliny's attack on Greek doctors and medicine (described in Nutton's chapter); and Pliny's preference for old Roman rustic simplicity may have seemed to Leoniceno another area in which Pliny was dangerously close to being barbarian. Perhaps too, Pliny's jaundiced view of 'Greek vanity (compare the **vanitas Graecae** of Greek astronomy, p.187 above) recalled to Leoniceno contemporary scoffing, by the academics, at the elegant **graecitas** of his group of Hellenists. Leoniceno's aim was to defend Hellenism as much as to belittle Pliny.

In Leoniceno´s view these shortcomings of Pliny became manifest in the **Natural History** in two principal ways. The root of the problem was Pliny´s lack of philosophy which, said Leoniceno, was the cause of Pliny not practising an adequate scientific method. The results of this were several categories of errors and confusion of fact of the text of the **Natural History: vicinitas nominum**, confusion of similar names of dissimilar things (**cissos** and **kisthos** being the **locus classicus**); **aequivocatio**, ambiguity, were a single name might suggest to the unwary compiler more than one thing; a single thing with more than one name, each taken by the hasty encyclopedist to represent another thing; and similarity between things taken rashly as identity.(40)

The method that would have avoided such errors, and in which Pliny was deficient was, said Leoniceno, the best scientific method of the Greeks, based on the superiority of sense observation over reason, and of knowledge over (written) opinion. In practising the method (said Leoniceno), large numbers of observations were brought together to form a single statement, which was then divided in accordance with its now apparent natural articulations to reveal truth. According to Leoniceno the best practitioner of the method had been Socrates, but it was Aristotle who had used it to the greatest extent (with some difficulty however in the zoological works). Likewise Theophrastos, the philosophical successor of Aristotle and the literary source for Pliny, was a skilful practitioner of the method, unrecognised by Pliny. And of course, Galen likewise earned Leoniceno´s praise, for in using the method he was philosophical, medical and Greek.

Leoniceno demonstrated his ability to live up to his own ideal as a philosophical, medical and eloquent scholar in much of what he wrote; and particularly in his treatise(41) on the ´three doctrines´ announced so tersely by Galen at the beginning of the **Ars Parva** that they were subject thereafter to much commentary. Here Leoniceno does indeed deal with the technical matter of logical forms and arguments in a very lucid way. In doing so he is remedying what he saw as defects in the academic treatment, particularly that of the commentaries. He may have been thinking of the commentary on this text by Gentile da Foligno, whom Leoniceno often describes as one of most important of the **iuniores**, the recent (that is, medieval) and barbaric commentators. Whether or not he had Gentile in mind, the latter's commentary(42) is characteristically medieval, and his discussion is abbreviated, unrelieved by example, highly technical and less considerate to the reader than Leoniceno's. But of course Gentile expected his readers to be entirely familiar with the kinds of technical detail and the presentation, and he can address them with all scholarly rigour and comprehensiveness. Leoniceno on the other hand knew that his Hellenists were on the whole nervous of the technicalities of the scholasticism of Gentile's day and of the academic treatment of their own, and he has to lead them by the hand, lighting the way with eloquence and providing easy examples to show how the methods worked.

The defence of Pliny

From what has been said above it can be seen that in attacking Pliny Leoniceno was putting into operation his programme for a Hellenistic invasion of academic territory. He could attack Pliny on medical matters (the identification of simples), philosophical (scientific method) and linguistic (confusion of terms). We need not be surprised that the academics (for example Berengario) resented this invasion, and those who (like Collenuccio) defended Pliny did so as Leoniceno had attacked him, that is, at a level deeper than the factual accuracy of details: that Pliny was a kind of author worthy of defence. And even more relevant to our interest is that the academics' reply was determined partly by the kind of author they thought Leoniceno was.

This is clear from Collenuccio's defence of Pliny against Leoniceno.(43) Even in its external appearance - black letter, double columns - Collenuccio's text is clearly a product of the schools, resembling for example the nearly contemporary anatomy text of Zerbi(44) and the weighty folios of commentary on Avicenna printed in Venice for the Italian medical schools.(45) Leoniceno and the Hellenists were always careful to have their words printed in a plain roman uncial or in italic, without columns. Collenuccio's academic subject was law, which like medicine, could only accept so much humanism and which by its very nature (it was Roman law) could be less readily Hellenised than medicine (where the Greek authors were important). Collenuccio does not pretend, he says, to study 'eloquence' (Greek) or to have a detailed knowledge of medicine: he modestly says he is versed "only in the most illiterate of letters, since I am a lawyer".(46) Indeed, Collenuccio groups himself with the **scholastici**(47) who urged him to reply to Leoniceno, and like these academics he suspected Leoniceno of an excessive zeal for things Greek.

It was as an academic that Collenuccio resented Leoniceno's attempt to extend the disciplinary boundaries of Hellenism. He recognised these boundaries, and knew that he would himself risk criticism in straying too far from his own professional field of law into those where he had no special knowledge, "using his scythe in a foreign field" as he expressed it. But the Hellenists' attack could be resisted by taking the initiative and altering the boundaries in favour of the academic and technical subjects. Collenuccio argued that one philosophy should embrace all the "arts, disciplines and letters". As a lawyer speaking from the stronghold of technical argument ("dialectic and philosophy"), he saw 'eloquence' and 'letters' as something to be brought within the grasp of the academics.

Naturally Collenuccio arranges his defence of Pliny in a legalistic way, first appointing himself the "patron" or advocate of Pliny. The main force of his 'case for the defence' of Pliny - and it was echoed by others who disagreed with Leoniceno - was not so much that the attack was incorrect in the disputed details, but that it was **unfair.** We should here pause to remind ourselves that the principal model for conducting an argument and discovering truth was the disputation, the structure of which was so thoroughly absorbed by university-trained men that it perhaps even unconsciously determined their conception of what constituted proper discussion and proof. The essence of the disputation, and of the legal procedures with which Collenuccio was familiar in court, was that the argument went from one side to the other until a resolution was reached. But as Collenuccio reminded his readers, Pliny had been dead for more than a thousand years, and unlike the disputant or litigant was **not there to defend himself.** What was involved was not simple injustice, but that the argument could not reach a satisfactory conclusion, and truth discovered, without one party being present to make **distinctiones** and to offer, and resolve the **quaestiones** and **dubia** that were the necessary stages of the **disputatio.** "I wish that Gentile were alive, so that he could answer my **quaestiones** and **dubia!**" exclaimed Leoniceno on an anatomical matter.(48) But Gentile, like Pliny, being dead, the argument could only proceed with an adopted Patron to speak for the absent disputant: Benedetti in the anatomical matter, as we shall see, and Collenuccio in the present. Collenuccio´s models are Cicero and Crassus, **prisci** but of course Roman advocates. The unfairness of Leoniceno´s attack on Pliny is contrasted by Collenuccio with the strict legal procedures by which a fair judge always defends the rights of even an absent defendant to a fair trial. Moreover, adds Collenuccio, even in cases of confessed crime (even if Pliny sometimes **is** wrong) the defendant escapes punishment if he is sufficiently useful to, or a great ornament of, society. Pliny of course - and everyone who defended him did so partly on these grounds - was a great ornament of **Latin** culture, which Collenuccio and others called the **Res Latina.** (49)

The **res Latina** - the term seems to be a conscious reaction against the **Graecitas(50)** of the Hellenists - involved the academic subjects that Leoniceno was urging his fellow Hellenists to invade. In the later dispute for and against Pliny, Leoniceno, his followers and the academics further illustrate the battle lines that were drawn up. Leoniceno´s anonymous pupil and defender, the ´Roman Physician´, felt he had scored a particular triumph when, in line with Leoniceno´s programme, he maintained his defence of Leoniceno´s account of the three doctrines of the **Ars Parva**, not only before the modern **scholastici**, but in the terms of their teachers who, the Roman Physician confesses, were very learned men.(51) These teachers included the ´old expositor´ of Avicenna, Gentile da Foligno, the ´new expositor´, Jacobus de Partibus, and ´the Monk´ or Turrisanus, the **plusquam commentator** on the **Ars Parva.**(52)

These medieval figures were very much part of the tradition of Latin scholarship of the academics, and their commentaries were well known and were printed in the early sixteenth century. Broadly, the Hellenists wished to avoid the commentators; and in the scorn with which they used the words the Monk´ and ´monkish´ in general(53), there is a hint of the difference between the pre-Christian philosophy of their intellectual heroes and the superstitious religiosity they saw in the medieval Latins.

That the ´Roman Physician´ found a minor triumph in matching the learning of the medieval scholastics reflects a common feeling among the humanists and Hellenists that the medieval commentary was not only inelegant but formidable. The medieval medical commentary had a very rigid and complex form and its formal **expositio** section, at its most elaborate, could reduce a bulky text like that of the **Canon** of Avicenna to a series of statements so short that each could be treated as the proposition of a syllogism and so exposed to the whole apparatus of argument. The **expositor** did this without summary or omission of the text, and his purpose was to **expose** the flow of author´s argument in its entirety.(54) Medieval medical commentaries could be twenty times as long as the text, and to one not brought up on them as a staple diet of education it was (and is) a difficult business to get ´inside´ them. The humanists and Hellenists did not want to do so. Leoniceno, mocking the successive quotations of an early stage of the **expositio** as **"...primam ibi, secundam ibi, tertiam ibi..."** argued that the technique (by which the commentator divided his text) rather broke up the text and argument than allowing it to speak for itself. Turrisanus´ **expositio** similarly offended Leoniceno´s Roman pupil, and Leoniceno called it "all **ostensio** and no use".(55) But the medical men in the universities still read the great commentaries and even, like Berengario in Bologna, composed new works in commentary form. They found the **periti Elleni** elegant but unwilling or unable to cope with the technical matter and techniques of medicine and philosophy, and dismissed them as grammarians: Leoniceno´s Roman Pupil, attempting to be as medical and philosophical as his teacher, felt the insult keenly. Barbaro, who brought out an edition of the **Natural History,** resented being dismissed by the scholastics of Padua under their leader, the "Ape of Padua" (said Barbaro) as one of the **insensissimi** Hellenists, who were to be avoided.(56)

Pliny and the anatomists

It was observed at the beginning of this chapter that the **Natural History** was, for the medical men of the renaissance, a source not only of accounts of items of **materia medica,** but of Latin anatomical terminology. Leoniceno´s criticisms of Pliny were as sharp in this field as in the other. But again, not all anatomists were Hellenists of Leoniceno´s kind; and the practice of dissection was common enough to provide physical criteria for the resolution of disputes about terminology.

As he was advocating the Hellenisation of medicine, Leoniceno resented the attempt of a medical man to ´usurp´ the function of the literary man in emending the text of, and in defending Pliny. Leoniceno bitterly attacked the ´medical Patron of Pliny´, whose duties, he claimed, should be to try to understand the workings of nature, not to meddle with texts: the Patron had not only published an edition of the **Natural History**, but had written an anatomical textbook embodying Plinian errors. Leoniceno´s rhetoric of invective included the device of denying the Patron the dignity of a name, but from the quotations he makes of his opponent´s anatomical opinions, we can identify him as Alessandro Benedetti.(57)

In using the terms **patronus** and **cliens**, Leoniceno may be going beyond the legal use Collenuccio made of the terms when he made himself Pliny´s **patronus**, advocate. When Leoniceno called Benedetti ´Patron´, and when his Roman pupil used the term for the modern Turrisanists, it was meant as an insult. What they may have had in mind was the civil patron-client relationship of ancient Rome, in which the patron, generally rich or noble, fed and protected the client, who may have been poor, a non-citizen or a freed slave. The benefits to the client were obvious; and the patron gained prestige by the number of his clients, and could call upon their services. But the relationship was binding, and the patron was obliged to protect the client irrespective of the merit of the client´s opinions; nor could civil or legal patrons and clients sue each other. Perhaps Leoniceno saw Pliny as a client, deficient in true scholarship but nevertheless necessarily defended by Benedetti, the better informed patron, committed right or wrong to his client.

Leoniceno differed from Benedetti principally on the place to be given to Pliny and Latin culture in the classical revival of the renaissance. This difference is highlighted by the fact that in many things Benedetti appears to have shared the ideals of the Hellenists. He practised medicine in Greek speaking areas for sixteen years, and knew the language; he was a member of a circle of Hellenists who supported and advised each other; and he declared that the Greeks were the true founders of all medicine. In dedicating his **Anatomice** to the emperor Maximilian, the **humanissimus princeps**, he promised to guide him through the terminology as Pollux had guided Commodus: the learned Greek scholar informing the powerful Roman emperor. In this dedication, moreover, he declares that anatomy is a purely Greek matter, and it is clear that he is rescuing a **prisca anatomia** from the clutches of later barbarians who claim the Greeks´ renown as the discoverers of medicine. He anticipates some criticism from the academics on this question, but dismisses it in advance, talking over their heads directly to his prince.

But apart from the obvious Hellenism of the **Anatomice**, Benedetti embraced also the **res Latina.** He believed (with Leoniceno) that eloquence should enter the technicalities of medicine, but for him eloquence included Latin, and the **externa lingua** used by those without eloquence was the vernacular, or barbaric Latin, or Arabic. Greek and Roman dignity were both pristine and both to be rescued. They differed, of course, for the Roman virtue of **gravitas** did not seize readily upon the subtleties of Greek theory, and so (Benedetti implies) medicine remained Greek. In Benedetti´s prefatory material in the **Natural History**, the **Anatomice** and his collection of medical aphorisms, we miss the urgent tone of the Byzantine writers, the sense of Greek identity. For Benedetti, Greece was purely classical and had long ceased to exist; but there **was** continuity with ancient Rome: not only did the educated in Pliny´s time speak the same language as the educated in Benedetti´s, but Pliny was Italian, even (Benedetti believed) from Benedetti´s own town, Verona. The title and the preface of Benedetti´s edition of the Natural History hail Pliny as ´our citizen´.

In practice Benedetti´s anatomical debt to Pliny was limited to terminology. Like Pliny, Benedetti listed the sources he was using and it is clear that the anatomical information, the description of structure, was taken from the Greek authors. The Latin authors are used - because Benedetti is writing in Latin - to supply good Latin names for the parts thus described. Most of the discussions that arose among the anatomists over Plinian terminology concerned the structures of the throat and the superficial parts of the face. There were also discussions on the oddities of animals and man as reported by Pliny, particularly where the **Natural History** differed from Aristotle´s zoological works.

In addition to the humanist Benedetti, we can profitably glance at Berengario da Carpi, whom Leoniceno and Fallopio regarded as the greatest anatomist of the time.(58) Berengario was an academic: he had had an early surgical training from his father, a late humanist-Hellenist education from Aldo Manuzio and then a formal medical training in the university of Bologna. He had a taste for the elegant and antique, but wrote with a businesslike Latin that was closer to that of the medieval surgeons than to Cicero. He used to great effect the humanists´ tools of philology and historical criticism, but did so also on Arabic texts. He admired Galen above all authors but was immensely well read in Avicenna and the commentators, and indeed cast his own anatomical work in the form of a commentary. He strove for a purity of terminology, but accepted uncorrupted Arab words as perfectly satisfactory technical terms. He approved of the efforts of the "learned Hellenists" (in whose number he held Leoniceno and his Roman pupil) to establish a sound anatomical terminology, but he attacked them for avoiding the difficult business of true (academic) scholarship by hiding behind the elegance of ´good letters´; he even took the battle into Leoniceno´s camp in accusing him of mistranslating from the Greek. Berengario was, in short, a good example of an academic practitioner of the medicine of the early sixteenth century, which had absorbed what it could of Western humanism and which was felt by its practitioners to be distinct from the newer Hellenism.(59)

Berengario´s personal interpretation of anatomy was to lay great stress on the role of sense observation, and so his criterion for assessing the written authorities was whether the authors had used observation or had been simply **aggregatores**, putting books together from other books. In this way too Berengario saw himself and his science as distinct from most of his scholastic forbears (but he still called himself and his colleagues **scholastici**). Lastly Berengario, in company with most medical men of his time, although allowing that philosophy had strong claims on the fundamentals of medical thinking, nevertheless marked out a professional territory in which medical questions could only be answered by medical answers.

How did Berengario react to Pliny? When looking for references to Pliny in the writings of the academic anatomists, we should remember that part of the function of writing anatomy books, and particularly the sort that Berengario wrote, was to report to the reader what was to be found in the authorities. This was the first stage of an assessment of opinions, followed by the objections and resolution. The use of Pliny by the anatomist does not reflect an ´influence´ of Pliny upon him, and an uncritical presentation of Pliny's statements does not imply acceptance until the final resolution. While Pliny is often quoted on anatomical terminology, this is only partly that the anatomist has found a preferred classical usage; it is partly also that the renaissance author is providing a guide to classical usage for his reader. Much the same is true of the early sixteenth-century works on natural history or zoology: although often seen as examples of nascent sciences struggling against the influence of the ancients, their authors were as much seeking to use nature as a guide to the authors as the authors as a guide to nature.(60) In both cases it seemed as if there was an objective reality - the structure of the body and the animated world, respectively - against which one could check Pliny's meaning, terminology and accuracy. (Again, we see in the renaissance the beginning of the kind of practical evaluation of Pliny that appears in Rottlander's chapter in this book.) Thus Berengario saw that Pliny had used terms for the top of the windpipe, and for the top of the gullet in man, that other authors had used interchanged. As authors sympathetic to Pliny, Berengario and Benedetti(61) distinguish, record and adopt Pliny's usage; unsympathetic, Leoniceno(62) accused Pliny of not a mere terminological confusion, but of the gross anatomical error of confusing the two structures, that is, a windpipe that descended to the stomach and a gullet terminating in the lungs. What view was taken of Pliny, here again, depended not on the text of the **Natural History** (which was not in question), nor here directly on the evidence of the dissected corpse, but on the cultural background of the reader and, indeed, of the writer of the **Natural History**.

Conclusio totius operis

The bulk of this book consists of specialist assessments of Pliny's **Natural History** in various subject areas. Common to them all is the admission that Pliny as collector of very many items of information did not have the expert's understanding or precision, or indeed, purposes.

This assessement itself has a history. This chapter has described how such a history began, with Leoniceno's attack on Pliny's confusing some medical simples, which is parallelled by Scarborough's critique of Pliny in the chapter on pharmacology and Morton's on botany, which elaborate on the causes given by Leoniceno for Pliny's errors: his misreading of his Greek sources. Secondly, it can be shown that Berengario da Carpi performed dissections of the human body in order to resolve ambiguities, locate corrupt passages and emend the text of his ancient anatomical sources, and that he used this knowledge in assessing both Pliny´s and Leoniceno´s remarks on anatomical topics. This technique of matching Pliny´s descriptions with re-creations of the physical phenomena with which he was concerned is employed by the German translation group. Here, too, archaeology offers physical objects related to the processes that Pliny describes. The temptation evident here to use something as reliable as an artfact or a modern descriptive science as a yardstick to measure Pliny´s accuracy is also apparent in Healy´s chapter on metals and mineralogy. Any danger of an over-confident use of an approach of this sort is avoided in Greenaway´s chapter on chemical tests, which are located in the context of quality-testing in a commercial world. The Hellenists´ opinion of the **Natural History** as a secondary and rather graceless text has continued to inform classical scholarship at least up until the time of Norden, as Locher allows in his chapter. In yet another area, Eastwood has described how Plinian astronomical theory was increasingly found unsatisfactory in the renaissance; a tradition of criticism of which Pedersen´s chapter is a modern example.

In a number of ways, then, this book continues an historical assessment of Pliny that began in the renaissance. The result of specialist enquiries into the **Natural History** must necessarily be as diverse as the topics to which Pliny addressed himself, and lack of a cohering argument is a complaint that the commentators have raised against the **Natural History**. Yet overall there is a characteristic Plinian approach, certainly in comparison with that of his Greek sources. Pliny´s topic is nature as the theatre of man´s actions, nature as Designed. It is not the search for natural-philosophical causes, as in Aristotle´s zoology or Theophrastus´ botany, and not a categorical exercise or a catalogue of things from which to draw out inductions. Pliny´s biological knowledge is that important to man. The stars are consulted not as embodying perfection but as a guide to the agricultural seasons. His description of quality-testing of natural and manufactured substances, and his rejection of sophistical Greek medicine, to say nothing of his search for a simple, reliable and preferably Roman diet and **materia medica** all tell the same story. It was not just that man´s needs and concerns defined what was important in nature (see the chapters by Pedersen, Locher and Morton), but that nature was providential to the point of being divine. It was the providence of nature that led to Pliny´s physics replacing Aristotle´s in Milich´s Wittenberg, and its divinity that caused Philemon Holland to have doctrinal qualms about translating the **Natural History.** (This may serve as a reminder that the attractiveness of Pliny´s books on nature to every potential reader (and therefore their ´influence´) depended, more than simply on the utility or factual accuracy of their contents, on the existing conceptions of the reader, whether religious (Milich and Holland), cultural (Leoniceno), or academic (Berengario).

NOTES

1. In looking for progressive change in the renaissance, historians of medicine have commonly focussed on Vesalius and his attack on Galen. The result has been to pre-judge the period we are dealing with here. See for example C D O´Malley, **Andreas Vesalius of Brussels, 1514-1564**, University of California Press (the standard biography); L R Lind, **Pre-Vesalian Anatomy**, Philadelphia, 1975, and Thorndike´s account of the attack of Pliny: L Thorndike, **History of Magic and Experimental Science**, vol.4, Columbia University Press, 1934, p. 593.

2. The **Natural History** was known in the middle ages, and mss. of the eleventh century survive: H le Bonniec, **Bibliographie de l´Histoire Naturelle de Pline**, Paris, 1946, p. 23. G S Sarton, **The Appreciation of Ancient and Medieval Science during the Renaissance (1450-1600)**, Philadelphia, University of Pennsylvania Press, 1955, counts fifteen incunable editions, three in the Italian vernacular. Eleven of these editions came from Venice, the work of nine different printers. Four commentaries were printed in the same period. At least 43 editions appeared during the course of the sixteenth century.

3. W Turner, **A New Herball**, London, 1551, dedication. On Turner in general, see C Raven, **English Naturalists from Neckham to Ray**, Cambridge University Press, 1947.

4. Convenient accounts can be found in Thorndike (1934), by Bylebyl, "Leoniceno", **Dictionary of Scientific Biography** (DSB) ed. C C Gi-

llespie, New York, 1970 and A Castiglioni, "The school of Ferrara and the controversy on Pliny", in E Underwood, ed., **Science, Medicine and History**, Oxford University Press, 1953, vol. 1, pp. 269-279.

5. Rome, 1492-3

6. P Collenuccio, **Pliniana Defensio Pandulfi Collenuccii Pisaurensis Iuriconsulti adversus Nicolai Leoniceni Accusationem**, Ferrara, no date (?late 1492-early 1493).

7. N Leoniceno, **De Plinii et plurium aliorum Medicorum in Medicina Erroribus**, Ferrara, 1509.

8. N Leoniceno, **De Morbo Gallico** (first ed. Venice, 1497) in **Opuscula**, Basel, 1532, pp.111r - 112r

9. Useful sources here are N Siraisi, **Arts and Sciences at Padua. The Studium of Padua before 1350**, Toronto, 1973; Q Skinner, **The Foundations of Modern Political Thought**, 2 vols., Cambridge, 1978 (I am indebted to Dr A R Cunningham for drawing my attention to this) and P O Kristeller, **Renaissance Thought and its Sources**, New York, 1979.

10. Kristeller (1979) p. 22

11. This evidence is presented in my chapter on Berengario da Carpi and anatomical commentary in A Wear, R French and I Lonie, **The Medical Renaissance of the Sixteenth Century**, Cambridge, 1985.

12. The discussion is found in the proemium to Gentile´s exposition of book 3 of the **Canon** of Avicenna. This was printed in Venice in about 1505 and again in 1522.

13. Kristeller (1979) p. 29.

14. D J Geanokoplos, **Greek Scholars in Venice**, Harvard University Press, 1962, p. 24

15. D J Geanokoplos, **Interaction of the "Sibling" Byzantine and Western Cultures in the Middle Ages and Renaissance, 1300 - 1600**, Yale University Press, p. 248

16. Geanokoplos gives the text.

17. Berengario da Carpi, **Commentaria cum amplissimis Additionibus super Anatomia Mundini**, Bologna, 1521; Gabriele de Zerbi, **Liber Anathomie Corporis Humani et singulorum Membrorum illius**, Venice, 1502. Both use the term **periti Elleni** (in various spellings).

18. Geanokoplos, "Sibling", p. 191

19. Ibid.,p.192

20. See note 11

21. For example Gentile da Foligno in his proemium to his commentary to book 3 of the **Canon** (note 21).

22. Avicenna´s natural philosophical works could be arranged in an order similar to that adopted in the universities for the Aristotelian treatises. See the **Avicenne perhypatetici: philosophi ac medicorum facile primi opera in lucem redacta: ac nuper quantum ars niti potuit per canonicos emendata,** Venice, 1508 (Frankfurt, 1961)

23. **C Plinii Liber Secundus, de Mundi Historia cum erudito commentario V. Cl. Jacobi Milichii,** without notice of place or date; "now revised from the public lectures of the University of Wittemberg". See notes 143-5 in Eastwood´s chapter.

24. Milich (note 23) dedication.

25. R Browning, **The Byzantine Empire**, London, 1980, p. 181

26. The Hellenists commonly regarded themselves as drinking from the ´pure founts´ of Greek wisdom and eloquence, while the barbarians wallowed in ´turbid waters´, phrases used for example by Erasmus, the anatomist Sylvius and Leoniceno´s Roman pupil. On eloquence and the Hellenists´ image of themselves as a group, see Leoniceno´s letter to Politian at the beginning of the **De Erroribus**, Menochius´ letter to Leoniceno (Leoniceno´s **Opscula,** p. 55r) and Leoniceno´s reply, the letters between Leoniceno´s Roman pupil and Bonaciolus (**Opuscula** pp.146r-v) and the text of the **Antisophista** which follows, particularly pp. 147r, 170v.

27. For example Leoniceno´s pupil speaks of literary studies being pursued more by "private men" than by professional teachers. The anonymous **Antisophista** is included (p.146r) in the **Opuscula.**

28. His position is stated at the beginning of the whole Pliny controversy, in the letter to Politian.

29. **Opuscula,** p.65r

30. **Opuscula,** p.22v

31. **Opuscula,** p.39v

32. **Opuscula,** p.55r

33. **Opuscula,** pp. 55r and 61v; **De Erroribus** (ed. of 1509).

34. See for example A Benedetti, **Historia Corporis Humani; sive Anatomice,** Venice 1502, dedication; Leoniceno´s Roman pupil in his **Antisophista** (**Opuscula,** p. 146v); Benedetti to Marcus Sanutus (prefatory material to Benedetti´s **Aphorisms**, included with the **Anatomice** of 1502).

35. Very often the trio Galen, Dioscorides and Paulus (Aegineta) are Leoniceno´s preferred authors; for example **Opuscula** p.9v

36. **Opuscula,** p. 1v

37. Book three of the **De Erroribus**, that is, the letter to Tottus: **Opuscula**, p. 22v
38. **Opuscula**, , pp.22v.ff
39. In the address to Politian at the beginning of **De Erroribus**.
40. **Opuscula**, pp,2r,3r,3v,5r,16v
41. Leoniceno´s **De Tribus Doctrinis** was published in the **Opuscula** of 1532 and in (Turrisanus) **Plusquam Commentum in Parvam Galeni Artem** , Venice, 1557, p. 241
42. In **Plusquam Commentum** (1557).
43. See note 6.
44. That is, Zerbi (1502).
45. See note 12.
46. The **Defensio** is unpaginated: this remark appears at sign. aii.
47. A **scholasticus** was a teacher or pupil in a **studium**. The term was used at first without a pejorative sense by the Hellenists (the Roman pupil of Leoniceno calls Montanus and his teacher **scholastici** (**Opuscula** pp. 173ff.) and Berengario and Collenuccio as academics call themselves and their colleagues by the same term. See also note 11.
48. **Opuscula**, p.44r
49. Collenuccio used the phrase twice and attributes it to Barbarus (sign. fiii).
50. Leoniceno defends himself against a charge of affectation of **Graecitas** when he introduced the Greek term **epiglossis** to correct the confusion that followed Pliny´s description of the structures of the throat.
51. **Opuscula**, p.173
52. Leoniceno, **Opuscula**, pp.29v, 43r; the Roman pupil, **Opuscula**, p. 172r
53. Leoniceno´s Roman pupil in particular attacks "the Paduan Sophist" as a **cliens** of Turrisanus, "The Monk": **Opuscula**, pp.158r, 168v. Bonaciolus makes a more general attack on monks, but both are discussing the three doctrines of Galen, and Turrisanus is intended by both. (**Opuscula**, p.156v.)
54. See note 11.
55. **Opuscula**, p.5v
56. Leoniceno´s Roman pupil reports the exchange: **Opuscula**, pp. 146v, 147r.
57. A Benedetti, ed., **C Plinii Secundi Veronensis Historiae Naturalis Libri XXXVII**, Venice, 1513. For the anatomy see note 31.
58. Leoniceno defended himself against the critics of his translations of Galen, including Berengario, in his **Contra suos Obtrectatores Apo-**

logia (published in the **Opuscula** and also separately, Venice, 1522). Falloppio considered Berengario to be the man who initiated the anatomical revolution concluded by Vesalius.

59. See note 11.

60. This purpose is seen for example in the prefatory material of the various works of Gesner, William Turner and Edward Wotton.

61. **Anatomice,** p.5r

62. **Opuscula,** p.35r

XII

The Languages of William Harvey's Natural Philosophy

INTRODUCTION

FOR 300 years before William Harvey's time the language of natural philosophy had been Latin. In the schools, it continued to be taught in Latin until it vanished in its Aristotelian form not long after Harvey had died. Outside the schools, the forces that eventually led to the disappearance of Aristotelian natural philosophy also encouraged authors who were composing an alternative to it to write in the vernacular. Galileo is a luminous example. Gassendi's sceptical vernacular critique of Harvey is, in contrast, an example that has lain in the dark for a long time, but an example nevertheless.[1] One need hardly do more than mention Boyle as a third example to make the point.[2]

Harvey's work supplies some hints as to the forces at work in this change. He lived at a time when the change was becoming manifest. Galileo was at work before Harvey published on the heart and blood, and Boyle, a generation younger than Harvey, took Harvey's own work as a contribution to the new philosophy. It was a change then that took

1. S. S. [Gassendi], *Discours Sceptique sur la Passage du Chyle & sur le Mouvement du Coeur,* Leiden: Jean Maire, 1648. The identity of Gassendi as the author is revealed in his story of the demonstration of the septal pores at Aix en Provence; in any case, the identity of the author as Gassendi was known at the time to Riolan. See J. Riolan [the younger], *Notationes in Tractatum clarissimi D D Petri Gassendi . . . de Circulatione Sanguinis,* no date, in eod., *Tractatus de Motu Sanguinis eiusque Circulatione Vera, ex Doctrinae Hippocratis,* Paris, 1652. For the story of Aix, see P. Gassendi (1648) p. 83 and his *Opera Omnia,* 6 vols., Florence, 1727, p. 218.

2. It is true, of course, that Newton published only in Latin and that other scholars such as Glisson used English more than Harvey. The point of this paper is not to make comparisons but to investigate one person's usage. I am grateful to my colleague Dr. Andrew Cunningham for reading through the draft of this paper and making useful comments.

ISSN 0022-5045 VOLUME 49 PAGES 24 TO 51

place partly in Harvey's lifetime, and it is of interest to see that Harvey, although he always published in Latin, yet used a proportion of English in his notes for the Lumleian lectures on anatomy, the lectures on the motion of animals, and those on the muscles. Examination of this use of English shows that Harvey used his native language in certain circumstances only. This in turn illuminates how he thought about his natural philosophy. If we can re-establish how Harvey used his bilinguality, we can perhaps gain some insight into how he used his natural philosophy. There may even be hints that add to our wider picture of how natural philosophy, and the language in which it was expressed, changed in the seventeenth century.

LATIN AND THE VERNACULAR

In English society of Harvey's day, Latin was used at certain times for certain purposes. The language of government in action was English. When the College of Physicians wrote to the king or the Court wrote to the College, they did so in English. The Privy Council also wrote to the College in English. Harvey's marriage licence and his tax assessment were in the vernacular. Permissions to stay in London over the winter were given in English. The language of politics was English: preferments were pursued at Court in English; and if the Attourney General wrote to you, he did so in English.[3]

But Latin remained important, and its use signified where power lay in society. At the lowest level, Latin formulae indicate controlling mechanisms, as when a book in English on surgery carries an *imprimatur* in Latin.[4] Correspondence with the monarch or the Court normally carried a date in Latin and the same date expressed as the year of the current reign, just as the Roman chronologers dated events by the reign of the emperors. As Royal Physician, Harvey signed authorizations in this form for the purchase of drugs. At a higher level, Latin was used more extensively. Enactments of law were dated similarly, and of course formal proclamations, charters, and so on were in Latin. The Court Calendar (noting such things as the appointment of Royal Physicians) was also in Latin. The professions also used Latin. While the surgeons, as tradesmen, kept their records in English, the College of Physicians

3. These details can be found in G. Keynes, *The Life of William Harvey* (Oxford: Clarendon, 1978), esp. chapters 3–5.

4. For example, Richard Wiseman, *Several Chirurgical Treatises*, 2nd ed. (London: R. Norton and J. Macock, 1686), carries what amounts to a licence to print by the president and three censors of the Royal College of Physicians.

kept theirs partly in Latin.[5] The College had good professional reasons to conduct their external business in Latin, for it helped to preserve their monopoly of medical learning and practice. They accordingly examined candidates for membership in Latin, and those who sought a simple surgical licence, in English.[6] Medical prescriptions were always in Latin. Hospitals were places where physicians and surgeons interacted professionally, and Harvey, physician to St. Bartholomew's, wrote out a list of regulations for the surgeons in English, under a Latin date. He would of course have spoken to his patients and the surgeons (like Woodall) in English. The Latin heading and date of the hospital's appointment of Harvey likewise give a formality and authority to an English document. The universities managed almost all their business in Latin. While the Master of Sidney Sussex wrote to Harvey in English (under a Latin date), the Merton College record of Harvey's address to the Fellows is in Latin.[7]

In other words, in Harvey's world the use of Latin was associated with social authority. It was also the international and ancient language of authorial authority, where the *auctor* had *auctoritas*. During the earlier part of the Renaissance, when the place of Aristotle as Philosopher to the Church was threatened by the Hellenists' Plato, and Latin as the language of culture by Greek, there was a reactionary defence of Latin culture. Its apologists called it the *res Latina*, and it often included the traditional school subjects, their commentators, and their source, Aristotle:[8] it was an attempt to reassert authority. During part of his education, Harvey had been a paying guest in a world where one addressed God in Latin and where the church expressed God's will for one in the same language: the ultimate authority.

LATIN AND NATURAL PHILOSOPHY

Harvey had put together his natural philosophy largely in Cambridge and Padua. It was based on Aristotle; and Paduan Aristotelianism has received some distinguished historical attention.[9] But this was not the

5. See for example the quotations from the annals of the College made by Duane H. D. Roller, *The De Magnete of William Gilbert* (Amsterdam: Menno Hertzberger, 1959), p. 80; see also p. 84.

6. Many of these details are to be found in Keynes, (n. 3) *Harvey*; for examinations in Latin and English, see chapter 16.

7. Ibid., pp. 274, 302.

8. See my discussion in "Pliny and renaissance medicine" in R. K. French and F. Greenaway, eds, *Science in the Early Roman Empire* (London, Croom Helm, 1986).

9. For a summary of Paduan scholarship from Randall onward, see C. Schmitt's collected essays, *Studies in Renaissance Philosophy and Science* (London: Variorum Reprints, 1981) and *Reappraisals in Renaissance Thought* (London: Variorum Reprints, 1989). For medicine at Padua see J. Bylebyl, "The school of Padua: humanistic medicine in the sixteenth century," in C. Webster ed., *Health, Medicine and Mortality in the Sixteenth Century* (Cambridge: Cambridge University Press, 1979), pp. 335–70.

dialectical Aristotle, or the Aristotle of the physical works and thus of traditional school natural philosophy. In Padua, where they now preferred to "listen" to Aristotle himself through improved texts and *auscultationes*, they were also reading Aristotle's books on animals. These were the *Historia Animalium* and the *De Partibus Animalium*, as well as the smaller works on the generation and motion of animals. In particular, Harvey's teacher, Fabricius of Aquapendente, was teachng animal anatomy from Aristotle (much to the irritation of his German students, who wanted medical and surgical human anatomy for professional purposes). What Fabricius seems to have realized was that Aristotle's "History of Animals" was a collection of data that was of necessity incomplete (it did not exclude any category of animal and could not therefore say everything about them) and that the "Parts of Animals" was a way of handling that data that provided true causal knowledge of the differences between the "parts," but which was again incomplete because there were always more parts, more correlations, and so more causes. Aristotle says so.

Fabricius[10] and his pupil Harvey thus had a program of *research*. This was new. Universities were places where knowledge was refined or laundered, depending on its source. Generation of new knowledge was not expected. Harvey's program of research led him accidentally to the circulation of the blood, and we can follow some of that discovery in his notes for his anatomy lectures. But we can understand more about his research if we look first at a project that was not upset by an unexpected discovery and which was in any case more circumscribed.

THE LOCAL MOTION OF ANIMALS

This project was the series of lectures on the local motion of animals, which seem related to those on the anatomy of the muscles. This was a research project in the sense intended above. Aristotle had provided a set of philosophical principles about motion in general—their application to the physical world is the topic of the whole cursus of the *libri naturales* and the substance of university natural philosophy—and had indicated how these acted in animals. Yet Aristotle was in ignorance of both nerve and muscle, the very agents of animal motion. Harvey contrived to suggest that Aristotle had not been ignorant in this way,[11] but not even

10. See A. R. Cunningham, "Fabricius and the 'Aristotle project' in anatomical teaching and research in Padua" in *The Medical Renaissance of the Sixteenth Century*, ed. A. Wear, R.K. French and I. Lonie (Cambridge: Cambridge University Press, 1985), pp. 195–222.

11. Historians owe a great debt to Gweneth Whitteridge for the transcriptions and translations of Harvey's works on anatomy. The most important of these for our purposes is *The Anatomical Lectures of William Harvey. Prelectiones Anatomiae Universalis. De Musculis*, ed., with an introduction, transla-

such an Aristotelian as Harvey could deny the greatly superior knowledge of Galen on these topics, to say nothing of his sophisticated experiments. Harvey as a medical man knew his Galen; but he also believed in Aristotelian methods and wished to extend them into an area where Harvey's medical knowledge suggested they might go.

Harvey accordingly begins with Aristotle's physical principles, that is, the kinds of and conditions for motion. These are well known to historians: generation, growth, corruption, alteration, and so on; the Mover and the Moved, Nature as the principle of motion, the *primum mobile.* The motion of animals fits this scheme in that an (unmoved) Good or Evil is the subject of their Appetite and moves the animal to pursuit or avoidance. All things in Nature, says Harvey,[12] believing he is following Aristotle, desire the Good, and the Good for the animal is to seek food and drink, cooling respiration, generation of its kind, and so on.

These are the *causes* of animal motion, and Harvey is writing at a philosophical level about causal knowledge. The physical principles just mentioned are the grand principles of his natural philosophy, and Harvey writes about them in Latin. Certainly he seems to have been writing a formal lecture series, probably for the College of Physicians, for which delivery in Latin might have been expected (but English became frequent for such affairs in Harvey's lifetime). He may possibly have been thinking about ultimate publication, and so had another reason to write in Latin. But, despite this, there is good evidence that Harvey was so familiar with Latin that he essentially thought in Latin. Latin is a much more economical language than English, and thus suitable for notes and concise expression. Harvey presumably took notes from lectures in Cambridge and Padua and for the whole period of his education would have been trained to work in Latin. It was therefore natural that, when writing notes for his own lectures, he should have used Latin for its immediate purposes as well as for its economy of words. *Circumvallent* would have needed an English phrase to translate: there is some pressure to make notes in Latin whatever the destination language. Moreover, his notes to himself (and so not part of the lecture or intended publication) are often in Latin—for

tion and notes by G. Whitteridge (Edinburgh and London: E. and S. Livingstone, 1964). In this paper reference is made to Whitteridge's pagination (henceforth W) and to the foliation of Harvey's mss. This begins anew for *De Musculis* at W 347. Second is W. Harvey, *De Locali Motu Animalium 1627*, ed., trans. and introduced by G. Whitteridge (Cambridge: Cambridge University Press, 1959) (henceforth W (1959). For Aristotle's "knowledge" of the nerves see f.86r W (1959) 64.

12. f.70r W (1959) 14.

example, in the anatomy lectures Harvey wrote a bracketed note for himself to do more work on presentation and decide whether the emulgent veins and other structures can be seen without removing the intestines: *NB NB Quere an emulgentes et vena et arteria magna, item testiculi, manifestari possunt relictis intestinis.* If not, then Harvey reminds himself to insert a discussion of the viscera: *Si non hic inserenda de visceribus. . . .*[13] In another note, he reminds himself (with another NB NB) to discuss the dangers of wounds on the abdomen.[14] Moreover, when he breaks into English, often enough the structure of the sentence, its prepositions, conjunctions, and verb are Latin. Characteristic is his discussion of the purposes and co-ordination of movements: *Motus acquiritur et ab anima et appetitu cooncitatur, ut playing of the lute, dancing, speaking; partim one finger, one foote, one letter, deinde coniungit et tanquam unum imperat et ultro tanquam signo dato.*[15] To illustrate tonic motion of the muscles he has . . . *manere tonico: Δ miluo vento, trowt torrente.*[16] (A better example of the Latin structure of the sentence is where, in the anatomy lectures, he says of the size of the spleen in animals *ut WH semper in a barble et partim in a goose.*[17] Likewise, discussing the relative heat of creatures and the position of the genitalia, *Contra apparent elephant et porpos, hedghogg; hott creatures habent intus.*)[18] So habitual was Latin for an early seventeenth-century natural philosopher that the pertinent question is why Harvey departed from it.

Having set up the principles of motion in philosophical terms, Harvey narrows himself down to the kinds of motion relevant to his topic. He discusses voluntary motion, motion of the parts, mode of progression, and so on. Then he discusses the local source of motion within the animal, the Mover and the Moved, appetite, purpose, and related matters. It is heavily natural-philosophical, and Harvey, quoting the page number of a contemporary edition of Aristotle, uses very little English. He goes on to distinguish different Movers, the different kinds of limb that produce different kinds of motion, and what it is that remains immobile. This is all at the philosophical level. This means he is close to Aristotle and still distant from English, from particulars of observation, and from Galen. Then, nearly half way through the text, he introduces the subject of muscle. He does so with a formal accessus: name, defini-

13. f.21v W 92.
14. f.23r W 98.
15. f.116v, W (1959) 146.
16. ff.86r, 103v; W (1959) 64.
17. f.35r W 132.
18. f.51r W 186.

tion, parts (similar and organic), quantity, position, figure, etc., actions, diseases, and uses. Because this ends with purpose—"uses"—it is as near as the anatomist could get to demonstrative knowledge, and Harvey is still deep in his natural-philosophical exposition. Now too we have Galen and many other medical authorities on the nature and the parts of muscle. The English begins to creep in as Harvey finds images to illustrate this or that characteristic of the parts of muscle. Δ *partridge*[19] illustrates how tendon degenerates into cartilaginous bone. Querying whether the branches of a tendon do go entirely through a muscle (as Fabricius held), Harvey has more images: *WH Δ chorda, a cable, in medio in fila divisa, Δ rush.* He soon comes to the appearance of tendons and uses his native language more readily. Δ *sene, carpenters hands. Yeonge and nimble, oud and strong. Δ bel rope. A cable. . . .* [20]

Harvey does not discuss nerves formally until chapter fifteen. That is, his text to this point has been structured by first principles, largely from Aristotle, then by his discussion of muscles as the agents of motion, partly from Galen, and now has reached the nerves as the controllers of motion and is in Galenic and medical territory. English is used sparingly. It becomes frequent, almost a flood, when Harvey's method of exposition reaches the particular action of the different muscles and particularly how they interact to produce a whole motion. *medium inter agere and making: sedendo, saltando tripudiis, dancing in any part . . . nodding . . . membra movere mollis: tipto dancing. Item motuum diversorum unio. Δ sweteing in payne. Δ spiralis linea vel circularis absque rectis. Shite by degrees not by squirts.*[21] He was particularly taken with the co-ordination of muscles in rhythmic actions, like playing instruments and dancing. Δ *play on the organe, virgenals. Ut idem ab eodem ita instrumento ad instrumentum yt speakes because this key putt down that putt down because of than motion of the finger, arme, ope ex Harmina illorum musculorum.*[22] None of this could be adequately expressed in Latin, and nor could the co-ordinated motions of muscles by which purposeful actions were achieved in civil and military life. The *masons, briclayers carpenters* were like those with different tasks in the army, *hors, foote shel pichers, pioners, worke marshal, defenders, assault, secundum rithmum et unionem quando cum quibus* and those on stage: *Chorus, musicians, base, treble; sum sing, sum dance, sum act.*

19. f.89r W (1959) 76.
20. ff.91v, 92r W (1959) 82.
21. f.113v W(1959) 142.
22. f.115v W (1959) 14.

This disposition of the vernacular is quite general throughout Harvey's notes. It is entirely consistent with his view of natural philosophy. The first principles of nature are those given by Aristotle and which Harvey satisfied himself gave the best explanation of natural things. They were taught and expressed in a language that boys like Harvey had learned from their earliest education and which was the language of all teaching from the age of, at the latest, fourteen. The Latin of natural philosophy bristled with technical terms, the resonances of which were the intellectual world and authority within it. Harvey never doubted that Aristotle's apparatus of forms, matter, substance, causes, and so on gave a powerful explanation of the first principles of the natural world, nature's *archai*. But Aristotle's undertaking in the animal books was, as Harvey learned in Padua, incomplete. Aristotle could not have encountered and described all animals. Harvey may have realized that the fauna and flora of Aristotle's Greece (and perhaps also Alexander the Great's India) were different from that of Kent and Cambridgeshire, where Harvey had been educated. Certainly Harvey's own knowledge of animals was unusually extensive and included many that Aristotle and the Latin writers did not mention, at least to Harvey's knowledge. His very common mentioning of animals in the vernacular represents two things. First, it is an extension of the Aristotelian program of listing differences to kinds of animals that Aristotle had not described. Second, it is a listing of *particulars* that serve to exemplify the general, or *universal*, principles announced by Aristotle.

So in both cases Harvey is extending the formal and Latin principles of a program of natural philosophy into a range of vernacular particulars of observation that exemplify them. In addition, he is adding to his own interpretation of a broadly Aristotelian undertaking. Harvey gave great importance to knowledge gained directly by the senses. This may have been because he could give no formal, causal, and demonstrative proof of the circulation of the blood and instead emphasized his experimental results. It may be, as he later claimed,[23] that a universal could be generated directly from sensation. For whatever reason, it is clear that he saw the power of a graphic and vernacular image, example, or analogy in giving strength to those examples he listed in the vernacular and which illustrate the general principles of his natural philosophy. Where the *validity* of his natural philosophy rested in the authority of Aristotle and the tradition of the Latin language in which he was presented in the schools, yet the

23. See the introduction to *De Generatione Animalium*.

immediacy of the sensory image, the particular, that both illustrated the first principles of natural philosophy and—Harvey came to argue—provided a kind of universal knowledge itself, resided in the power of the vernacular.

An important point in relation to this, and one which can be seen most clearly in the lectures on muscles, is that Harvey used four signs in connection with the observed particulars. Where he used the sign X, it meant that he disagreed with what was said in this or that author, and often enough Harvey gives his own opinion in preference. Wherever he does this he marks it with his monogram WH, and this seems always to indicate personal, autopsical, observation of particulars. He also used NB and a small triangle, Δ, to draw attention to particular points that are not necessarily original to him.[24] These are his personal Determinations[25] of a disputed question or possibly sometimes a novelty without precedent. Elsewhere too, these signs are designate words containing a higher proportion of English than the rest of the text (but of course very often introduce Latin only). They represent, then, the experiential knowledge of particulars that are the basis and the examples of Harvey's personal vision of natural philosophy. They—and particularly those marked by the WH sign—are the vernacular that supplies and illustrates his Latin first principles.

The same pattern of exposition is followed in the subsequent chapters of the discussion of animal motion. Harvey usually begins with a statement of a general principle of motion, perhaps quoting the *Physics* or *De Motu Animalium*, and ultimately reaches observations that illustrate it. Where the "principles" of natural motion are closer to the categories of observation than to fundamental physics, as was the case with the differences between flight, swimming, and walking, Harvey fairly rapidly reaches the point where his own experience in the vernacular is appropriate: *motu tonico Mr Barsons busard on a fowle* is an example of "tonic motion" in the claws.

In contrast, in the following chapter, the fourth, Harvey returns to the principles of mover, moved, and nature as the source of motion, and quotes Aristotle's *Physics* and the *De Motu Animalium*, giving the page numbers of a contemporary edition. The object is to explain the important Aristotelian categories of appetition, the pursuit of Good, and the

24. The triangle may mean "demonstration": Whitteridge, (n. 11) *Anatomical Lectures*, p. xxii.

25. A "determination" was the act by which a master concluded a disputation between students, and so decided upon the truth at stake.

fulfilment of Purpose, and the vernacular is unnecessary. Likewise, in chapter five Harvey is explaining the important categories of "movers", the form, the soul, and nature. With a trivial exception, the vernacular is not needed.

To summarize to this point, it seems to be general that Harvey expressed the principles of his natural philosophy in Latin and the particulars from which it was built and the examples that illustrated it, often in English. It was partly because they gave an immediacy that was in line with his sensualist epistemology, and partly because he was addressing an English audience and wished to convince them. It is also general that when dealing with technical aspects of anatomy he used only Latin, because it was a subject that had a vast Latin literature with a fully developed vocabulary where English had scarcely any of either. Anatomy rested firmly on natural philosophy (which is almost the same as saying on theoretical medicine), and it was expressed best in Latin.

THE ANATOMY OF THE MUSCLES

The lectures on the muscles are in some senses a special case in Harvey's writing. They present a uniform category within anatomy as a whole, and Harvey could adopt a uniform mode of presentation. There are few basic philosophical principles, and an important function of Harvey's treatment is to list all the muscles in the body, giving their "philosophical" and medical Latin name followed shortly by their vernacular names—certainly the biggest category of English words. Perhaps this is intended in some way for surgeons, but on the whole the lectures on muscles seem to contain less English than those "on the whole of anatomy" (which contain just over eight per cent English). Characteristically, Harvey first gives the Latin name of the muscle, then a reason for its name, the vernacular equivalent as his personal contribution, its anatomical relations, and then perhaps an illustrative vernacular phrase. *SERRATUS MAJOR latus carneus. WH great jagged muscle. Oritur: scapulae basis interiori, carnosus. WH Δ shoulder of mutton* is typical.[26]

In discussing muscles and their tendons and the bones they act on, Harvey naturally uses mechanical analogies that would have provided powerful images for his contemporaries. *WH a straw cable . . . WH a cable of threedes . . .* (*ut WH a cable ex filis*) are used to illustrate what is meant

26. f. 2v W 348. Compare 8v W 370: *ROTUNDUS, pestle muscle, the first cut of a showlder of mutton; carnosus crassus teres* and 9v, W 372 *SUBSCAPULARIS IMMERSUS the inward plate muscle that is cut crosswise in the rosting.*

by "tendon."[27] Here too Harvey has drawn little diagrams of mechanical things, presumably for reproduction at the lecture, illustrating the insertion of tendons into bones: *Unde insertio fibrarum altior et altior. WH can hardier stay. Δ tressels, too narrow; pedestal of a pillar. Unde natura docet usual angle.*[28] He makes comparisons between the strength and the nature of the part: *omnino propter robur aequipollet eius magnitudine crassitities. WH a little iron barr to a great peece of timber.*[29]

THE USE OF ENGLISH

Within the general scheme of things outlined above, there seems to be a number of conditions that govern Harvey's use of English. They are best seen perhaps in the notes for the Lumleian anatomy lectures, where Harvey ranges over a richer field than in the anatomy of muscles and the local motion of animals.

(i) He sometimes seems to engage in a *technical* vernacular. We may suppose that the details of medical and surgical practice were handled in a professional language. In St. Bartholomew's Hospital and when talking to or lecturing to surgeons, Harvey must have used English. The Lumleian lectures were originally intended to be partly in English for the benefit of surgeons. Things seemed to have changed by Harvey's time, and there is not much evidence from the notes for the anatomy lectures that Harvey was devoting a quarter of the hour's lecture to English, as originally envisaged. But, when he routinely gives an English equivalent of the Latin when describing every muscle in the relevant notes, he perhaps had an audience in mind that was partly more comfortable in English.

Perhaps *absunpta mucca per tres dies ante generatur sickish windiness* includes a phrase of medical vernacular, and certainly *Item hernia carnosa ex sarcosi, a fungous flesh or parenchyma, vulgo carnosity* indicates a conscious reference to a technical English.[30] Harvey also used *prowde flesh* as a technical term, either to emphasize the normal differences between bone, flesh, and cartilage, or to illustrate the light texture of the lungs, but most perhaps in connection with the pathological fungous flesh just mentioned: [Of the spermatic duct] *Aliquando spongiosoa, prowd flesh, swell, ut sequatur ischuria. It is easyly felt and as easyly inflamed; be tender and seare by using*

27. f.20r W 389.
28. f.21v W 400.
29. f.44v W 448.
30. f.28v, W 53v; f.28v W 114; f.53r W 194.

searing candle and streyning bleed of every little touch. Hinc the terrible dissease caruncula but many decipiuntur hac quae naturalis yett somtime swell as Sir Thomas Hardy.[31] So here Harvey has been tempted into English by a technical vernacular of pathological states and surgical procedures. Certainly the latter would not have encouraged expression in a natural-philosophical language.

More examples can be found in the discussion of the local motion of animals, where Harvey has reached, on his formal rote of observables, the diseases muscles are heir to. This is naturally less philosophical, more medical, and more observational. The English expresses the technical Latin and provides a vehicle for personal observation.

1. Resolutio, ded palsey
2. Tremor, shaking palsy
3. Convulsio, epilepticis, histericis pueris; strabismo occulo; risus sardonicus, [Harvey's] unkle Will. Halte dying.
5. Cramp, flatulenta convulsio, Δ planta pedis . . .
6. Twinges, palpitatio, convulsio a twitches cum levi dolore et punctione vel cum nullo, Δ WH potius Mr. Rants ey.
7. Pulsus palpitatio . . . mise creeping, flittering flees a stupore.
10. Crick cum tentat movere . . . differt a cramp.[32]

Harvey seems to have found a particular difficulty in choosing a Latin equivalent for "cramp." We see here his concern with cramp in the sole of the foot, and how it differs from "crick." He wondered too about what caused it. *NB WH the crampe et pedis. WH the cramp nullibi ubi non sit tendo. An quia vicinus nervus comprimitur? unde in the neck complex.* And *Vide ductum nervi quarti ante. Ubi tiptoe inseritur, decussatim tendine huius. WH an ista decussatio the cramp?*[33] *An . . . crampe, a flatu.*[34] Cramp was often regarded as a kind of gout, and Harvey may here have in mind a very personal and painful particular of sense observation, for he suffered from gout.[35] In trying to find the Latin name for it, he was faced with the same problem as that faced by historians of medicine in trying to identify ancient diseases. Harvey was bound to use the vernacular.

(ii) He cites a number of animals that do not appear in Aristotle.[36] In

31. f.57r W 142; prowde fleshe: f.38r W 202, f.81v W 278.

32. ff.105r-v W (1959) 124. For the case of Mr Rant's eyelid, see also f.97v and 95v W (1959) 102: it seems to have had a constant tremulous motion.

33. ff.57v, 58r-v: W 474, 476.

34. f.97v W (1959) 100.

35. See Keynes, (n. 3) *Harvey*, p. 435 for Aubrey's story of how Harvey alleviated his gout by cold.

36. On Harvey's use of animals, see F. J. Cole, "Harvey's animals," *J.Hist.Med.Allied Sci.*, 1957, *12* 106–13, and Whitteridge's introduction to the anatomy lectures.

using the vernacular names for these, Harvey is not only extending the range of particulars on which his Aristotelian method is being exercised, but is vernacularizing the natural philosophy involved for his audience. Commenting on a dictum of Aristotle that small-bodied animals have loose bowels, Harvey adds a non-Aristotelian particular about their motion: *Vero diutius non stare; waddle like a puffin.*[37] Discussing animals with mobile skin, Harvey adds animals not in his Aristotelian sources: *Qibusdam motu voluntario, porcupin, hedghog, turkey, coctoo, ruff bird in the ballad.*[38] It is very unlikely that the yellowhammer, lapwing, hedge-sparrow, and the various game birds that Harvey mentions[39] could have been identified with any certainty in Aristotle's texts. In fact, Harvey seems often to have thought about his animals, even when there existed a good Latin equivalent term for them, in English. Where the particulars rather than the principles of his "Aristotle project" were concerned, a major part of it was a vernacular affair. He uses *weesel, powlcatt, catt,* and *stote* as if there were no Latin equivalents.[40] It would have been difficult too to identify confidently in the text of Aristotle the fish so familiar to Harvey: the *plays, soals, hering, whiting, redfish, mopp, roch, flownders, barble, mackerel, sea hors, smelt.*[41] Harvey's *ratt* and *mows* constitutes a "distinction"[42] of the classical *mus*, which covered both kinds of animal. When Harvey is discussing the attachment of the limbs to the thorax in different animals (*aliis prominens ut pedes sint coniunctiores ut geyhownd*), he is very close to a locus in Aristotle, but is giving as an example a breed of dog unknown to Aristotle. In contrast (and in the same place), when he is discussing broad *kinds* of animals, Harvey often uses the Latin as representing a more philosophical category or genus. Thus here he says that birds in general have deep chests: *Avibus carinatum as the shippe keele, tanquam pes to sitt on decumbere . . .* [43] Likewise "man" in general for Harvey is a category of obvious natural-philosophical and anatomical importance,

37. f.7v W 28.

38. f.11v W 44. Harvey continues with the effect of lack of sleep on the skin of the human face. *Hominibus: vigiliis, manè lord how you look! as gamesters; sick leane dog; begger sick, eriguntur pili horridi.*

39. *avibus partridg, quailes fesant* f.51v W 188: note again that "birds" as a *genus* are in the philosophical Latin. *woodcock,* f.34r W 130 (also *vide sparrow hawk, milvis, owle, columbis, goos, duck*). Note also f.26v W 108 and f.13r W 52.

40. f.23r W 98; f.26r W104; f.f.34v W 132; f.38r W 144; f.81r W 274.

41. f.23r W 98; f.26v W 108; ff.31r–v W 120; f.34v W 130; f.38r W 142; f.60r W 212; f.73r W 250.

42. Harvey's was a dialectical *distinctio* that drew out different meanings of the same term. The technique was of the essence in the school disputation and aimed to show that the defendant's meaning of the term was inconsistent with his conclusion. For Harvey's rats and mice see f.17v W 74; f.20r W 86; f.29 (following W's numeration) W 116.

43. f.61r–v W 214 greyhownd also 234.

and Harvey uses *homo*, not the vernacular. This distinction between the particular and the general is seen for example in his discussion of the position of the genital organs: *ibi testiculi minus fixi, homine, hares, ratts; ubi contra minori natibus appensi, boare, vel intus ut avibus, mulieribus.* And *modo foras modo intus, ratts, hare. Intus ad renes, aves, embrione cervi; ad lumbos ginney coney; grampos and a porpos intra abdomen . . .* [44] The philosophical importance of *homo* was that man was the measure of all things, the text, while all else was a commentary. Harvey does not mean that animals were of interest only inasfar as they illustrated man, which was the position of Galen and the doctors, for Harvey's Aristotle project gave importance to knowledge of animals themselves. Rather, Harvey had in mind that man was the best known philosophically: like other anatomists Harvey was claiming that anatomy had a philosophical before a medical purpose.[45] *Homo* thus subsumes *mulier* and both fit into the philosophical apparatus more readily than *man*.

Harvey was celebrated in his lifetime for this knowledge of animals. Even those who disagreed with him acknowledged his reputation in this respect.[46] One of his favorite animals was the rat, which was no doubt readily available in early seventeenth-century London. He on several occasions mentions his dissection of a rat that had died as a result of swallowing glass, where he found inflamed scratches in its intestines: *WH ratt poysoned vitro, long scratches inflamed.*[47] Of the organs of generation, Harvey says *Of all creatures ratts have these parts most playnly delineated and curiously made, unde puto tam potentes generatione. Unde non orire putredine ut vulgo, quia Natura nil facit frustra, praecipue tam eleganter.*[48] Clearly his English serves to express his sensory observations, and in an animal ambiguously named in the ancient literature and so identifiable only in the vernacular. His Latin takes up the philosophical question of purpose of the organs (for "generation") and the disputed question of whether

44. f.50v–51r W 186.

45. f.81v W (1959) 50: *homo enim the text, the other the comment.* It was standard among the anatomists to give a religious and philosophical purpose for anatomy above a medical purpose. An exception, perhaps because he did not have time to write a full introduction (his book was published posthumously) was R. Colombo, *De Re Anatomica* (Venice: Nicholas Beuilacqua, 1559).

46. One of Harvey's first opponents was James Primrose, who disagreed with Harvey's use of animals, but saw that others were impressed. See his *Exercitationes, at Animadversiones in librum, De Motu Cordis, et Circulatione Sanguinis adversus Guilielmum Harveium Medicum Reqium, et Anatomes in Collegio Londinensi Professorem* (London: G. Jones, 1630) p.54.

47. f.30r W 116. Compare *Ulceratus, long scratches quale in a rat vitro*, f.56v W 202. Harvey also used the rat in investigating the brain and nerves: ff.93 v, 95v W 324, 334.

48. f.53r W 192 Harvey also expresses facts of observation in other English remarks here: *In a ratt like infinit little guts and Figure in a ratt ut intestina convoluta.* 53v.

rats are generated from putrefaction. Even though it was *vulgo*, commonly, (and therefore not philosophically) thought that rats were indeed the product of putrefaction, it was a question often discussed in the Latin literature, and Harvey keeps to his philosophical language, especially as his argument involves the fundamental philosophical principle that Nature does nothing in vain.

Sometimes Harvey uses Latin and English names interchangeably, like *goose* and *anser,*[49] or *hors* and *equus*, even when the Latin occurs in a sentence otherwise largely English. It is of course always the vernacular when Harvey has non-classical breeds and uses of horse, like *tracehors, coach hors* and *carthors.*[50] Discussing disorders of the gut, Harvey has an unusual concentration of English: *Humida* [*sc.* guts] *relaxantur, wett parchment or lether, flatulent; exemplo cattle going to grass, equo loose belly fundament swabby gutts croake and wallop. Aliquibus magis frigida quam humida tardas digestiones quia obstructa muccae copia et sensus defectus. Omnes isti ut equi faynt and without spirit.*[51] Here again is a series of images and sounds of animals that Harvey can evoke for his audience more forcibly than by the use of Latin.

In one case Harvey discusses an animal only recently known in his culture and therefore without a Latin name. It is the *ginneyconey*, apparently our "guineapig"[52] but for him in the same way a "kind" of rabbit, *coney.*

(iii) There are many cases where the vernacular simply carries more weight than a Latin alternative. This may be because the Latin equivalent (as in the case of animals) was unknown; or because the vernacular was so much better known and awakened personal memories in the audience that the Latin could never supply. Harvey's audience knew exactly what he meant when he talked about pudding and gravy, and bread and cheese;[53] any Latin equivalent was purely verbal. Harvey talked about pudding in an entirely typical way. His subject is "fat" *pinguedo*, a major subheading in the part of the anatomy lectures that deals with the "similar" parts of the body. The similar parts were those defined by Aristotle as homogeneous, incapable of being resolved into parts by division.

49. f. 11v W 44; f. 19v W 84; f. 30v W 118; f. 34r W 130.
50. f. 109r W (1959) 132.
51. f. 29r W 114.
52. Whitteridge, (n. 11) *Anatomical Lectures*, p.lxii.
53. *A man hold utrinque oute bread and cheese* (to illustrate the actions of the muscles of the arms) f. 22r W 402.

They were of major importance in philosophical and synthetic[54] presentations of anatomy, and Harvey divides up his treatment in a formal *accessus* of *situs, quantitas, sunstantia et passiones, generatio, problemata*. Having thus set up the matter philosophically and having discussed Nature's purposes for fat, Harvey can descend to particulars and discuss the appearance of fat in different animals. When he says *Unde yeong goose etc, like a pudding, unde ould geese dripp awaye,*[55] he is supplying a vivid and homely image of cooking unlikely to be matched in the Latin authors. The kinds of fat were discussed among the anatomists, and a large number of classical words were found to carry refinements of the basic term.[56] But Harvey's vernacular supplies more, some of which the ancient world did not know, like *cake sope*. Nor would it be easy to find classical terms with the immediacy of *tallow, gravey* or even *pasti italici*.[57] The anatomists also disputed about the origin of fat (was it caused by heat or cold?), and, as it is a philosophical problem, Harvey uses Latin. But there is room again for English for the particulars of observation of the animals and men who lose fat through excessive venery—*ut omnia animalia, crest fallen, pin buttockt*.[58]

Many of the basic Saxon words of Harvey's vernacular must have carried an impact that was not carried by the Latin equivalents. Indeed, Latin as a philosophical language came to be preferred for its power to provide *euphemisms* to hide the impact of such words; and we generally now use Latin-based words to mean exactly what Harvey meant by his direct English. *Homines . . . quando multum potant urina; drunk to bed, piss free* illustrates the action of the kidneys.[59] Thus Harvey uses *urina* in a medical context and the vernacular for matters of observation; thus also (for the composition of urine) *Eadem materia sive omnibus est urina enim ut lixivium; coperas or alome aqua heat and putt into a vessell will candy unde omnibus urinis eiiciunt such a gravelly fur and crust; all pissing corners yeallow.*[60] (Note that chemical operations also invite English.) *Ut hens ars* explains

54. A synthetic presentation of anatomy, usually employed in teaching, especially in the absence of a body, was to begin with the "similar" (homogeneous) parts of the body and "put them together" to explain the constitution of the organic parts and finally the whole body. One could begin with the bones, as Vesalius did, and thus have another rationale of presentation in addition.

55. f. 13r W 52.

56. See for example Jacopo Berengario da Carpi, *Commentaria cum amplissimis Additionibus super Anatomia Mundini* (Bologna: Hieronymus de Benedictis, 1521), f. 53v.

57. f. 13v W 54.

58. f. 14r W 58.

59. f. 43v W 160.

60. f. 54v W 196.

the action of sphincters.[61] When Harvey bluntly told Aubrey that the new philosophers were *shitt-breeches*,[62] he may have been using the language of the tap-room in a man-to-man conversation about the neoterics who in Harvey's view were anything but philosophical, but it was not a language that was excluded from formal lectures: *shite by degrees.*[63]

Occasionally Harvey uses English measures. While the medical drachms and scruples would have been expressed in Latin, larger measures naturally called for English, particularly when the result of observation. Harvey had observed, presumably in St. Bartholomew's, a patient who generated a large amount of pus. *Apostema ingens per multos menses ex pure foetidissimo, two or three gallons, et aqua cum viscosis panniculis convolutis, as glew stepened in water or isonglass; regressus hospitali.*[64] Note again that the analogy that illuminates the sensory observation is also in the vernacular. It would have been difficult to find a classical term for glue or isinglass.

A subcategory here is English idiom and proverbs, which clearly carried greater impact than a Latin equivalent. Discussing the order of nobility of the organs and their consequent position, Harvey says *quia inferiores ordinis iecori locum cedunt; quia ut macrocosmo the weakest to the wall.* The physiognomical observation that those with thick necks are *hedstrong* is also an English commonplace. Is *To steal Jupiters fulmen*[65] an English or Latin proverb? Sometimes Harvey puts brackets round his English phrases: (*unde stumble att a straw and lep over the block*) is part of this treatment and looks like another proverb (he is explaining the actions of muscles).[66]

To bracket off the vernacular in this fashion is akin to the device of using *Anglice*[67] or (with other authors) *Gallice* to indicate to readers that a break in the continuity of the Latin was about to occur. Harvey sometimes uses *vulgo* for the same purpose. But he uses it too to introduce vulgar notions, commonly held by the mass of uneducated people and necessarily not philosophical. When he says *unde gobbi animosi audaces praesertim loquela quia vulgo ther hart nerer the tong*, he is explaining that the common opinion is that dwarves are spirited in their speech because their hearts (traditionally conceived as the center of emotion and expression)

61. f.27r W 108.
62. Keynes, (n. 3) *Harvey*, p. 434.
63. f.113v W (1959) 142.
64. f.39v W 148.
65. f.106v W (1959) 126.
66. f.22r W 94; 64r W 222; 50v W 460.
67. Harvey has *reynes anglice, licet renes altiores.* f.9r W 34.

are nearer their tongues. But Harvey the medical man and philosopher cannot admit such a vulgar notion and at once gives the correct, philosophical cause in Latin and its result in English: *Sed WH a maiore copia caloris more bowld and prompt.*[68]

The vernacular also carries more weight on a number of occasions when Harvey is explicitly using examples, that is, particulars of observation that support some general principle. The control of the motion of food through the gut is illustrated by *Exemplo: lead bullet, drink standing hed, rise a medice colice incassum.*[69] On the other hand, *exemplo: cutting on the finger*[70] seems to refer to a surgical technique of cutting for the stone of the bladder, and so has an additional reason for the vernacular.

(iv) The process complementary to awakening images in the minds of his audience is Harvey's use of his *own* personal recollections to give the audience a share in the immediacy of his vernacular. His audience would have felt the force of the story of the boy on Holborn bridge—he had a beard on one side of his face only—even if they had not seen him themselves. There was no point at all in telling the story in Latin. The *man behind Covent Garden,* [with a rupture] *bigger than his belly* is a story in English for the same reasons. Perhaps the boy was a beggar, displaying a peculiarity for professional reasons. Likewise *Nan Gunter etc* seems to refer to a well known spectacle of a woman able to stick pins into herself without pain (Harvey thought she had made her skin thick). Was she the same as *The mad woman pins in her arme?*[71] Harvey probably expected that his audience would be familiar with these spectacles and certainly with the London landmarks. Perhaps they knew the *bird att St James* that seemed to have a skin disease; they would certainly take Harvey's point that the intestine was a single channel with different names along the route, like *From Powles to Leden hale one way but many names as Cheape, Powtry etc.*[72]

Harvey also often uses English for his reports on his patients and here too is presenting personal recollections with added force. Many of them are well-connected or noble. Harvey is practicing a form of validation by "jury" practiced by anatomists and doctors since Galen, and its impact—that he has proved himself to or (in Harvey's case mostly) upon

68. f.62r W 216.
69. f.20r W 86.
70. f.20v W 88.
71. f.11v W 46.
72. f.12r W 48 and f.20v W 88. As Whitteridge observes, the second of these may have been a recognized device: Vesalius treats the streets of Paris in the same way.

notable witnesses—depends on the audience's knowledge of the society in which these things counted. Latin would have been wrong. *Sir Will Rigdon all yellow* may have been related to Harvey and may have been dissected by him after death.[73] Probably too *FEL . . . inflammatum . . . Sir James Crosby* also came under Harvey's knife.[74] Lord Chichester (a peculiarity of the bladder), Sir Thomas Hardy, Lord Clark, Lord Carey, Sir Robert Sherly, and Lady Hervey (all with some sexual peculiarity) all may have been explored *post mortem* by Harvey.[75] Harvey saw the value of such stories: *yett these storeys are cited but they are rare, yet sufficient to testefy.* Here he has given a number of them on the topic of suffocation, some of them from the ancient world and some from a recent anatomist, all in Latin. Harvey's own story is about how the chest can still be in motion and suffocation occur through poisoned air. [The motion of] *pulmonum si naturalis primo pulmones torpent vel concidunt, chincough, aura venenata, licet agitatum pectus non sequuntur ut by the opening of a fitt choked, ut corn heapes in Apulgia, et diing crye Oh! my breath is gone! agitando pectus ex industria Δ WH; Δ Mistress Fisher.*[76] Likewise, *WH scoller of Cambridge* is a personal story from Harvey about a case of suffocation from fumes from a fire, sandwiched between similar stories from antiquity in Latin.[77]

(v) A major category of Harvey's use of English is where the Latin was quite incapable of supplying what he intended. Again, because he was addressing an English audience, powerful images drawn from seventeenth-century English society could neither be foregone nor Latinized. He uses the images of bear-baiting, cockfighting, and acrobats, *tumblers*, to illustrate the action of the muscles.[78] These belonged to seventeenth-century society as much as the ruff, which provided an analogy for a portion of the intestines and the mesentery,[79] leaden bullets (which manage to pass through the intestines),[80]girls who lace their waists too tightly and disturb the guts, the compass,[81] and the printing press.[82] Nothing could be less classical than the instrument to which Harvey compares the stomach, the bagpipes.[83] Nothing could be more English than *spring or*

73. Lady Croft is mentioned by Harvey in the same place: f. 19r W 82.
74. f. 21r W 90.
75. f. 54v W 196; f. 57r W 202; f. 59r W 208; f. 60r W 212; f. 63v W 220.
76. f. 84v W 288.
77. f. 85v W 292.
78. f. 14v W 62.
79. W 84, 88. See also f. 8r W 370 (the muscles) for the damage done by ruff-supports, *pickedilles*.
80. f. 20r W 86; f. 26v W 106.
81. f. 113v W (1959) 140.
82. W 72, W 86.
83. f. 32r W 122.

summer overclowded nothing ripens.[84] *Item dog by the fier*[85] is an English rather than classical image, entirely appropriate for an overclouded spring. Witches too were part of seventeenth-century life, and Harvey was called on to examine some for witches' marks.[86] When he says, in commenting on the grateful warmth of animals, *Unde catus vetuli, David puella; unde catt a witch quia petit to yeong people,*[87] he has slipped from his normal Latin and turned *catus* into *catt* because his mind has moved from a classical language and a biblical story to his own world in which cats were witches' familiars. Strings of the lute, an instrument well known in the seventeenth century, provide Harvey with analogies for parts of the body, and he used garters to indicate an anatomical location;[88] neither could be expressed adequately in Latin.

Another part of seventeenth-century life that lacked a classical vocabulary was technology. In explaining how some parts of the genital organs serve to keep others separate, Harvey can use *ut instar textricium ponderum* for "weavers' weights" because the ancients had such things. But Harvey refers also to the production of articles of silk and bone lace in which, as in ropemaking, the threads have to be kept apart lest, in Harvey's elegant term, they *intertangle.*[89] Silk was not used in ancient Greece or Rome, and we may suppose that the images of devices used for making silk, lace, and ropes that Harvey is invoking could not be matched in Latin. To take another example, it is well known that an important part of seventeenth-century technology was the water-pump; although ancient pumps had valves, Harvey more naturally turns to those of his own times when adding to the original notes a brief later announcement explaining how the circulating blood crosses the heart. *WH constat per fabricam cordis sanguis per pulmones in aortam perpetuo transferi as by two clackes of a water bellows to rays water.*[90]

When Harvey added this, he had perhaps already completed the manuscript of *De Motu Cordis.*[91] At all events, he had long since made the discovery of the circulation and had promoted it and defended it in a formal—Latin—way. The vernacular addition looks like a rider to the

84. f.502 W 184.
85. f.27r W 110.
86. Keynes, (n. 3) *Harvey*, p. 206.
87. f.30r W 116.
88. f.21v W 400; f.44r W 446; f.47r W 452.
89. f.50v W 186: Δ *ut instar textricium ponderum evenly to stretch lest longi meatus intertangle,* Δ *making ropes, twining of silk, making bone lace, without that they would run together and intertangle.* Cf f.20v W 88 (of the function of the mesentery) *Quia intertangle, quia fall downe on a heap.*
90. f.80v W 272.
91. Whitteridge dates it to about 1627: see (n. 11) *Anatomical Lectures*, note b, p. 272.

formal Latin argument, intended to catch the audience's attention with a striking image. The formal Latin argument was a good strategy for Harvey in the published work. It was a language that was understood across the whole of Europe, and, in choosing to have his book printed in Frankfurt, Harvey was making sure that it was available for the Book Fair. Harvey was probably more concerned with reaching a wide audience than with any financial reward of selling lots of copies, but he not only had to reach a wide audience, but to convince them. Here Latin had its advantages. It was the language of philosophy, of demonstration, of rhetoric, and of proof. Harvey uses it for all these. It was the language of the medical experiment, a central part of Harvey's natural philosophy and derived from an anatomical tradition going back through Fabricius, Colombo, and Vesalius to Galen (whom the medical men read in Latin translations).

The same strategy was also good for Harvey's first discovery, that of the forceful systole, which was announced, promoted, and defended in the anatomy lectures themselves with an extended Latin argument. Having done so, he illustrated it by the image of inflating a glove: if not technological, this image is at least more appropriate for Harvey's time than for the ancient world, and Harvey accordingly uses English. [Of the heart] *Actio: thus relaxed receyves blood, contracted scuppes it over. Universum corpus arteriae respondet as my breth in a glove.*[92]

Two points arise from Harvey's use of English here. First, the advantage of the vernacular was that Harvey did not have to struggle with an entirely inappropriate vocabulary in which terms had connotations that themselves argued against Harvey's case. *Systole*, from the Greek, meant "contraction," but, for Galen and most doctors of the seventeenth century, it was a *passive* contraction. To argue for an active systole in Latin, would have looked like a contradiction in terms. Correspondingly, *diastole* was conventionally an active expansion and only to Harvey the passive result of blood flowing into the heart, and Harvey's use of the Latinized Greek would have been equally confusing. This is why, when he used Latin when he came to write *De Motu Cordis*, he had to spend some time explaining the terminology of the matter, and how he differed from Colombo and from the common opinion.

The second point about Harvey's use of English here is that these advantages of the vernacular come only when Harvey wanted a striking

92. f.79v W 272.

image to round off an extended Latin argument, a rider like the interpolated *two clackes of a water bellows.*[93] If Harvey's argument was to be serious, it had to be a Latin argument. Occasionally, as when Harvey reports on the experiment of removing the heart of animals, the experiment is given in Latin, the observed particulars of the result in English. *Exempto corde frogg scipps, eele crawle, dogg ambulat.*[94] The same division of labor in languages is apparent in Harvey's other report of this experiment in the lectures on the local motion of animals: *NB tamen WH a frogg Δ exempto corde movetur, vulnerato cerebro immobilis. An ex spiritibus remanentibus ut anguilla vita.*[95] While the experimental animal as an object of sensory experience is *frogg*, "frogs" as *kinds* of animals in a philosophical context are *rania.*

Perhaps the vernacular in Δ *a cockes hed off ligatis arteriis et respiratione dato loco, motus perseverant. . . .*[96] is because the cock is an individual animal, an observed particular, and not a philosophical category; but here *hed off* is exactly equivalent to *ligatis arteriis* as an experimental procedure without any indication of why Harvey should have chosen English. Much more often than this, indeed, the whole of the experimental protocol is in Latin. When presenting the forceful systole, the major discovery of the anatomy lectures, Harvey writes in Latin from the moment he addresses the question of the motion of the heart. He describes how he watched and felt the heart as it pulsated. He pierced the heart and pulmonary artery to observe when blood was ejected. He cut the heart into pieces and saw a continued motion and felt the dying pulsations in the auricles of the bird an hour after the animal died. He discusses the experiments of Colombo and Vesalius. He announces his resultant new discovery, the forceful systole (it is combined with the transit of blood across the lungs). On average, in the number of words used in all this, we would have expected some scattered English phrases or sentences adding up to about a small paragraph. But, apart from three uses of the breath-in-glove image and a reference to the lungs of a woodcock, there are none. The argument is firmly within the language of the rationalist, medical, and experimental tradition. We do not meet English for about twenty pages until Harvey adds the rider we have met to the conclusion of the argument.

In addition to technology, chemistry was another field where Harvey

93. At f.62v W 216 Harvey uses the image of the bellows to explain how air is drawn into the lungs in respiration. Again the term *clack* has no Latin equivalent.

94. f.73v W 252. Cf. ff.73v, 100v W (1959) 28 and 111.

95. f.100v W (1959) 110.

96. f.98r W (1959) 104.

used English because of the absence of appropriate Latin terms. We have already seen one example of this. When Harvey says *unde Natura divers offices et diversa instrumenta, velut chemistria in elixum divers heates, vessels, furnaces to draw away the phlemge, rayse the spirit, extract oyle, fermentate and prepare, circulate and perfect,* he is using English because chemistry was a recent branch of knowledge and had no ancient vocabulary. Harvey was perhaps unwilling to use the chemists' Latin neologisms and certainly would not have admitted their principles into his own Latin natural philosophy: for him chemistry was not philosophical and could not be expressed in philosophical language.[97]

A big subgroup in this fifth section is where Harvey uses English *analogies* to expand, illustrate, and explain what the Latin means. The principle is again the same, that the intellectul *structure*, of the natural philosophy as of the sentence, is Latin, and that of the illustrative particulars is in the vernacular and, based on English seventeenth-century life, more emphatic in meaning. When Harvey uses the analogy of *foot-ball; decumbit dormiat dextro; turn on the toe, lepp, hop,*[98] he is extending the meaning of the Latin into the vernacular particulars. The English analogies are often introduced by a Latin rather than an English conjunction: *ut a lute string* he says of the vas deferens; *WH ut cotton to kepe a jewell* illustrates the protective function of parenchyma; *In a purpos* [the diaphragm] *longissimum uti a sayle.*[99] Often where the analogy is introduced with an English word it is outside classical knowledge, like *Huius tricuspides duo a bishops mitre* (of the mitral valves)[100] and the *East Indy bezar in the liver of a goate.* This is in his list of pathological appearances of the liver, where English occurs often, such as *absessus like an eagle stone.*[101] Of the pathological state of the spleen, he notes *maxime sanguine refertissimus ut bagg of blood.*[102] Other analogies must have come more readily from the English than from the Latin: *like unshorne velvet* (the villous inside surface of the bladder and stomach), *kidney beenes* (the shape of the kidney), and *swollen like pudding.*[103]

By the use of English in analogy, then, Harvey could bring into his argument meanings and images not otherwise available. His philosophi-

97. f.24v W 100. For Harvey's dislike of chemistry, see Keynes, (n. 3) *Harvey,* p. 372.
98. f.8r W 30.
99. f.49r W 180, f.38r W 142; f.69v W 238.
100. f.75v W 260.
101. f.40r W 148.
102. f.39r W 144.
103. f.55r W 189; f.28r W 112; f.24r W 166; f.60r W 210.

cal language remained Latin. There may however be an exception to this. Harvey was not fond of reworking old anatomical controversies (which some textbooks of his time made a point of handling) but could not avoid the differences between the philosophers and physicians on the question of the central organ of the body. First, the doctors, as followers of Galen, held that the veins arose from the liver, the organ of nutrition. The philosophers preferred the Aristotelian view that the heart, as the central organ of the body, was the source of the veins. To have discussed the matter in Latin would have been to supply authority for the view that Harvey opposed. In the anatomy lectures, in the middle of a long Latin section on the liver and its relationship to the veins, he breaks into English. *WH yf I coud shew what I have seene yt were att an end betwene physicians et philosophos.*[104] Perhaps this summarizes an English-language attempt to dismiss an opposing philosophy. Second, the other part of this question was the status of the brain. If the heart was central, as the philosophers insisted, how was it, as Galen had shown with sophisticated experiments (directed against the Aristotelians), that the brain controlled motion, consciousness, and life? The Aristotelian Harvey, the discoverer of the forceful systole and pulse, had extra reason to defend a heart-centered Aristotelian microcosm. By using the vernacular, Harvey seems to want to distance himself from a dispute that was unphilosophical in that it threatened his own, natural-philosophical (rather than medical) view of the centrality of the heart. A properly philosophical language was one that supported *his* philosophy. His considered use of vernacular analogies at the end of the lectures on the local motion of animals may be evidence of this. At least, they are an extended example of his use of English analogies. Here, in a section headed *Similitudo Analogica*, he deals with the question of the central organ of the body. As an Aristotelian he wanted it to be the heart, but as a physician he could not ignore Galen's extensive and experimental knowledge of the brain and nerves. He tried therefore, in using vernacular analogies, to push the question to a proper resolution by using terms that did not have either scholastic or Galenic resonances. Perhaps (says he, putting the opposing case first) the brain is like the *mester del choro. Nervi timekeepers and prompters, dancers. Musculi actores, cantatores, dancers.* The *maestro*, in charge of the chorus, actors, and dancers, is an image Harvey probably picked up in Italy; he uses it four times at least.

Or perhaps the brain is an architect? Then *Nervi praepositi, surveiors.*

104. f.33r W 126.

Ramuli clerkes of every worke. Perhaps a nautical analogy is better? *An cerebrum master. Spinae his mate. Nervi botesweynes. Musculi saylers.* Then Harvey gives his preferred analogies, with the heart central. *An WH potius Cor imperator, rex. Cerebrum iudex sarieant maior, praepositus marching . . . Ramuli decuriones, constables, corporals.* Or the heart is the architect, *Nervuli controwlers, prompters, directors. An cor captayne, factor, owner, primus motor. Cerebrum master of the ship, primum mobile, sol. Nervi masters mates, boys, officers. . . .*[105]

A minor subgroup is where he provides a Latin term and its English equivalent, as a translation rather than analogy, to ensure that his audience understands. He gives the English name of all the nuscles, uses both "pancreas" and "sweetbread," and translates *inflammatur* [as] *chapped, sore,* and *carinatum* as *like the keel of a ship.*[106] *Vesica urina, blather*[107] is a Latin-English pair. Another is *canna pulmonum, wind pipe.*[108]

(v) Colors are notoriously difficult to translate.[109] It is not absolutely clear that Harvey saw this, but he does often use English for colors. This is entirely consistent with his use of English as a whole, for it is another way in which he gives immediacy to the sensory observation of particulars. In the terms of his Latin natural philosophy, colors were generally "accidents" of things, not relating to causal principles or leading to true knowledge. But, when he came to discuss how knowledge is produced (in the preliminary material of *De Generatione Animalium*),[110] he claimed that direct visual experience of a particular could lead to a kind of universal in the mind which remained there after the senses were directed elsewhere and which was used as a basis of further judgment. The example he chose was the color yellow. So, in expressing his colors in English, Harvey is giving power and precision to particulars which were of direct use in the intellectual processes of his natural philosophy. Such a Latin term as *flavus* could never mean as much to Harvey or his audience as *Unde Sir Will Rigdon all yellow* from bile, or (of the gall bladder) *Color: darke yellow, alii black, alii rusty, item greenish blewish,* or (of other organs) *straw color* or *inter pale yellow* and *light red.* His description of the pathological appearance of the lungs is a characteristic example of how he used

105. f.117v–118r W (1959) 150.
106. f.21r W 90; f.58v W 208; f.9r W 34.
107. f.54v W 196.
108. f.65v W 226.
109. Indeed we have to "translate" obsolete terms like Harvey's *watchet*; it is light blue. f.24v W 102; f.39r W 146.
110. W Harvey, *Disputations touching the Generation of Animals*, trans. G. Whitteridge (Oxford: Blackwell, 1981), pp. 10–17.

Latin for the technical terms of his trade and its system of knowledge and the vernacular for the particulars of sensory knowledge: *3° morbosis swarty purple blewish ut peripneumonia, sanguine refertissimi; a duskey ash color, a a durty greye, ledish in apostemate absque et cum venis livescentibus; more white and yellow, cley color contracti.*[111] A considerable number of Harvey's remarks about the color of organs relate to pathological states, in which Harvey had a special interest. Again we can see the importance of sensory particulars, and in a subject that Harvey wanted to treat in a new way. He thought that Riolan's work on the subject[112] paid too little attention to the contrast between the healthy and the pathological, a sensory business. Harvey observes of a healthy liver *Homine sano somwhat russet, iron grey,* but that, in those who are cachectic, *foras watchet etiam porraceus plumbeus* (the color of leeks and lead). Several such observations on pathological livers were based on Harvey's post-mortem dissections.

1. Iecur vidi russet hard contracted absque sanguine, yeallow cankret substance venis. Primo a febri pleno corpore obeso, Sir Rigdon, secundo extenuato cum felle magno fluente ut urina et calculis referto; ab ictero ambo. WH quo casu magis puto ab ictero longo, caliditate concrescit materia, quam contra icterus a calculis.
2. Item russetish ingente et durum plane scirrus tumor, absque pene sanguine, aspera superficie.
3. Between russet and purple, as bigg as an ox-liver, Jhon Bracey extinctum.
4. Beginning to be discoloured, Joan Jhonson mortua ex febre maligna et haemorhogica post quartanum.[113]

Again we see that the technical details of medicine as a system of knowledge are expressed in Latin, while the particulars of sensory observation and the personal details of the victims of disease are in English. When dealing with the different colors of the skin, Harvey deals with races of man and parts of the world outside the knowledge and vocabulary of the ancients, and necessarily uses English. *Color varius: white and fayer; pale; darker Hispanus, tanned, sunburnt; tawny Mores, Fess, gypsy colored, cole black Abisin, Congo; ash color East Indyes; olive color West Indyes, betwene green sunburnt and black.*[114]

(vii) An unexpected category is where Harvey uses English for stories from antiquity. The presumption is that he read them in Latin, and indeed

111. f.38r W 144; f.40v W 148; f.45v W 170; f.82r W 280.
112. J. Riolan, *Encheiridium Anatomicum and Pathologicum*, (Leiden, 1649).
113. ff.39r–v W 146.
114. f.12v W 48–50.

he quotes a Latin historian; but Alexander the Great's drinking competition perhaps sounded better in English. In quoting stories of ancient and modern prowess at the table to illustrate the greater size of the stomach in antiquity, Harvey was perhaps seeking a moment of light relief in the middle of a dissection. At all events, his words read best without analysis.

Quantitas ventriculi; ingenti quantitate ventriculos fuisse quosdam helluones, gourmandisers, drunkers. Historiae veteres novae plurimae. Ex Vopisco, phago Aurelii favorit eate a boare, a mutton and a pigg. WH Wilkinson of Cambridg, pigg of the spitt. Milo Crotoniates 20 lbs carnis at a meale, eate the bull the next day. Athlete: Aristoteles, prae copia alimenti, in mensa dicuntur 20lbs. Att Hollingborne he that eats bollough livers. Of drunkerds non minor fama. Alexander sett a prise, many fell, many died; Promachus victor dicitur potasse quatuor congii, soe 20 quarts and better. Torquatus tricongius, Ciceronis filius bicongius. Syracusans drinke untill an egg hatched. Persi games, matches and prises for drink. Romans quot litere in ther mistris name.[115]

CONCLUSION

We have seen that Harvey used English in a number of ways that related to his natural philosophy. Perhaps chief amongst them was to supply images—particulars—of sensory observation. In contrast, his philosophy, with its general principles, remained firmly Latin. So did his experimental procedure, which drew partly from the long tradition of Latin Galenism. For all his anatomical novelties, Harvey's natural philosophy remained a thing of the schools, expressed in a language common to universities from Rostock to Rome. It was common, too, to the College of Physicians and its formal lectures. Addressing an English audience, there Harvey found it appropriate to use English to give emphasis and strength to his natural philosophy. It was not an attempt to replace Latin. But things were changing in Harvey's lifetime.[116] Traditional school natural philosophy continued to be taught in the universities throughout his life, whether it was the entirely traditional study of the *octo physicorum* or the "new Aristotle" of the *auscultationes*. But increasingly a new class of student was coming up to the universities who did not need degrees and did not therefore have to obey statutes. If they chose to study natural philosophy with their tutors, it might have been Cartesian rather than Aristotelian. Outside the universities, many sought an alternative to

115. f.31r W 120.

116. On these changes, see my *William Harvey's Natural Philosophy*, Cambridge University Press, forthcoming (1994).

Aristotelian natural philosophy. What they replaced it with was generally some form of particulate and mechanical world view. Because this was new, it was often appropriate to express it in a language that did not have the resonances of traditional natural philosophy. Descartes in the *Discourse on Method* used his native language to avoid sounding scholastic and to employ all the vividness of the vernacular that Harvey had gained when supplying his images and analogies from sense perception in *his* vernacular. Of course, the impact of Descartes' vernacular was limited largely to France, and, when Descartes wanted to reach an international audience, he was bound to express himself in Latin. He also used Latin in his attempt to have himself adopted in place of Aristotle within the universities as The Philosopher. The case of the use of the vernacular with Descartes is very different from that of Harvey.

Harvey's natural philosophy, which he defended in the preface to the book on the generation of animals, was not influential and shared the fate of school natural philosophy. In contrast, within his lifetime Harvey's experiments became an important model for the Experimental Philosophy, both inside and outside the universities. It was particularly important for those now suspicious of natural-philosophical "systems." Descartes had built a new system of the world to replace the old, but it was increasingly seen to have suffered from the same faults as the old: any great rationalist system must be vitiated by the uncertainty of human reason. The sceptics and the men who now wanted above all to avoid contentious rational systems of the world turned to the "matter of fact" of experimental results. These, as particulars of sensory perception, could often be best expressed in the vernacular, as Harvey had done. But now there was no background of a great rationalist structure of natural philosophy, and the Experimental Philosophers often set out not only their experimental observations in their vernacular, but also the experiment itself and whatever conclusions they wished to draw from them. To such people, natural philosophy no longer needed Latin.

INDEX